Who cares?

When he retired in 1994, Peter Bruggen, MB ChB (Edinburgh, 1957) DRCOG DCH FRCPsych, had a national reputation in his field. He had been consultant psychiatrist at the specialist Hill End Adolescent Unit for 25 years and at the Tavistock Clinic for 20 of them. He had also been one of the first medical directors of a trust in the NHS reforms.

He had published two books, *Surviving Adolescence* and *Helping Families* (both with Charles O'Brian and both published by Faber and Faber). His journal publications included papers on the value of authority with adolescents, open communication in management, and audit.

His most quoted papers include seven with Sandy Bourne, published in the *BMJ*, on the secret allocation of millions of pounds of distinction award money to consultants; one with Charles O'Brian in *Family Process*, on practising circular questions in the car; and one with Amanda Ackworth in *The Journal of Family Therapy*, on work at the death bed.

Since he retired, Peter Bruggen has interviewed 100 NHS staff. They have told him what they have not told others. In bringing their stories to public view in this book, he is exposing something of crucial importance for us all.

Who Cares?

True stories of the NHS reforms

Dr Peter Bruggen

JON CARPENTER

First published 1997 by Jon Carpenter Publishing,
The Spendlove Centre, Charlbury OX7 3PQ
☎ 01608 811969
Please write or phone for our catalogue

The right of Peter Bruggen to be identified as author of this work has been
asserted in accordance with the Copyright, Designs and Patents Act 1988

ISBN 1 897766 32 7

Printed and bound in England by J W Arrowsmith Ltd., Bristol

Contents

Acknowledgements   vi

Introduction   1

1 Starting out as a manager in the NHS   18

2 The manager, the new structure and the meetings   20

3 Managers: five who were out of the NHS   36

4 'Three hours to clear your desk'   61

5 The administrators   77

6 The medical director   85

7 The GPs who were not fundholders   102

8 The fundholding GP   110

9 The country doctors   121

10 The general nurse   128

11 Community care and the district nurse   136

12 The health visitors   144

13 The unhappy dentists   152

14 Mental health: hospital and community   163

15 'To support you, I am suspending you'   179

16 Work in the children's ward   194

17 That 'phone tap': what *did* happen?   210

18 Leicester Royal Infirmary: a place that works?   218

19 Occupational health, occupational hazard   232

20 Bureaucracy and managing   235

21 Life with the purchasers   256

22 Regional authorities and the NHS Executive   268

23 Sexism in NHS management   282

24 How many patients? 'I'd rather die at home'   285

25 Conclusion   293

Appendix I Just a bit more paperwork   300

Appendix II Bibliography   305

Index   308

Abbreviations   314

Acknowledgements

Alice, Camilla, Emma and Joan for practical, supervisory, editorial help and inspiration.

Joanna Lal, Deborah Leembruggen, Kathryn Redway and Esther Whitby, who know something of these things, for advice on getting my ideas together and writing another book.

Luna Restaurant, Chalk Farm Road, for being the best place for some meetings, reading and editing.

Jill Champkins, who typed and gave ideas; and encouraged me to do more myself.

Many friends who scouted, read, edited; but whom I shall not name.

Those who spoke on the telephone and often did so at length.

The hundred who met me and shared their stories. I agreed not to name them, but to them is the greatest debt.

Readers may write to the author c/o the publisher (Jon Carpenter Publishing, The Spendlove Centre, Charlbury OX7 3PQ), or e-mail him at pbruggen @cableinet.co.uk.

Introduction

'I felt as if the floor and the furniture and all the people I knew or had ever known had disappeared. I should have been accelerating downwards, faster and faster, as I fell into a great hole, but I was not falling at all. I was standing still, so I felt unreal. I was suspended.' (Manager)

'When I was offered 'retirement in the interests of service' I signed an agreement to withhold my experience in the NHS.' (Consultant)

'If you want to get on here, say that you are enthusiastic about the trust's strategy.' (Charge Nurse)

'I know that everyone on the team, including myself, was at times sobbing.' (Consultant)

The National Health Service is writhing in agony. I was gasping at the end of my last two years at work before my retirement at 60. During those two years I rarely slept through the night. I had headaches and other psychosomatic complaints. Although my retirement date had been chosen well in advance, I told my family and close colleagues that I might not last out; that any day I might resign. I cried for those that I was leaving behind to struggle in the mess.

I comforted myself with thinking that I might write up my experiences for publication. I even made a very few notes in my diary. When I mentioned this to some colleagues they immediately told me that they hoped I would widen the subject, because they still felt so firmly gagged.

They said that there might be a story to tell.

It was not only the individuals who felt gagged and were very silent but also the organisations. With occasional exceptional outbursts, both my own union and professional body, the British Medical Association (BMA) and the others had been remarkably silent on the experience of working the NHS reforms. Even the 'Personal View' weekly column in the *British Medical Journal*

(*BMJ*), in which doctors' disclosures are very common, has been silent on what it has felt like to be suspended, moved out of one's office, told to rewrite a business plan or to shed staff.

The 'old' National Health Service

I commend the clear account of the history of the health services of the UK in the third edition of Rudolf Klein's *The New Politics of the NHS* (1995), but for this introduction I risk a more personal review.

My background to the NHS and the reforms

I remember the start of the NHS in 1948. My father, who was a GP, jokingly complained that he was having to stop being a doctor and would become a civil servant. It was not true of course for the GPs remained independent contractors. After a few more jokes on politically raised expectations (the patient who walked into the surgery on the first day to demand her injection of penicillin and the one who rang for a telephone consultation after swallowing a prune stone), my father became a dedicated supporter of the NHS.

(Many years later, with the advent of the trusts and reforms, I was to look up old copies of the *BMJ* of around the time of the start of the NHS. There was a remarkable similarity between the ways in which Mr Bevan and Mr Waldegrave, the respective politicians, addressed the doctors in open letters and between the contents of the correspondence columns. Except, of course, that the doctors had 'changed sides' and had come to be defenders of the 'old' NHS.)

It was always being changed, reorganised or reformed, one way or another, as the practices of medicine, nursing and all the other disciplines were also changing. The first 'reform' that I remember was soon after I left school when Mr Justice Danckwerts was called in by the government to help reconsider how much money the doctors should be getting, bearing in mind what they seemed to be earning before the second world war and the wider changes in incomes since then. It was decided that the GPs were not being paid enough money and so my family got more: a second car, uncommon in those days. It was a secondhand brown Austin with gear lever on the steering column.

As a medical student from 1951 to 1957, I found everyone assumed the NHS was there to stay and its being a good thing was never challenged. But I was influenced by the prevailing status of hospital practice. Most of what I was taught came with a shouted statement that hospital was best: the really bright people worked in them and the real excitement was there. The newly appointed professor of general practice, one of the first in the country, was regarded as an oddity.

Soon it was apparent that the high-profile, high-technology parts of the hospital services, and some new hospitals, were taking an increasing part of the NHS money. With that shift, almost with every turn of it, they were also taking more control. The more things were going the way of the big spending specialties, the more that trend continued. There were various attempts to move the balance of power and money away from the ever more absorbing hospital services and back to general practitioners and others working 'in the community', but there was little success.

The merging of government departments

There had been a Ministry of Health for ages, at least since shortly after the first world war. In 1968, after much debate, there was a merger to create the Department of Health and Social Security, led by senior civil servants of a new generation who had not been leaders at the time of the setting up of the NHS. In 1974, with more changes, this Department of Health and Social Security sent instructions and money to the local authorities and to the newly formed regional health authorities. Both of those bodies had influence on the new area health authorities. The regional health authorities were given more executive power than the earlier regional hospital boards, and they had greater involvement of doctors in them. They held the purse strings over the area health authorities, which were at the same level and had the same boundaries as the family practitioner committees, the GPs' administrative organisation. The family practitioner committees got their money direct from the government department. The area health authorities sent money and instruction down to the district management teams who ran the hospitals and the specialist services and were supposed to be kept in check, a bit, by the community health councils.

Within the hospital services, communication was to be from whatever nursing or medical structure there was to the hospital management team to the district management team to the area health authority to the regional health authority. Of course it did not work like that and there were many noisy, influential people who could hop over a layer or two, upwards or downwards.

Fewer tiers again

To improve on that, in 1982 the area health authorities were abolished. The Department of Health and Social Security sent money and instruction to the regional health authorities and to the family practitioner committees. The regional health authorities did the same with the district health authorities. The community health councils were still there to keep in check the district health authorities and the hospitals; and the local authorities continued their vaguer relationships with the district health authority and the Department of Health and Social Security.

Those who organised this change and those who succeeded in getting jobs in the new management structure thought that it worked a bit better, but there were still problems with some people being able to get more for their patch by shouting louder.

People continued to complain of not having enough money, and from time to time the government said it was throwing more money at the service. More people were getting prepared to say that there would never be enough money.

There continued to be a national forum for making the 'best' decisions on the allocation of resources, how many beds there should be for this or that, or how many specialists of whatever sort for so many hundred thousand of the population. The professional bodies and the government seemed to collude in the idea that it was possible to get such an exercise right.

Management and the loss of the ideal of universalising the best

The year following the abolition of the area health authorities had the government appoint Sir Roy Griffiths, Sainsbury's managing director, to lead a management inquiry. It was Griffiths and his report that created the now famous sentence, 'If Florence Nightingale were carrying her lamp through the corridors of the NHS today she would almost certainly be searching for the people in charge.' What was required, Sir Roy concluded, was good general management from top to bottom: general managers accountable for getting things done.

These ideas were not quite as new as they were made out to be at the time (I remember hearing the one about who is in charge from John Bowlby when I was a senior registrar in 1966). But this time they were given prominence and the government listened. Perhaps it was what they wanted to hear.

Many things followed rapidly.

The resource management initiative gave clinical departments a budget, a clinical director or manager and let them get on with it. They were not to be rescued.

As general management was pushed, for the first time significant numbers of people were attracted from outside the NHS to join this management core. Higher salaries were available for top management. The first fixed term contracts came in and with them the first rumours of 'Clear your desk and clear out.'

But it was not enough. The NHS was still seen as heavily political and politicians, perhaps of all parties, had a longing for getting such an organisa tion, of which the general population had unreasonable and unrealistic expectations, right off the political agenda. More money was still being demanded and 'Foul!' was still being shouted.

It still seemed impossible to control. The population was continuing to age, with a rise in the proportion of dependent people. Medical advances were continuing to become more expensive (the treatment for angina in 1948 cost pennies per week, now everybody knows that some people can have expen sive surgery for that condition).

A new look was announced to those cabinet members who had not been in on the discussion, and to the rest of the country, during a *Panorama* inter- view with Mrs Thatcher in January 1988. A year later the white paper *Working for Patients* was published.

I welcomed the bold heralding of this revolution because I thought the whole thing needed a very good shake up. I thought doctors did have too much power and did not use it well. They had learned to manage all sorts of elabo- rate interventions and treatments; but not outpatient clinics or waiting lists.

The high-spending and high-tech specialties of medicine were always good at convincing managers that they were the ones who should never have a smaller slice of the cake, and often a rather bigger one. There was something about the threat of a coronary thrombosis, a brain tumour or a major phys- ical accident that could be guaranteed to bring out the feelings of not wanting to deny oneself, or somebody else, the very latest that is available in tech- nology. When it came to arguments in meetings or committees, primary care, preventive measures, conservative management and any of the other things seen at the 'soft' end of medicine always lost out to the high-tech, dramatic, expensive interventions.

In the early 1980s I was convinced by some colleagues that the idea that the best could ever be available for everybody was one of the most ridiculous of myths. I was given two reasons for this. First, it would mean that everything was equal and as a species we have been very bad at ever getting equality. Second, I was told that there were estimated to be a hundred people in the world who had their own personal coronary care unit: a team of skilled professionals with cardiac resuscitation equipment, drips, monitors and all the high-power electrical gadgetry which features in many a TV serial. 'Should that be available to all?' my friends asked me. I was given a picture of everybody in the street being followed by his or her own team of ten professionals with all their equipment; and every member of each team having a similar retinue, and so on.

The reforms: my summary
The announcement

Remember that a lot happened at once and then very quickly after that. Not even all the cabinet knew of the idea before Mrs. Thatcher spoke on the *Panorama* show. I heard from one senior manager that it was widely said in their circles that at least one of the health politicians did not understand the reforms. They were changing some things and we would all see what happened.

One of my friends told me of a summons to all the doctors from a manager in the hospital in which she worked. They met in the old style 'doctors' quarters'. The doctors had still not seen a copy of *Working for Patients*, but the manager had been sent a video and had been asked to show it to them. It opened with the Prime Minister, Mrs. Thatcher, speaking to camera. She was followed by the Secretary of State for Health. The other thing that my friend remembered of that meeting was how quickly something happened that was later to become commonplace: division among the doctors. There was a majority who thought that the whole idea was half-baked and dangerous, and a minority who thought that it all sounded, at least, interesting. And already, those were strongly expressed views.

I welcomed the idea of the trusts. That they would be able to put extra earnings back into their own business, pay their own staff what they decided, control their own budgets and transfer money from one heading to another without being stopped or interfered with by heavy bureaucracy.

I thought that the idea of a purchasing authority whose job it was to determine the needs for treatment in the community, and then purchase the services from whatsoever provider they chose, was brilliant. At a stroke it could deal with one of the main paralysing muddles of the old area and regional health authorities and could give the public health department something really useful to do.

Although the idea of separating purchaser from provider flew into most peoples' consciousness with the white paper, it does have a history from suggestions made by A. C. Enthoven (1985).

Most brilliant of all may have been giving back power to the general practitioners. Their status was lower than that of doctors in the hospitals, although it waxed and waned. The founding of the Royal College of General

Practitioners and some changes in funding and postgraduate training made it more of a specialty and more attractive. But GPs were still being pushed around by the hospitals, with consultants acting as specialists who decided what was best for the GPs' patients, and what were the best plans.

Purchaser or purchasers, singular or plural?

Most documents and speech refer to the organisation in the singular ('the purchaser wants'), but because the plural is also often used, in the stories I have sometimes done likewise. What follows is how I understand the word and the development of the function. Sorry it comes out so complicated: after involving five people in telephone consultations, this is the best I could do...

The reforms created purchasing *health authorities*, called *purchasers*. For each former district there was a health authority with the job of assessing the needs of the populace and buying services from providers. Most of the purchasing authorities worked the same areas as the previous district health authorities; many had several of the same staff and some had the same offices.

They purchased the services from the providers, who were turning into trusts. They did not dispense all the money for services, however, because GP fundholding was starting and those practices were doing their own purchasing of some services.

GP fundholding practices had two main sources of money. The family health service authorities (FHSAs) gave them money for the doctors, nurses, receptionists etc., while the health authority transferred that amount of its budget which represented each practice's share for services payable by fundholding. As the reforms progressed the number of those services grew. Money for the fundholding manager and for other fundholding management costs (secretarial time and equipment) also came from that source.

How boundaries and responsibilities were drawn up meant that most of the new trusts had one main purchaser, but may or may not have sought some contracts or extra contractual referrals (ECRs) from elsewhere. Some trusts, however, had two or more main purchasers — for example where a district general hospital had in the past served an area which was later administratively divided into two purchaser domains. (Chapter 9 gives an example.)

The next evolution was *merging*. Purchasers merged, as for example the purchasers for one county combining. (And trusts merged or refined their divisions and boundaries: examples include paediatrics going into a community services trust along with other child and family services, or a big and a small hospital joining, merging, or one taking the other over.)

In 1996, after GP fundholding had expanded and the FHSAs had fewer non-fundholding practices to manage, the government combined the FHSAs and the health authorities (the purchasers) into new, larger, purchasing authorities.

These purchasing authorities give out money. Some goes to all GP practices (the old FHSA role). More goes to the fundholding practices who give most of it to providers whom they pay to carry out services. Some goes direct to providers whom the other, non fundholding, GPs commission to provide services. This can be represented by a diagram:

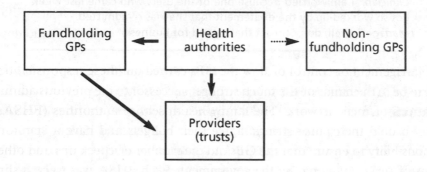

When a consultant talks of 'the purchaser', it may indicate that the directorate in which he or she works (but not necessarily the trust as a whole) has one main purchaser.

When a consultant uses the plural, 'purchasers', it may indicate that the directorate has more than one main purchasing authority and/or lots of GP fundholders.

Or it may be a bit of both, or people may be a bit confused, in which case both versions of the word are used.

When the word is used with a reverence usually reserved for those holding a particular sort of authority, or when it is invoked as a threat, remember that purchasers and providers are not in fact in a managerial hierarchical relationship. It is simply that money shapes the service and that market forces are powerful.

The real gate-keepers: the GP fundholders

The consultants were the gate-keepers within the hospitals themselves. They decided who was admitted and who was discharged, and that was the main expense for hospitals. But they were the gate-keepers only for the people who came to their notice.

Fundholding reached a higher level of gate-keeping, the general practitioner. Under fundholding agreements the general practitioners were to be given 'their' population's share of the funding of the hospital (or part of it), for them to spend as they wished.

The days of the specialist surgeon arguing how many new and very expensive operations they should do were to be numbered. The general practitioners could decide what proportion of their budget they wished to spend on that

And because the general practitioners were close to the individual patients and their families, they would also have more influence.

Clinician: I am worried because one of the users who came last week got so worked up by the excitement that she was re admitted

Manager. Well, don't forget that's good for business

Management or control of how the GPs carried out these responsibilities was to be in the hands of the much stronger successor to the previous administrations of their network. The family health service authorities (FHSAs) were to hold their purse strings, agree their budgets and have a statutory responsibility to ensure that the GPs did the number of check ups and other items of service required by the government. Each FHSA was to be a slim sized, managerial body. And those GP practices that were to change their status to that of fundholding were to manage their own budgets and 'their' part of the funding of the hospital (provider trust) services.

Who first thought of fundholding GPs?

Kenneth Clarke said he had thought up the idea of GP fundholding while he was on holiday in Spain, but it was not quite like that.

There is a section on 'The origins of the idea' in a King's Fund Institute's 1992 Research Report No. 12 on fundholding by Glennerster, Matsaganis and Owens. They said the idea had been discussed in a meeting at the Office of Health Economics in 1984 and gave references to George Teeling-Smith and Alan Maynard (1985 and 1986 respectively). It was then dropped from draft documents until Kenneth Clarke, who had been a junior minister at the Department and may have heard some of the discussions, became Secretary of State and pushed it forward.

I checked this with Mr Clarke who does not deny that he came across many ideas when he was a health minister in the early 1980s; but pointed out that nothing was happening to reform the position of GPs in the purchaser/provider system when he returned to the Department as Secretary of State. When it did happen, it was the 'fruit' of his holiday in Spain, which was then worked up in the Department.

I found a much earlier reference. In 1973, in a colourfully entitled book (Need your doctor be so useless?), Andrew Malleson described his idea of how health centres (with GP leadership) should run:

A health centre is made to pay out of its own budget for the care that its back-up hospital provides for the centre's patients. The back-up hospital therefore receives its funds from its satellite health centres in proportion to the work that it does for them. Not only does this arrangement discourage a health centre from insisting that its unwanted patients are kept in hospital, but it also makes it possible for the health centre to decide how much money is to be spent on hospital treatments and how much on other kinds of medical care.

So maybe Andrew Malleson broadcast his idea when not many people were listening and maybe Kenneth Clarke was listening to discussions more than some thought.

Consultants' contracts: another master power stroke

For years consultants had the special relationship embodied in a contract with the regional hospital board or the regional health authority. They were chosen at regional committees. They were paid by regional departments. Their travel expenses came from a regional purse. They were protected by elaborate and costly procedures if anyone wanted to get rid of them. If they considered that their appointment was being unfairly ended they had a right to send a 'full statement of the facts' to the Secretary of State.

There had been various attempts to clip these wings but, as with so many of the earlier endeavours to make change in the massive institution, not much had come of them.

With the spirit of the reforms, it was easy. Trusts were to have the power to appoint consultants and terms could be negotiated individually. True, some things did remain, notably in the constitution of the appointment committees: regional health authorities would send representatives after having agreed the advertisement and job description; and the universities were still to be represented.

Consultants like me, appointed under the old system, still seemed to have the right of appeal to the Secretary of State, and kept their indefinite contracts. But, with more young ones appointed, the special relationship and status had gone. Doctors (and the BMA) could now be included in the trust's own review machinery of salaries and wages, terms and conditions, as any other workers.

On the whole, trusts have been very cautious in making policy changes in terms and conditions of service, but individual contracts for consultants have become quite common. These have covered salary increment, extra payment (e.g. for a set number of discretionary sessions per month in return for a commit ment to do them 'as required'), removal expenses and, less commonly fixed length of time to the contract. Many consultants have gone along with such individual contracts, while some have been worried by this dividing of the profession.

Many of the troubles between consultants and managers, some of which are described in this book, can be seen in terms of adjustments in this power balance, or in the vicissitudes of this change.

Stronger management and the market

Value for money. No one could be relied upon to cut costs unless they could see immediate advantages to doing so. That was the resource manage ment argument, but it was not good enough. Additional to that came the 'market'. Giving GPs and other purchasers (the district health authorities) the responsibility to define needs and find the best value treatment available brought competition in. The hospital that was doing an operation or another treatment for £x would be inclined to reduce the figure if a neighbour was charging less.

Alongside this went the Griffiths-style enthusiasm for firm and direct management, but many times over more powerfully. The origins of this were partly in the 'management initiative' in government service of the 1980s and some may have been inspired by the personal style of the Prime Minister, Mrs. Thatcher (see the review I quote in Chapter 25). Interpretations have varied, from the fairly common 'managers should manage' to, in one place at least, 'FIFO', which stood for, 'Fit in or...'

Audit

Not a new word or idea, but wonderful how the government used it.

Think of an event in a hospital and how you would like it to be done. Say, the arrival at an accident and emergency department: being seen by a clinical person within 5 minutes and by a doctor within 20; or the telling of bad news: in privacy, with chairs for everyone and not in a rush. Work out 'indicators of good practice' which are clear, concrete and measurable. Have someone on the team follow up a month's events and work out in how many instances the indicators of good practice were met. Examine in more detail the incidents where they were not met. What can be learned and how can performance be improved? Check again, in a few months' time.

Audits should be short, achievable and relevant.

One of the first papers I remember reading on audit was different, but nonetheless heartwarming. It described a group of hospital consultant physicians watching video recordings of themselves seeing patients. All had been arranged with careful explanations and informed consent. The physicians discussed the videos with the 'rule' that anything might be said and that offence, if ever experienced, was not to be considered as intended.

One of the first audits that I was involved with was on how we did physical examinations on adolescents. Working out the indicators of good practice led to a modification of practice; and the problems that had prompted us to choose the subject went away. That led to one of the three audit papers of which I was a co-author.

The government said audit was a good thing and every consultant had to be doing it (an opportunity for management to check on this.) Consultants had to do audit (one session, or half day, was supposed to be given over to it) and had to have some link with an audit meeting to ensure peer review. How this could degenerate in practice is described in Chapter 14.

Initiatives

Extra money was allocated from time to time for special purposes. The treatment of AIDS is one example. Waiting list eradication is another.

Waiting list money came from two routes.

Centrally, some was allocated for special initiatives in those specialties which had a history of long waiting times. It was used by hospitals or trusts to 'hire in' staff (or pay consultants extra sessions) to work on Saturday mornings or other extra time. Sometimes there was little extra payment to be made by the management, for the nurses would be there anyway and the 'hotel' side of the hospital was always being run. Sometimes, the cash went to private hospitals to do some of the work.

GP fundholders also could take 'waiting list initiatives'. I came across this first in child and adolescent psychiatry. Some clinics received 'once off', or 'twice off', payments of £10,000-£20,000 from GP fundholders for them to take on, by way of short term contract, a family therapist, social worker, or member of another discipline, to work on reducing the waiting list. Some trusts were slow in taking up such offers and so were some clinics. One person told me there were anxieties over how much it might become a two tier system. Yet many of these contracts seemed to work well and even the person with the short term work seemed more pleased with that than with none at all. Market forces were wending their ways.

The Patient's Charter and the voice of the consumer

For years the British patient had tolerated delay and being kept in the dark.

The Patient's Charter rode on the bandwagon of consumerism and openness (for example the Access to Information Act which gave each of us some rights over what notes were kept on us).

With the charter, standards were laid down by the government and the rate at which these were to be approached. Waiting lists of more than so many months or years were not to be tolerated, letters from GPs requesting appointments were to be answered within a certain time, summaries were to be sent out also within a certain time of someone being discharged from hospital.

Consumers were to be consulted more.

The government ordered change and change quickly. Departments of quality control sprang up and worked alongside those involved in audit to check on how well things were being done and how well patients were being treated.

Strong objections were raised quickly by the clinical professions: they said this was a random (not randomised), uncontrolled, unplanned, unscientific experiment. But in fact some of the really great investigative energy and skill of staff was being redirected, away from dry academic subjects to those obviously relevant to all.

Progress in approaching, meeting, or extending quality standards became a routine subject dealt with in annual reports, statements to managers or visitors; or in petitions for funds.

What neither the audit nor the charter initiatives dealt with was the position of the departments which already did not keep people waiting, had no waiting list and did consult consumers. Here, market forces had an interesting effect: some of these places were advised to develop a waiting list.

All in all, a terrible indictment of how the medical profession had been inward looking over many years. It took a tantrum from a government (or a prime minister) to get them to deflect their energy from research and paper publishing, which was often irrelevant to patient care, into listening to their consumers. Some said that rarely were troubles better deserved.

How I got the stories

I was well in the network before I retired. As a medical director of a trust and as a consultant psychiatrist of a specialised unit, I met many people. I attended three meetings of medical directors, one with the Secretary of State for Health and one with the Chief Medical Officer of the Department of

Health. I met chief executives: from trusts, purchasing authorities and regional health authorities.

I met doctors from many specialties and members of other disciplines. I met fellow executive and non-executive directors of the trust in which I worked. Over the last five years I must have met 15 chief executives.

But in fact, little of my own story is included in this book, although my own experiences and conversations enabled me to tune in very rapidly to what others told me.

Making contacts

While I got in touch with a few people whom I had read of in the press, most of my contacts came by word of mouth.

People asked me what I was doing in my retirement and I told them that I was collecting stories on working in the NHS reforms. I did not say that I was looking for problems or bad news. It followed from that. Some suggested names of others I should contact. Some came up to me themselves and said they wanted to talk to me.

I made no public announcement and nor did anyone make one on my behalf at any meeting.

I saw most of the people for between and hour and an hour and a half. We met at their homes or offices, occasionally my home, twice in restaurants and twice on railway stations. Three people I saw twice and one person I saw three times; but the remainder, once. With three exceptions, I used public transport. I met a hundred people.

While a few of the proposed arrangements for meetings fizzled out, I experienced no downright refusals.

Some of the people I met were tired or in tears. Some told of having been off work with breakdowns or with serious physical illness. Some told of family problems and of being on antidepressants or tranquillisers.

Two had been convicted for the illegal possession of drugs. One of these had been in prison and the other, by the skin of their teeth, had avoided it. Both had been clinicians turned to management.

Some asked me if it was all right for them to talk to me. Some thanked me for letting them talk to me. While I wrote and thanked everybody within a few days of the interview, some had already written to me. Some described the telling of their story as a therapeutic experience.

I failed to find very few of my informants when publishing was getting near. Otherwise all saw a late draft of the chapter or part of the chapter to which their interview contributed. Some made useful comments on the text, worked on it and gave extra information.

What is included in this book is included with their permission.

These are stories. Other things have been written in different styles and more will follow. For an excellent initial assessment, see Ray Robinson and Julian Le Grand's *Evaluating the NHS Reforms* (1994). Many interesting publications come from Stephen Harrison and colleagues from the Nuffield Institute for Health in Leeds (for example, 1991 and 1994).

Who were the informants?

A few of the people who looked at drafts of chapters left me with an uncomfortable anxiety. Would I appear as a shielder of dead wood? This is the last thing I would want to happen and would be an ironic swan song for me retiring from the NHS. I was no shielder of dead wood and was firmly in the authority camp. I wrote two papers on the use of authority with adolescents and, 15 years ago, a management paper which referred to discussing in a meeting the wish for one member of staff, who was present, to resign. I was used to people (including myself) being told what others expected them to do, and this being checked on. Later, as a medical director of a trust, I played my authority part in disciplinary procedures and in confronting staff with the unacceptability of their behaviour.

I accepted that with strong management in the reforms, some very uncomfortable things would happen precisely because it had been so mismanaged before. (Chapter 21 gives an example of controlling a consultant.) I have always accepted that some people had to go.

As for getting doctors to go, there has been clumsiness for years. Some of the fuss over suspended doctors is because so many of them have been found 'not guilty' by the tribunals that have deliberated, often a year or two after suspension started. There is a book on how to discipline doctors but it does not seem to be widely known and, if it had been, perhaps some of these stories might not have happened. (There is a curious thing about this book, two copies of which have been in my hands. One, which I was given, was by Tony Bunbury and Angus McGregor, published in 1988. The other looks more or less the same, even to the same photograph of stethoscope and envelope on the cover, but has a few extra sections. It was published in 1995 but, biggest difference of all, has different authors (Swift and Scotland). The second pair of authors make no reference to the first. I do not understand it, but wonder if disciplining doctors is too difficult to be seen to be associated with for long.)

It was also suggested to me that I might have picked up some people who were precipitated into management and then did not like it or could not do it. I have come across tales of those with no experience in the health or related services, or with lower status clinical roles, being brought in, subsequently to flounder over the tops of clinicians. I have not included any such as central players, although some on the sidelines may fit. Some of the people I met had been in their jobs a long time; some had been recently appointed; some had been head-hunted.

This book is not about how the NHS should be run, nor about finding villains, goodies or baddies. It is about a process. But, if you still have any doubt and think that I may write only of hard-done-by inadequates who should never have been selected for responsible jobs, then first try Chapter 22.

The management structures: why can't I be clearer?

Several readers of early drafts had difficulty in following who was who and where decisions were being made. They suggested that I head each section with a management structure diagram; and that I should be more consistent in style, by giving everyone a name.

I have given the matter, as has been so often said, careful consideration. I have heard the objections and suggestions made. I agree that the stories would be easier to follow if, in some circumstances, the suggestions were carried out. I have made some changes.

I think that diagrams often give an impression of clarity and certainty where neither is really present in the minds of the people concerned. I experienced too much of this myself and have heard too much of it from others.

I know of trusts where one management structure and profile presented in the annual report belies what is public knowledge. One group, accorded a twentieth of space in such documents, may be bringing in nearly half of the income of the trust and may be openly negotiating with another trust for assimilation. Senior managers going to public meetings may be informed of what is going to be presented, not by their peers for they have been excluded from the inner circle, but by some of those not on the diagrams at all.

Therefore, most of my text I have not altered. A 'higher level' of understanding dictates that it stays as it is. It really is confusing. Some of the key players really are vaguely known. It is not always clear to anyone where the final decisions are being made. Management structures vary more widely than ever in the NHS and some were changing during the time of the stories. I have tried to present them as clearly as I can, but that is what it is like. It is often difficult for those who are there to understand what is happening, except that it changes from day to day. What is clear is confusion and fear. Please bear with some of the unclarity as I try to communicate with you.

Openness, confidentiality and anonymity

People's anxiety to speak out is fuelled by many factors, not least of which is loyalty. Additionally some feel trapped by the fears of how it might affect their security and livelihood, working with systems of bonuses, performance related pay, time limited contracts, distinction awards (for consultants). They fear it might make things more difficult for themselves or their colleagues And they are tired.

In most of the stories I have omitted identifying information and I have changed names (sometimes several times, so as not to have too many of one name and I dread an unintentional indiscretion). Sometimes I have run two or three people's stories into one, thus protecting and concealing the identities of informants while protecting and exposing the truth of the experiences they shared with me.

On 29th August 1994, Virginia Bottomley, when she was Secretary of State for Health, said in a BBC interview on *The World at One* that she wanted much more openness.

At the beginning of 1995 there were two important public letters. I quote the second first. On 17th February, in *The Guardian*, Gerald Malone, Minister of State for Health, wrote that the NHS was then more open and accountable than ever.

On 21st January, in the *BMJ*, Alan Langlands, chief executive of the NHS Executive, wrote of the responsibility which people working within the service had to help the culture of openness.

I hope that this book helps.

Chapter 1

Starting out as a manager in the NHS: Frances' story

I remember the first days of my first job, as well as the first days of a few other jobs. Firmly in my mind are memories of several key, influential events. I wanted to start this book with the story of someone starting out in the NHS.

Ten days after she started her first job, Frances' own manager was sacked, apparently on the spot. No notice. He was just informed. There was a heads of department meeting called the next day to explain what had happened, but Frances did not go because she did not realise that she was a 'head of department' and nobody had told her.

Frances had recently graduated. She was interested in the NHS and in management. She was to manage the outpatient department of a wing in a big hospital. It was a new job. She was responsible for the reception area, the clinical areas, the medical records and all the outpatients' appointments. She was also to produce whatever statistics were required by management.

She did not see her first manager again. They had no goodbye. She was told by his manager, whose base was in an office four miles away, to carry on. He was sure that she would manage.

Changes since the interview

Frances now found that she had an extra task to do which had not been mentioned at her interview and which was not included in the job description she had been shown. It had been decided between her interview and the date of her starting. A centralised 'patient administration system' was being implemented throughout the trust and Frances was to bring her department into line. She was pleased to be valued highly enough to be entrusted with the task of introducing this new system.

Previously, new outpatient appointments had been made by the secretaries of the consultants concerned and this applied to other appointments too. Now this was taken over by Frances. Additionally she had to manage two assistants, one of whom was a nurse by training, and the other a nursing assistant. It was not clear to Frances whether the one who was the nurse was meant to work as a nurse or as a manager. The only answer she could get to that question was that it was for her to work out; and it was clear that she was going to be judged on it.

The role of scapegoat

So Frances became everybody's scapegoat. She could not arrange for appointments to be sent with the efficiency of the medical secretaries. The support staff thought that most of the ills of their working day were brought upon them by their new manager. With her own manager suddenly gone and no one to support her, when things were difficult for the support staff she could not support them. Notes always go missing from records and records departments (busy clinical workers take them suddenly to deal with a telephone call or an urgent referral and they do not put them back), but the medical records department will be held to account. And now it had a new scapegoat.

So Frances was tackling this while also trying to bring in the patient administration system. And with her own line manager being a few miles away.

She did take one problem in the team to the manager in what was called a supervision group. She described how the support worker, who was the nurse by training, was spending a great deal of time befriending and caring for the patients. This meant that filing and sorting out appointments had to be done by the other assistant and Frances herself. The senior manager very clearly saw this as a petty squabble for her to manage and showed no more interest.

She so rarely saw her own manager that she was getting hardly any feedback at all, and most of the comments she did get from him were negative. She became worried and felt depressed. She withdrew socially and other relationships became more difficult. She was often in tears. She had fantasies of crashing her car so as not to have to come to work.

She went to the occupational health department and saw a counsellor who said that the position was very simple and clear. It was impossible and she should get out.

The first internal move

But she could not get out. Eight months after she had started in her first job, another new service manager was in post and the department moved to another part of the building along with all the other outpatient clinics.

The budget was clearer and she could manage it. Architecturally, the new place was more open-plan; fewer barriers and more vulnerability.

A distressed patient, a new referral, became threatening, stood over Frances and shouted. He continued to shout. The other staff kept away. The new service manager was nowhere to be seen or heard. Some other patients and relatives were in the back of the room. She felt utterly exposed and useless, stuck in a goldfish bowl with everyone watching her. Somehow, eventually, she managed to help the person to calm down and to organise a convenient time for an appointment. She thought it was all over and that she was through, when the person started to shout again. This time one of the support team did come in and she was able to hand over to them while she took as dignified leave as possible and went into a back room to recover. The first thing she did was to burst into tears. One of the clinical staff, who had just turned up, offered to accompany her to the service manager where at least she could discuss what had happened. She accepted this offer, but on arrival at the service manager's office, was astounded to hear him say that he had passed by the area and heard the noise. He then added, 'I thought you handled it very well.' That was not what she wanted to hear. At the very least she wanted to discuss how she could have handled it better and how she might prevent such a thing happening in the future. Most of all she wanted him to have come in himself, but that, she dare not say to him.

She received no advice on how to handle such incidents in future.

A few weeks later Frances was being addressed by somebody with an obvious difficulty in English. The person also had a history of considerable violence, known to all the other staff but not yet to Frances, for scapegoats are the last to be told. Suddenly, Frances was being screamed at and threatened. She ran before there was time for all of the memories of the previous incident to overwhelm her. She rushed into the nearest office with someone in it in order to recover. Later she spoke to the union rep who was not very helpful, but did say that she should get some supervision. When she asked the service manager for the supervision, he said that what had happened was just what she should expect if she worked with those sorts of client groups. (The union rep subsequently suggested that she should have reminded him that the staff working with other client groups, whom the service manager obviously did not expect to behave threateningly, were not paid less than she was.)

She took a new problem to supervision. One of the support staff seemed to be working even fewer of her contracted hours than a few weeks ago and when Frances confronted her over it, she said that she did not intend to work her full hours. But all the service manager suggested was, 'Kick her into shape.'

Three weeks later, there was another case of a young new employee working in the department with whom there were many difficulties. The most simple performance targets were not met. His behaviour improved and then deteriorated again. After the second time of pointing this out and a confrontation over leave arrangements, 'formal procedures' were started. A counselling session was arranged with Frances, the service manager (her supervisor), the new person and his union rep. Was this to be Frances' initiation into 'macho' management? She was not looking forward to it. In fact it became just another session of personal attacks by the new member of staff on Frances, and all the while the service manager let this happen, agreeing that it might be right that she could be getting stressed and taking it out on her juniors.

Appraisal and a new contract

A few days after this event Frances reported on her own appraisal. She was told that the conclusion was that she was capable of being a good manager, but should work on the conflict between her wish to be a manager and wish to be a carer.

Shortly after that somewhat reassuring appraisal, somebody from one of the other departments wrote a letter to the service manager accusing Frances of gross inefficiency in not being able to get files. The letter named one of the support staff as the only one who was any good (in fact it was that person who had not been able to get the particular file that provoked this complaint). Frances learned of this letter when her service manager called her in and showed it to her. Her stress level had been getting worse, she was developing abdominal pains with increasing frequency, for which she had consulted her GP. This complaint seemed like the last straw.

The suggestion the service manager made was that she take another job with a clearer contract, and he offered to arrange this in another sector.

Two weeks later Frances started a six-months contract as manager for a day and residential care unit for elderly people. The clinical manager of this was a nurse who was very supportive when Frances arrived in fresh panic on the first day, developing the first full-blown migraine of her life. It seemed to be her response to the relief of stress. She had heard of this happening with other people

It was to be her 'own' department. A secretary was brought in from another part of the hospital: a competent older woman, who then left very quickly and went into the private sector.

Frances enjoyed the new job. Her stress level and symptoms went down. She demonstrated that she was able to resolve administrative problems. She organised the office. She set up systems for all the things which the staff had to manage. She enjoyed the casual but frequent meetings with the patients, who would often wander into the office or with whom she would sit for a time to relieve some of the clinical staff.

The job description

Frances was invited to write the first draft of her new job description. Clearly the job combined two roles: of manager and carer. The human resources department said this was impossible (she was to organise trips for the residents and care staff to go on, but not to go on them herself). She did continue to do both things. This went well, until after 12 months in that post, the unit was running out of new things for her to organise or to create a system for. She was then told very firmly by her manager not to do any more patient care but to do one day a week in the administration of another one of the locality centres.

Meanwhile, in the second new management structure since Frances had started her first job, a new service manager was in post. The management hierarchy within which she was working appeared as follows:

The service manager who had sent Frances there had the authority to do just that. It was to him that she was managerially accountable. It was he who could sack her.

Frances was immediately accountable to the clinical manager of the day and residential care unit to which she had just moved.

The clinical manager was accountable to the service manager.

The service manager managed the clinical managers of several units and had responsibility for them.

In her own particular job, Frances had no one to supervise, in contrast with having had the two people to manage when she had first joined the NHS. In all but salary it was an effective demotion.

Within that structure, Frances started on a new and disturbing sort of relationship, such as she had heard described by people working in other places. Frances had four different sorts of experience of the new service manager:

- being totally ignored by him as they passed each other in the corridor or one entered a room occupied by the other;
- being ignored while others were acknowledged, so that if the manager entered a room occupied by several people, or if several entered one occu-

pied by the manager, each would be greeted in turn by name, except Frances to whom no reference would be made at all;

- receiving messages from his secretary: 'He has asked me to tell you to take minutes of today's meeting';
- being spoken to in barked commands

Frances did not mind taking minutes of a meeting. It was something to do, but when she asked more about her role at that meeting she was told not to speak.

Why do nothing? Frances decided to sit quiet, with the hope of getting out gracefully as soon as possible. Right from the start she had been determined not to leave her first job too early for the appearance of her CV. As time went by, she became increasingly convinced that while at least some of the managers wanted her to go, others considered that she was too small fry to bother about and, anyway, they reckoned that she would be gone soon enough. Frances herself thought the second assessment was pretty fair. On the whole, she was left well alone.

Meanwhile her role was being looked at more within the context of the total service. This made good sense to Frances who managed now to take a somewhat detached position: all discussion on the matter almost pointedly avoided asking what she, as holder of the post, felt. She was experiencing at first hand something else she had been told to expect in the NHS: that its employees would not be treated as human beings.

The service manager decided that the job should change and this did eventually happen.

New pressures: equipment and places

Meanwhile Frances noticed that the new word processor with a quieter printer which she had ordered, and which had been agreed almost as soon as she had started the new role, had not arrived. Because she was doing tables and spreadsheets in the centre and the old dot matrix which was there made so much noise that it really disrupted other people, this had been seen as a logical and 'cost effective' expense. Frances' expertise with computers had been welcomed and her role as word processor 'helper' throughout the whole department had even been formalised through the service manager's secretary.

Without suitable equipment, she had to move from place to place, and often from building to building, to get the use of a printer for the work which other people were appreciating very much. It was an exercise in tolerance to accept that the manager's own secretary was given a new machine and others were ordered and delivered for people in other posts even though no one had yet been appointed to them.

As Frances' personal goals became lower and lower (often it was enough to survive the day) she did not put energy into too much fury. Somehow she staggered on through the next months.

The new printer came 15 months later, and even the manager commented on its usefulness. (The old equipment was given to one of the secretaries somewhere else in the trust and she did not use it at all because of its noise.)

To work to the new job description required Frances to be on three sites each week:

- one whole day in a new department, although the people in that department, and Frances' own report, had concluded that only half a day was required;
- one day a week at the office of the service manager, where she covered the intercom and did filing; and
- three days in the original day and residential care unit for the elderly.

Because she was no longer supported by an immediate manager in the main centre, she felt that she could no longer initiate work there and the staff often felt let down. Because she was no longer allowed to do patient care tasks, when carers were stretched and stressed but Frances had nothing to do, she could not support them.

Eventually, Frances did have a new computer of her own in the place where she was most, but continued to use others in the other two places. Because there was often nothing like enough for her to do in the other two places where she spent just one day, she would take work round with her. This meant that the most up to date information on patients' filing was often on a floppy disk in Frances' hand as she went from place to place.

A new worry for her, which she managed to smile over, became the choice of what to wear in which place. Was there another thing she could get wrong here?

She agreed to start the new programme and to try it for a couple of months.

Trying to take some control

Frances felt she had been become an un-glorified ward and filing clerk with nothing like enough work to do. It was boring and tedious. Her headaches got worse. Her union rep suggested that she should take out a grievance against the senior manager.

Her GP advised her to take a week off work and offered her some sessions with the practice counsellor. She saw him once: his advice was the same as she had been given before. He said, 'Get out.'

When she got back to work there had been more changes. The service manager's part time secretary had resigned. To replace her, they had created two new full time posts, one to work half time in the manager's office and half time with a newly created clinical team, the other to work full time in quality management.

The new secretary in the service manager's office was to be given a greater bonus which brought her pay above what Frances had been getting. And she was given a new computer, over which Frances was shocked to realise she felt petty resentment.

When Frances told the service manager that she was going to take out a grievance it was the first time she felt that she ever got through to him. For a few minutes he looked shaken. And for a few minutes he actually asked her what she wanted him to do, but added that it would probably be impossible because the other jobs had by then been created. He appeared puzzled when Frances explained to him that she was being bored out of her mind, and received neither financial nor intrinsic rewards in the job. 'Was not the filing flattery?' she was asked.

Coping again and getting out

By this time Frances' part time management course, undertaken with the approval of the trust, was making more demands on her. For a time she found it hard to care even about her course and its work, but was determined to complete it because she saw it as her exit visa. Finding that she could bring some of the course work into one of her offices and that no one noticed gave her new lease of life.

She decided to put most of her energy into devising strategies to stop the boredom.

She stopped going to the service manager's office and found that not seeing him at all helped a great deal.

She created some more useful and interesting tasks to do at the main centre in which she worked.

She took pleasure in 'stealing' tiny involvement, even seconds, with patients.

She cleaned cabinets and re-sorted filing cabinets.

She managed to work occasionally with people that she respected.

For her successor's use she made lists of all the things she did. She was determined to have a successor as soon as possible.

She came in late and no one ever seemed to notice.

And as she found new ways to cope in those last few months, she wondered how she had got there in the first place. Was it she who was at fault? Had she had quite impossible and unrealistic expectations of her first job?

In the last weeks she was 'officially' four days a week at the centre which wanted her and one day a week at the other. Sometimes her work was finished by 11 am and there was nothing else to do. Then she would flagrantly help the residents with their lunches and their breakfasts.

She was told that, when she did leave, the post would be downgraded by two points.

She was being pushed out, but slowly. She felt uncomfortable doing a useless job when others were needed clinically. She had seen the nursing shifts reduced by a third in her two years and care was obviously inadequate. The money that was spent on her could be put to better use. She had suggested redundancy but this had been refused. Instead she was advised to resign, get her GP to write a letter saying that she had to leave because of mental health problems and then claim benefits.

Through the use of her strategies, Frances had got herself out of the victim role and therefore thoughts of pursuing the grievance were gone, but she did enjoy the memory of her service manager's face when she told him she was considering it.

Until the day she left she kept on thinking of the miserable waste of resources, money and herself. She tried again to work out when it had all started to go wrong. One key time was when she had produced a draft brochure on a proposal in the service. All the manager said was that it needed work doing on it. She immediately burst into tears. She felt that she could not face him again. She felt useless for having reacted like that and felt ridiculous being locked in a relationship of such fear with another person. She knew it was unnecessary and irrational, but she had no one to help her to work through it. It seemed that nobody was interested in making a change. But that was not the start. It went back to those first two weeks and to other people, when no one had offered to help her try to make sense of her manager being sacked and clearing his desk without saying goodbye to her. That was when she started to feel that nobody would have any interest in helping her to deal with what was beginning to happen to her.

Postscript

To be out was a relief in itself. But to be better paid, to feel valued and to be told that there were prospects of development of the service she was working in and of promotion for her? To be upgraded within 12 months and for some of the initiatives she had taken to be copied in other parts of the country? And for all of this to be happening in the public sector, and in a service similar to the one she had left with no job to go to? She had not dreamed that this could happen to her, but the last news I had of Frances, that was exactly what was happening.

Chapter 2

The manager, the new structure and the meetings: Fay's story

About a hundred people were assembled in the lecture theatre of a post-graduate centre of a Midlands hospital. Some were talking animatedly, some were silent. Some people were still coming in and the platform party was not yet complete. The man who used to be the general manager but had now become the first chief executive of the trust was there. The director of finance was there. The chief executive stood up, almost shyly, and held up his hands. When it was quiet enough he said that he was sorry to keep everybody waiting but a few were still coming in and the chairman and a couple more of the new executive directors should be joining them in a moment. In a cheerful way he finished with, 'Let's start in a few minutes,' and sat down again.

A few minutes later the chairman and some other people, whom most of the audience did not recognise, had joined the platform party, the murmuring quietened and the chief executive rose again.

'I thought we should meet, well just briefly, to mark what's happened. We have become a trust. I know you will have all heard this over the last couple of days, but I wanted us to have this meeting, well partly to say to all of you, 'Well done.' You are all the managers and the senior clinicians (and senior clinicians are managers these days) who have done a lot of work in licking our service into such good shape, that it was accepted in this wave of trusts.

'I thought it might be helpful just to spend a few minutes with the executive directors who can be here to say a little bit about their directorates and how they see the future.

'First how I see the future. I think it's going to be great. I think it's going to be very exciting and a lot of **hard** work and of course we are going to have to face changes, but as we all know things cannot stay the same. That's one thing we can be certain of.

'We don't know how it's going to work out. We do know that we will have much more responsibility ourselves. You will have much more responsibility for your areas and your directorates. We will have control of our own budget. We will be able to use our savings. And the energy that we put into improving our service and getting more business for it: well we will see the benefits come back to that service. But that does not mean to say that everything's going to be lovely. Remember, we are doing this for the first time. There are still challenges for us to face but that, I hope you will all agree with me, is part of the excitement.'

The chief executive then invited the chairman and some of the executive directors who were sharing the platform with him to address the meeting about their areas of development.

The chairman spoke about the hospital being blessed with extremely dedicated staff who shared common interests in the objectives and future of 'their hospital'. He said:

'With so much common ground between and involving staff at all levels, it seems to me there is reason to believe the way ahead is filled with common purpose.

'We all know about the constraints which face us and that very difficult tasks are involved in managing our affairs within them. Constraints, targets, objectives, call them what you will, they will be even more strictly focused towards each unit now than they have ever been in the past. We must nevertheless recognise that the other services which make up our new trust have achieved so far a great deal in overcoming some of the pressures imposed by past constraints. There have indeed been very positive responses in taking and implementing difficult decisions which otherwise would have been to our severe detriment.

'As we look forward we are fortunate to be staffed with well qualified people, in an effective and well structured organisation. As such we should be capable of responding to challenge.'

One by one the executive directors spoke about their valuable staff and the co-operation which they had achieved in creating their part of the proposal for the trust.

The personnel officer, now called director of human resources, concluded his speech by referring to the new management structure, before it was put on the screen:

'I would like to tell you that if any of you have any concerns about it, your concerns will be fully heard and dealt with on an individual basis through proper and established channels, as will groups who express any joint concern. Matters of concern to any of the representative groups will also be dealt with. I want you all to know that you will be listened to.'

The director of corporate affairs then put up a series of overheads about management structure, the past one and the one proposed for the future.

As the overall picture was presented and the departments identified, the members of the audience peered more intently.

An observation from the non-executive (lay) member of an investigating team:
'So far, the people who have been honest and said what they have done, have been penalised. It is like telling them to tell the truth but encouraging others to lie. Perhaps you need an extra policy.'

The senior medical clinicians, who also had management roles in supervising junior staff or leading a clinical team, were less directly affected, but for the others, something was very clear. It was about jobs. It was jobs. For most people in the room it meant that in a few months' time the job which they were currently doing would no longer exist. They had the choice between getting out or applying for one of the new jobs which had been presented on the screen. For a few people, this was not the position at all. Their jobs were clearly secure, for the immediate future. But they also had a choice: it was to do nothing and keep their job (and wonder how long that would be safe) or to apply for one of the 'new' jobs presented on the screen.

The audience had been attentive and quiet and even walked out quietly.

Later there was much discussion. What was made of the opening speeches? Most people said they did not understand them. Some said that there was nothing to understand and one said it was 'like listening to poetry'.

Among those in that meeting, the most frequently asked question over the next few days was, 'What are you going to do?' or 'Have you decided?' Each realised that she or he needed to know what others were planning in order to make an 'informed' decision.

So who were they?

One such person was Fay, a nurse manager who had spent all of her working life in the NHS. She had been the sister in charge of an innovative mixed medical ward, then the sister in charge of outpatient departments and later nursing officer of the accident and emergency department before moving to one of the first senior nurse management jobs in an earlier NHS reorganisation. She managed the outpatient department, the accident and emergency department and day surgery. In addition, she managed one of the first programmed investigation units in the country. It was a sort of medical equivalent of day surgery, a move to get away from the haphazard arrangements over investigations ('You should have investigation X done and then come back to see me after we have got the result.' 'Now we've got that result, I think you should have investigation B done, and come back to see me after we have got that result.'). The programmed investigations unit streamlined and co ordinated the process and even in the mid-1980s was open to the views of users, who were in those days still called patients.

Not for nothing, Fay had been told by her seniors that higher management's eyes were on her. An indication of her value was that she became project manager for the new genito-urinary medicine clinic. And then that job had expanded to take in medical records. So Fay was, at the time of the new trust, manager of most of the outpatient services and the medical records of the whole hospital. Here was one of those rare things in the NHS, a place where there was good communication between the medical records and the clinical departments.

Fay was experienced in managing, recruiting and interviewing staff. She had a part time secretary.

Realising that the new management structure did make sense, she also realised that just about every new management structure also made sense because, there being no perfection, each had its advantages. Each had its pros and cons. The meetings did not talk about the cons. She had to make a decision.

In deciding to make a 'strategic' application, that is to apply for the job she was most likely to get, Fay did research. She investigated who was happily accepting redundancy, applying for jobs elsewhere, applying for his or her own job. And she tried to work out what sort of people the new top managers wanted.

Fay applied for and got the management job of the accident and emergency department. This meant close relationships with medical as well as with nursing staff and it required taking over the management of the receptionists.

Past experience in co-ordinating relationships with the medical records and the clinical staff helped here.

Other people were not so lucky. Some went elsewhere, some waited for the redundancy deals, some tried and failed to get jobs they wanted, and were then made redundant. Some got jobs they did not really want or enjoy.

As a further empowered manager, Fay won funds for the accident and emergency department to be refurbished, and won the co-operation of staff in the introduction of a skill mix. That enabled money to be saved, which in turn allowed them to employ more night staff, which was safer, and to take on a new grade of health care workers who were dedicated and helpful. As in the previous job, she was on call, as a member of the senior management team, and the crises which that entailed were mostly to do with finding beds.

Trust confidence and a big new change

The trust appeared to go from strength to strength, but after two years there was talk of merger.

The applications for trust status at the start of the reforms had been based upon an idea about what was the 'right' size and composition for a trust. Now people were talking about a change due to the great success of the market forces. Trusts had to merge or they would submerge. There were meetings with other trusts. There were training days about managing merging. The senior managers spent most of their time working on merger proposals and merger negotiations. Everything else seemed to be put on hold.

The first person to get a new job and the first person to lose a job were the two chief executives of the neighbouring trusts. One stayed and one left. The method of appointment for these first posts led to much curiosity because all the consulting of users, carers and the workforce which had gone into many of the appointments of other people in the last two or three years did not seem to be happening. Wide discussions about job descriptions and informal meetings with applicants also did not seem to be happening. The reason given by the senior managers was that there simply was not time. Yes, the trust still had a equal opportunities policy, but sometimes there was not time.

The new executive directors were in post. Some of the old faces, some of the new. Nobody brought in from outside the trusts.

Next, the jobs immediately below those. What would the new trust's directorate be looking for?

In one area the acting manager made no bones about his wish to get a substantive post and his belief that what was being looked for was somebody who would get things done'.

One person who showed how to get things done was a fairly recently appointed sector manager, in a position senior to Fay. In one crisis meeting about beds in one part of the newly created, enlarged, trust, the manager said that because no junior doctor had been found that day for the accident and emergency department of the other part of the trust he would shut it for the weekend. This was to make more beds available. Fay did not understand the reasoning behind this seemingly drastic move, so he explained. With that department shut, fewer people would attend. Some would go in the other direction to departments in other districts. There would thus be fewer demands on beds for their trust. This happened. That manager was clearly seen as somebody who would 'get things done'

It was a few days later that Fay heard from a woman in the other accident and emergency department, that the senior manager in question had told phoned her at midday, well before the meeting, and told her to telephone the locum doctor who had been engaged to work that evening and tell her not to come. 'Getting things done' was more complicated than had been realised.

The executive directors were formally in post. One of them had been a nurse in the past and so there was 'a nurse on the Board'. Fay was told by one of the executive directors that there would be a job for her: one similar to the one she was doing, or he would support her for another one. But the other executive directors appeared more distant. They were clearly very busy managing the merger.

And Fay kept on wondering, how could two accident and emergency departments be kept going in one trust?

The lecture theatre again

For the next 'layer' there was another meeting but it was a smaller one this time and some people thought that in itself was significant. Most of the people attending had a better idea beforehand of the sort of structure being proposed. The meeting was run by the director of finance in the absence of the chief executive. He started by saying that some jobs were not being affected at all and gave examples, such as the head of the pharmacy at the hospital they were meeting in. Transparencies of the proposed new structure were displayed on the screen, statements were made, questions were asked, and answers were given.

When copies of the transparencies were requested, the director of finance said these would not be available yet. Several staff insisted that they needed them as soon as possible to start understanding all the implications. Some people were going away on holiday within days and needed the information with them. The concern was, the managers patiently explained, that some- body might show the planned structure to people from the other half of the newly merged trust, before they had their own meeting. Of course there was no reason for them not to see it in good time, and they would be shown it, but the managers did want to protect them from being given the piece of the paper without the meeting which gave all the explanations and could answer all the questions.

The discussion went on for some minutes and eventually the managers agreed to one of the photocopying machines being used immediately, so that staff who wished might take the information away.

On return from holiday, after the usual strategic considerations, Fay applied for the job managing the accident and emergency departments and the genito-urinary medicine clinic. As the person who had 'commissioned' the first genito-urinary medicine clinic, she applied with confidence.

Preliminary attempts at discussion about what staff might be required to run the departments and what management structure would be best, led to a curious response: 'That will be up to the person who gets the job to decide.' With the words of one of the directors (if she did not get this job she would be supported to get another) giving her confidence, Fay left her single appli- cation in.

The interviews

The interviews were on one day but the results would not be announced for a full week because a number of people had applied for more than one job. The task of the appointments committee was very difficult. They had to juggle and negotiate.

After the formal interviews the candidates felt their performances were still under close scrutiny. Each of them would meet, sometimes daily, members of the panel who, because they were still involved in discussions on the 'juggling', might be influenced if one of the people who had already been interviewed behaved in particular ways. But what ways? The final decision was made on one day of the following week, or so people were told, but the announcement was not made until the day after.

Most of the candidates gave themselves the most mundane tasks that day. Some were called over one after another and it was a day of rapid rumour: she must have got this job; he must have got that. Then some were summoned to the offices of the individual clinical directors, not the manager who had chaired the interview panel process. These meetings turned out to be mostly for telling people that they had not got jobs, though one was for the opposite purpose. They were certainly another example of 'We are doing this for the first time'. The clinical directors faltered, they stammered; two of them were in tears. They did not say they had been made to do it; they said they had wanted to give the message themselves and they were very sorry about it. Fay did not get a job and as she was told she felt some sense of relief that it was over and that she would have to go.

Some who did not get their jobs were offered six-month contracts to help the new person in by leading a particular project (the people offered these jobs did not commit themselves but in discussions with union representatives later they learnt that if they accepted they would lose their redundancy entitlements). Most declined. One was reminded that he could go to see the nemonai officer to discuss over and that remark led to one of the few examples of overt irritation in those painful meetings: 'How could I walk through the hospital in my present state?'

Telling the teams who was going to manage them was also done by the clinical directors. But, by that time, the teams already knew.

People who lost their jobs and who declined the six-month contract were offered the opportunity of going immediately, but all said that there were ends that they had to tie up, and so they did a few days more in their offices. Several accepted counselling through the staff health service.

In the two or three days that some went on working, other briefer encounters took place with the senior managers. One of Fay's friends was told that she had interviewed well, but the person that they appointed was younger (that meant cheaper) and had not already got one of the other jobs, so 'What were we to do with her?'

They were offered leaving events, salary in lieu of notice and some, whose age made it easy, got good pension deals.

Postscript

It was a year later that I met Fay. She had heard that one of the newly appointed project managers had gone nine months later. That had seemed to take one morning to happen.

For herself, Fay told me that it was such a relief not to have to go on trying to explain about patients to managers. They do not know about patients.

She was relieved to be away from the lies and from always having to say that things were all right. She no longer dreamed of reports and business plans.

Chapter 3

Managers: five who were out of the NHS

These stories are put together partly because each of the five managers had mentioned trying to make sense of why the really top leaders of the NHS were not staying there for long, and most were going before retirement age. They had not made sense of it, but had learnt a lesson: look to their own survival.

There were other observations common to them. Over 20 years ago, in 1974, when all five were young, the area health authorities were introduced in a coordinated way, with little redundancy. Most managers got something comparable to what they had before, or some sort of promotion.

Less than ten years later (1982) the area health authorities went, with a more vicious round of competition and displacement of individuals.

Three years later the general management initiative led to recruitment from outside the NHS. 'Market forces' required higher salaries, which were made available. In came fixed term contracts, and talk of 'Clear your desk and clear off'.

Following that, the latest reforms soon generated their own momentum with mergers between trusts and between purchasers. And with the government reducing the numbers doing the job, the staff left faced even less security.

They all spoke of their relationship with those they managed, especially their immediate juniors whom they sometimes found themselves treating in just the way they had been treated.

They coached these people in some of the patter to use in controlling clinicians ('This is trust policy', 'Is that what you heard me say?'). They taught them how to 'split' the clinicians into different groups, so that at least some were for the trust policies and change. Always to sound positive, definite and clear; to avoid the vagueness of consensus; and, even if they changed them later, to present clear and firm decisions.

Every reorganisation or merger had been time-consuming and sapped energy. A few appointments were made where 'very good reasons' precluded time for equal opportunity, race and sex discrimination procedures, or for consultation with colleagues and consumers. For all the other posts, everything else was looked into; application forms, interviews, appointment committees, consultations with colleagues, user and carer groups, and the composition and running of appointments committees.

Those who got the jobs were a bit more secure — until the next time. A change in the chairperson, bids for another merger from outside, or rumours of a merger between neighbouring organisations can shake it all up again. Performance review has given a sharper edge to tenure, as failure can be a disciplinary matter.

The temptation, especially for those approaching 50, is to cook books or fake research; falsified results can stay undetected for years as jobs are got elsewhere. Thus a senior manager whose performance review (and pension) depends on projects being completed in time and in good shape can easily make them look right. They do not even have to worry about disquiet among clinicians or other subordinates who can so easily be represented as squealing against change.

The rules of the competition

Some matters which used to be private had become very public. Nowadays, as soon as a merger or review was known, it was also known that the managers would be looking for jobs. Each knew the competition: their neighbours. On the one hand, openness (all in the same boat); on the other, secrecy (each trying to learn the other's intentions, without disclosing his or her own). Displays of confidence hid insecurity. Worry, poor sleep and illness were denied. They got on badly together.

Some principles for their continued survival:

- Think of the 'most sensible' option.

- Think much more widely, and laterally.

- Apply for jobs really wanted, or for ones higher management was very keen to fill.

- If in despair, apply for a lower rate in a different trust because that organisation will be under no obligation to continue their present high salaries and may reject some of its own people in favour of cheaper strangers.

- Accept psychometric testing or other procedures required by the senior management.

- Speak positively and with a smile.

They had never had so few people whom they could trust as in their last two years in the NHS.

One day somebody may do a thesis, going through the filing cabinets of a few trusts. They will uncover all the working parties, project groups, committees with their recommendations; all the grand schemes and plans which did not happen.

And they all said that they had lost friends.

Angela and Dennis

Angela and Dennis counted up for me. Between them they had four degrees and one MBA (Master of Business Administration). In the last five years they had been through a total of eight major management changes, three trust mergers and nine jobs. Neither of them had a job at the time they met me. They had two children.

They had met at university. Their first child was born six months after they had both graduated. They took a decision at that time that Dennis would continue to work full time and Angela part time, so that she might devote more of herself to their child to be and another, if that followed. After a few years, Angela followed Dennis into an NHS management career.

Ever since they had both been working full time in NHS management, they had shared the same bad dream, that they might one day be competing against each other. In fact they considered themselves lucky never to have worked as colleagues in the same management group because, as both of them observed, it is very difficult for managers to get on well together personally. They explained what they meant as their stories unfolded.

They were high-profile, high-achieving, highly ambitious. Angela did a second degree as an Open University student when the children were very small. Dennis did his second degree on a part time release from an earlier management job. His MBA had come later, but was also paid for by the NHS management. They were being groomed for higher things.

Dennis' had appeared the more straightforward course, so they told me his first.

Dennis

Back to the trust

The first thing that Dennis noticed on his return from doing the MBA was how packed the trust's offices had become. In the open-plan central area two narrow tracks could be found between piles of cardboard boxes. Several of the offices were shared or partitioned off since Dennis had last worked there. The old 'smoking room' which was little more than a large cupboard had been decommissioned, fumigated, painted, improved and fitted with a desk. It was occupied. The chief executive's personal secretary welcomed Dennis warmly and said that the chief would see him as soon as he was back from a meeting with consultants, which would finish before 9 o'clock.

Dennis made himself a cup of tea and sat in one of the passages.

The chief executive was as friendly as ever and very apologetic for keeping him waiting the extra half hour.

Things had heated up in the last months while Dennis had been away and they really needed him back. The chief executive did not know how things would settle down with the merger that was just under way, but was sure there would be a job for Dennis and that his skills were really needed. Meanwhile he wanted Dennis to pick up where he had left off. This was a project in the fields of diabetes and rehabilitation, but now over a much larger area. An appraisal and a proposal were required in three weeks. 'Can't stop now', as he rushed off to a meeting with the purchasers. 'Catch up with your news later'.

Dennis examined his resources. He had a contract which the chief's secretary had given him and the chair that he had to sit on. He had no room, no desk, no telephone and the files of all the information to do with the project on which he had to work were in the basement store.

But Dennis was a manager. He signed the contract. He told me that it had very little meaning, but that signing it was necessary for him to get his next pay cheque. By the end of the week he had a desk, half an office, a computer and all the files were upstairs again. They included the names and telephone numbers of most of the significant contacts.

That kept him going for the first two months. Then into the next reorganisation. Dennis was given a list of all the posts for which he could apply. Unfortunately every one of them had someone currently doing it. And Dennis knew every one of those people well.

Dennis went through the process but at each interview was told that he was not the most suitable candidate. So he became redundant, 'due to organisational change'.

Journeys and notice

Dennis got the next job fairly easily, but it was 64 miles away. He had to make long journeys each day, or he and Angela had to separate for several nights each week. It turned out to be a bit of both.

He was given a management task to do and he did it. He created a team and together that team did everything it was asked to do. They produced ideas, reports and, even within a few weeks, some changes in working practice. Some GPs told the chief executive that they were pleased with how the relationships with rehabilitation services had improved. The problem was isolation. Dennis was isolated from Angela and their children, one of whom was still living at home, and he and his team were isolated from other managers. They worked in two rooms in what had been the porter's lodge of the original hospital. The other rooms were occupied by what had been called the personnel department, but was now the department of human resources.

The other managers of comparable seniority all worked in the trust headquarters. It was very apparent that they met each other frequently. This was not only, Dennis explained to me, that they were making references to jokes or events at other parts of the day, but it was also obvious in how the agenda and meetings of the senior managers were handled. Before the first of these meetings Dennis had received the agenda and half an inch thickness of paper accompanying it. He read the papers, thought about the problems, and came up with ideas on some of them. When the first of these items came up on the agenda, Dennis, after a tactful silence for a few seconds, started to make his point. 'Oh don't worry Dennis,' the chief executive said, 'We sorted that one out yesterday afternoon.' Dennis described himself as having felt rather surprised but not particularly upset, but when this happened twice in subsequent meetings he did say something. He said it very gently and that all he was suggesting was that in future they could take items that had already been discussed and resolved off the agenda completely, and that anything left on the agenda should be discussed properly. No one said anything but the looks were cool.

The practice continued, so Dennis did mention it again, but he had learned from his experience in the meeting. He mentioned it in a rather lighthearted conversation with one of the executive directors while they were both waiting for another meeting to start. The other manager did not appear to take offence but said, 'Remember that sometimes it is best not to change things if they are already working.' Dennis was not sure if what was happening could really be called 'working' but decided to say no more.

Four weeks later the deputy chief executive came unannounced into his office.

'You are leaving. Now if you resign immediately we will give you good references and six months' salary. If you don't, we'll dismiss you.'

'When do I have to let you know?'

'Well, now.'

'I won't. I'll tell you tomorrow.'

Dennis said that he went immediately to see the personnel officer (director
of human resources) and as he sat down in his chair prepared himself not to
be surprised if he knew already. He did. Yes, he could fight it, take it to a
tribunal; and he might even win. But whether he won or lost, he would
labelled as a trouble-maker and might find it very difficult to get another job.

His friends and Angela said the same. He resigned the next day. Dennis
refused to leave on the day that they wanted him to go and instead got them
to agree to three months. With the tacit acceptance that there were certain
things that were not mentioned, he and his colleagues got on relatively well
in that time. He was glad that, in spite of his great powerlessness, he had taken
a stand twice: once on saying that he would give his answer the next day and
the other on negotiating for three months in which to finish the projects he
had started. And on the strength of the good references that they gave him,
he got a better paid job nearer to home.

Dennis went to a job with a health authority (purchaser), which really did
have the task of assessing the health care needs of the community and allocating the money supplied by government to buy the best services available
to meet the most important of those needs.

Boundaries had recently been refined and there had been an internal reorganisation. It was a time for high fantasy and rumour: 'Proposals have already
been made', 'Decisions have already been made.' 'There is a master plan.' It
was also a time for fine words. The chairman spoke them and the staff
bulletins wrote them. Individual programmes, personal development, the
organisation looking after people's futures. But again it appeared somewhat
more sympathetic an organisation than the trusts with their greater numbers
of staff. There were not hundreds of letters going round, which looked at first
glance to be so personal, but which a few minutes gossip disclosed as being
standard. There was not the same round of retirement parties with the apologies of the chairman and everybody wondering if he had ever been invited.

Six months into Dennis' new job at the end of a busy staff meeting, the
chief executive said she just wanted to mention that there would be a reorganisation of the whole team.

'You will be getting details,' she said as she got up to leave. But she was not
quite quick enough. She had to hear the question, 'What jobs will there be?'

To which she replied that she did not know.

Dennis had a private interview later. His position became clear. He was
nearly 50 and after 50 could take early retirement. While technically he could
apply for any of the jobs, there were fewer available than people already
employed in the organisation. The people below him in the hierarchy were

younger, and therefore more useful for longer, and cheaper. They must be offered the jobs first. Must? Yes. Market forces.

So Dennis became redundant again.

Angela

Angela's management career had taken her into the field of what used to be called 'mental handicap'. As the words changed to 'learning difficulties' and as the hospital in which she worked started to shed beds, she put an increasing amount of energy into links with the private sector because it was partly from that domain that they started to 'buy in' services. She also learned a great deal about raising money and being accountable for producing value for money.

She attended a few one-day, district-wide management seminars on change which were convened by the district general manager of the day to discuss the very first government white paper on the proposed reforms.

Some time later Angela learned that it had been her very active participation at those seminars that first caught the eye of the district general manager, whom she had not met personally. Subsequently her name came up his discussions with those in 'shadow' executive director roles in early pre-trust days. That led to her being 'head-hunted' for a new post to be set up to explore the feasibility of different types of contracts with both purchasers and sub-providers. It was an inspired political move, enabling as it did the senior managers in the area to back several horses at once. At least for a time; and as long as they were not too squeamish about the horses.

It was proposed that Angela be seconded to one of the new trusts on an 18-month contract with a review after nine months.

It was with great enthusiasm that Angela accepted the job. That was two years before our meeting. When we met, it was with great relief that she spoke of being out of it for six months.

Angela found the purchasers wanting to spend no money, make no decisions and be punitive. She found the trust, with all the people brought, bought or borrowed in, to be overmanaged and tripping over its own bureaucracy. She was amazed by the intensity of the in-fighting and the inability of the senior management to reduce their costs in any way except by rounding up scapegoats. As soon as she saw what was happening, Angela realised that as a seconded person she should be expecting to be a prime target.

Purchaser blight

Angela said that they used to call it 'planning blight' from the purchasers, who seemed capable of making only two clear decisions. The first was that there should be efficiency savings of 1 - 1½% in the first year. The second was that there should be cuts of 12% over two years, starting with the second year and with no change in the level of services provided.

In principle Angela had no objection to those objectives, but became alarmed when she realised that the purchasers were very unlikely to come to any agreement on the sort of services they wished to purchase. She related this to the relationship between the senior managers of the purchasers and the next or near but one level in the NHS hierarchy.

Many senior staff in the purchasers, Angela explained, had been fairly senior in local health authorities previously. Many of them knew each other. With the merging of the original purchasing authorities and the original providing authorities (trusts) in the area in which Angela went to work, personality differences became much more significant and clashes more frequent. Similarly within the departments and between purchasers and providers. To any request for dialogue with the purchasers Angela and her colleagues received the response, 'Purchasers must be allowed to purchase'.

Purchasing or politics

Unfortunately that was the one thing they were not able to do. Why? Because of political interference. They were working in a part of the country with a high national profile. Political interference was blatant.

I asked for an example. Angela told me that there had been an independent major review of some of the services which gave a very clear recommendation that there should be major closures. Logically this made sense. Following a particularly vociferous campaign by local people and a few nationals, the local MPs were brought in on the side of 'no closure'. Soon it was with the Department of Health and the Secretary of State. Eventually the purchasers were told (I was assured, really and truly 'instructed') by the Department of Health that they had to continue to purchase certain services from that group of provider units whose closure had been recommended by the independent review.

What price market forces there? The U-turn was blatant political interference with the previously hallowed market forces. This meant rethinking on behalf of both the purchasers and the providers. In that rethinking they seemed unable to make any other single decision. Effectively the purchaser and the provider organisations were paralysed.

Angela was made aware of this in her own personal niche by the lack of commitment of the money for her post from any side. For the purchasers, the trust and for Angela, this uncertainty continued for the nearly two years that she was there. The purchasers were kept unsure of Department of Health commitment, or interference; the trust, of the purchaser's intentions and commitment; and Angela, of the funding of her job and quite a bit more besides.

As with abuse cycles through generations, the purchasers seemed compelled to do what had been done to them. They made political decisions. They had a very rapid turnover of all staff and several precipitate and traumatic departures.

Angela noticed that when newcomers were brought into the purchasers, they would often start to revise plans previously made after lengthy negotiation and resolution. But for the managers in the trusts to change any plans required another concentrated process. They had to consult with the people directly involved and with the other senior managers. Several times that process in itself was given a six-month timetable, yet at the end of that, no firm decision was made because all the other senior managers had to be consulted. Decisions were delayed until all the directorates and senior managers' units were at the same level of advancement.

Similarly, the purchasers' intended timetable was also delayed. The general manager (later chief executive) of the purchasers publicly boasted that by September of 'Year One', the intentions for the year starting in the following April would be public and fixed. In fact, in some areas of the service, it was as much as 15 months later before a decision had been made. Please note, she said to me, that 15 months meant half a year into the next financial year before there was a clear definition of the service which the purchasers wanted.

It was with this group of people, the purchasers, that Angela was to negotiate. In fact she got on well with their negotiators and found them reasonable people. But in her two years in this post, she did not even set eyes on the chief executive.

Over-management, under-managing

Angela explained how money had been poured into the creation of the trust and how the new strong management got in the way of itself. Central government money had gone into the creation of high-powered directorate posts in strategic development, business development, human resources etc. There was money for the setting up of premises and offices. Information technology (IT) was 'in', so that anybody could have a computer (every single one from a batch of 30 on a particular office site was stolen six months later). New and individual paper headings, logos, signposting, notices and the upgrading of premises (tarting up offices).

Bringing into these high-powered posts the intelligent, dedicated and enlightened young managers created in itself a proliferation of management tasks. They met, consulted each other, consulted other people from outside the organisations. (Seeing my eyebrows rise at the last point, Angela said that it was like the professional colleges to which people are invited from abroad to give papers. In that academic sphere there is status in knowing people from other countries and hosting them here, with a pay-off in the reciprocal invitation to visit them.) So in the new management world there was a status for a director who brought in a prestigious consultant to run a training day for her staff. Most prestigious of all was when a manager was 'bought' by another trust to do a training day or consultation there. The distribution of memos, invitations, notices, consultative documents, and draft reports increased many times. The consumption of paper was never measured.

As a principal manager of a concern of this persuasion, Angela should have been negotiating directly with the purchasers. While in theory this was still expected of her, in practice her executive director had to be in agreement with proposals being negotiated, together with all the collateral managers of the other services, lest a unique contract with one should 'impact' on the others. Similarly, all the clinical leads within her own management sphere had to be brought in.

Angela explained more of the complexity of this, especially if all the people involved could not meet together. Proposals went into even more drafts. Negotiations went on everywhere and no one, it appeared, had the final say. It was a 'corporate trust', corporately insisting that all the contracts be negotiated alongside all the others.

Getting the complexity clearer

I was lost in the intricacy of this argument. I appreciated Angela's need to talk with the feeling which was quite apparent, but tried to get her to be more specific.

She took me again through the budgeting argument. The government said that the NHS must work within its budget. Trusts would have a budget through contracts with the purchasers, and had to work within this. Savings accrued could be ploughed back into the 'business'. It was the clearly expressed government intention at the start of the reforms that this principle should be pushed down into sector management. Many of the early trust propaganda meetings, which Angela had been to, spoke enthusiastically of the pleasures of management in running small units able to use their own savings. This was in sharp contrast with the bad old days of being able to do nothing of the sort, but making a grab for any surplus in the district's budget at the end of the financial year — to buy a new carpet.

When Angela started to negotiate a special contract for her own sector and a single variation in terms and conditions for one group of staff, she got their enthusiastic support. But the executive directors would not allow this to continue until they had had a study day to examine the possible implications for each directorate and implications for the trust as a whole and how it might affect its 'value' in a new round of mergers which were already in the air.

Through the delays caused by this, Angela lost both the individual contracts and the goodwill of her staff.

Who were those senior managers?

The chief executive of the trust was himself barely 40. He had recruited a group of young men to be directors and general managers. These people had mostly university or civil service backgrounds and no experience of working at the coal face.

This contrasts strongly with some other places I visited, for example Leicester Royal Infirmary, where most of the managers had grown up with the service. The people whom Angela met had been moving steadily in their careers before the sudden jump into this trust. They were well rewarded with high-profile jobs and salaries.

But their high salaries had a sting. There were few places for them to go. Many of them were trapped until they were kicked out. They were well versed in management theory, language and style, but of the intricacies of the health service they were innocents. Some had worked already in the private sector or had friends who were doing so now. They thought it would be as easy for them in the trust to understand enough of what was going on, but they had not appreciated the difference in size of the two organisations: size both of the hospitals themselves and of the management teams. (What Angela said reminded me of the boasts I had heard from those running private hospitals. To the visitor's question 'Where is the management block?' the answer was that there was none.)

So these smart-suited businessmen with clipboards and the latest articles in their briefcases were able to thrive in meetings on macho-style thrusting, and ego- or logic-driven rhetoric. Because they were so caught up in their rhetoric, and the excitement of their self-promotion, they could not question from a wider view. Angela reminded me of the story of the emperor's new clothes. In the NHS none dare comment on the pretend market, with its pretend freedom, pretend responsibility and pretend accountability.

Why she left

Angela had described chaos and frustration, but she still came across to me as an enthusiastic manager so I was still puzzled why she left.

She reminded me that the original deal which she had accepted with such enthusiasm had some things clear but some things left very vague, to be clarified later. I had been familiar with contracts which were deliberately kept vague and had had one myself for a few years. Sometimes they suit everyone immediately concerned, but are very difficult for people to understand. Above all, they work when people are getting on well enough together. Angela was seconded for 18 months and this was to have been reviewed at 9 months for the advertisement of a substantive post after that review if it was satisfactory.

The first review was in sharp contrast with the satisfaction that everybody had expressed with Angela's work during her first months. It was unhelpful and critically negative. Instead of being given the news that the substantive post would be advertised, Angela was offered a six-month extension of the secondment. She turned this down, expecting negotiations, but they said they could not negotiate. 'Could not'? Angela told me that when she did or said the things that she had seen her male colleagues do or say, acceptably and often successfully, she received a different reaction: she was described as somebody who 'went for the eyeballs', or 'liked to draw blood'.

Attempts at negotiation dragged on.

Meanwhile the purchasers' second decision, namely that there should be management cuts, had become trust policy. The domain of management became a battlefield, with no side but one's own. Each was protecting his or her own back while attempting to knife that of the others. Angela's secondment post was an obvious target because, more than any other, it was seen as 'denuding' the others. She explained that this was not simply a matter of money. If the seconded person was got rid of, then the empire of that person could be carved up between the others. There would be more for them to manage, and the more they could manage, the more they could feel secure.

One of the general managers suggested to Angela that they propose the merger of their two care groups as a 'pre-emptive' strategy. Angela was not sure what would happen to their jobs but in principle it seemed a good idea and she said she would think about it. Early the next morning she had a telephone call from one of the executive directors expressing concern at having heard from her peer, her fellow general manager, that she had been suggesting a merger between two of the centres. Angela explained that it was not her idea, but that she was quite prepared to consider it.

When she next met the manager in question she joked about it.

The following week the executive director had a letter from Angela's colleague suggesting that the two different care groups would not be able to work together well, expressing concern over the relationship with Angela and complaining about derogatory remarks. As happens in these affairs, Angela was then asked by the executive director, who was her own line manager, to explain. She had always got on well with her, so did not worry as she went to meet her. She explained why she thought the letter was a 'wind up', but agreed that its existence was a problem. She was asked for her own suggestion and gave one. Because the 'wind up' had worked, her colleague might be willing to withdraw the letter and the executive director could ask him to do that. He agreed and did make the request, but the manager did not comply. Both of them were in the office together with the executive director the following week.

Unlike any conflict resolution exercise in which Angela had been trained and would have used often in her role as a manager, hierarchical weight was thrown clearly behind her colleague in this meeting. Angela felt more strongly than ever before her status as a seconded person. There was no resolution. She was instructed not to speak to her colleague without the executive director being present and fortnightly meetings for this purpose were set up.

Money, too

At the same time as that episode took place, the financial constraints started to bite. While the definition of budgetary domain for each management sector had been made shortly before Angela's secondment, history had left its marks. Overspends and underspends of the past were inherited by the 'wrong' people. Angela was expected to manage the past overspend of the department, which had accrued while her predecessor was in charge, but when she did that and made some savings which led to an underspending, she was not to gain the benefit of that. In fact looking at the overall figure and extending backwards over the two years, her own service had been more or less in budget all the time.

Towards the end of the financial year most of the individual directors and managers were as civil and pleasant as ever with Angela to her face. However she found that things she required to be done, were not being done. More difficult was her discovery of meetings being held without her and decisions being made in those meetings without any statement in the minutes or memoranda acknowledging her absence. One of these meetings she discovered by accident when she happened to be in a different building and, in passing, enquired about one of her colleagues whom she was wanting to see briefly.

Angela told the chief executive that she could not go on and that there had to be a decision on her secondment. Unfortunately the chief executive appeared to be as beleaguered as the rest of them, struggling hard for survival. There followed another three months of hedging and delaying, while she herself was frantically trying to manage, keeping her staff enthusiastic enough to complete the plans, and create some action. And she was thinking every day how to cover her own back.

Still no action, so Angela wrote to the chief executive 'just to put it in writing'. Her position had become untenable. She wished him to create a substantive post to be advertised in open competition as had been agreed, or formally to end the secondment.

Angela was invited to meet the chief executive and the chairman. They went out for a drink. Five minutes of pleasantries. Fifteen minutes of uncomfortable general conversation ending with an overview of the restructuring of the management and what was called 'future planning'. Then the ever so slightly mumbled words, 'So there won't be a job.'

'You mean there won't be a job for me?'

'Yes, that is indeed what I mean,' the chairman nodded.

With clarity at last, Angela left as soon as she could.

So now we are both at home, she said.

I decided not to ask Angela if she had tried to go back to her old department in the trust which was the provider of services for those with learning difficulties. She had mentioned in passing that most of the old guard there, including the chief executive, had gone long ago and that the whole trust had been one of the first to merge with another to form a larger one and shed jobs.

Doris

In her enthusiasm for change and the new challenges, and with the conviction that the NHS needed to be caught by the scruff of its neck and given a good shaking, Doris got herself promoted into management. It was where the future lay. The job would be there. A contribution to make. Your own job may not exist much longer, you know. It's where all the bright people go.

So from her job in staff training, Doris volunteered to be seconded for 18 months into a bed management job at a busy district general hospital. This 9.00–5.00 job was newly created to deal with an old problem:

- no beds for emergencies;
- beds blocked by chronic cases;
- beds kept empty for surgeons' operating lists;
- beds 'bagged' by rogue clinicians;
- bed occupancy too low, or too high, too constant or too variable.

Doris was to juggle all of those. The specialists, particularly the surgeons, made it very uncomfortable for her. She pleased no one and her 9.00–5.00 hours stretched more and more. But there was surprising help from how creatively the management exploited the government's need for several well managed hospitals to take in any casualties from the Gulf War. This hospital became well prepared for dealing with those casualties which never arrived and Doris's contribution to the preparations were well appreciated, both by those who managed her and those whom she managed.

She had been bitten by the bug of management. When the first wave of the 'real' NHS reforms was rolling in, and there were advertisements for service managers, a 'new breed' of person, she applied. She was to be in the forefront of change.

Doris got the job and was one of the two new service managers of the acute sector of the district general hospital in another area. She knew that a service manager did more than manage staff, because the purchaser/provider split required such a person to deal with budgeting and contracts both for services (maintenance, personnel departments, etc.) and for the clinical 'product' (with GPs and the purchasing authorities). There was a lot of training to be gone through and Doris went through a lot of it: contracting, budgeting, managing, business planning, making service specifications, future planning, staff support and disciplinary procedures.

The first battle

Within Doris's sector there were four clinical directorates, which might have been any from accident and emergency, obstetrics and gynaecology, ear nose and throat surgery, orthopaedic surgery, genito-urinary surgery. Each of these clinical directorates had its own budget, competing interests and committed, powerful clinical directors. She had said she did not know how it would be possible to manage four clinical directorates and after six months, senior managers agreed. New posts were created and Doris was left with two clinical directorates to manage. She had to manage two lots of people and the services they ran. Among these groups the leader roles were held by consultants. They did not like being managed, having targets which they were expected to meet, and having to join in the process of negotiating contracts.

The senior managers did not seem to like things either, because management appeared to be crisis management. At first Doris blamed them for this, but very soon she learned that it was also how they, in their turn, were being treated by those above them.

An example of what would happen to Doris was that on a Friday afternoon she would be told that she had to produce a report on a particular matter by Monday. There was no point in saying that she could not or would not do this, because if any of them had tried that, they would be told that they had applied for the job, that the senior managers were having to jump also, and 'That's what life has changed to.'

The weekend would be dominated by getting that report done, and it was no sooner done than ignored. Soon another one would be demanded, and another crisis would have to be handled.

Doris had to fight for office space, for secretarial support, or for secretaries to be treated in a way that resulted in them staying.

Who controls the budget?

All this would have been bearable if Doris had been allowed to manage. She could keep the consultants and the other people in the clinical teams contented, working hard and co-operating with the reforms in the early days when they and she believed all they had heard on budget control. In this area the crucial thing was that the trusts and departments would be able to carry savings over from one year to the next and plough their savings back into improving their own services. So the people that Doris called 'my teams' were prepared to work harder to produce reports and plans and were prepared to accept the postponement of some staff appointments. They were prepared to accept all this because they trusted her to use the money saved to improve the departments and thereby the services they were providing for the patients.

They underspent their budget and when the figures came out they felt that they had achieved something very significant. However, some other sections in the trust did not underspend, they overspent, and the savings of Doris's directorship were promptly transferred to bail them out. Or to bail out the trust.

Doris had discovered new rules:

If you are good and work within your budget, you are praised.

If you are bad and overspend your budget, you are rewarded.

(I came upon several others who had worked out the new rules through what had often been a very painful learning experience. And some had said that there was a third, very important rule: *If you are praised, it won't be for long.*)

Within her own directorate, Doris's credibility fell. The clinical directors and their teams no longer trusted her.

On not being allowed to manage

One team had to move ward. The accommodation was old, in need of redecorating and 'refurbishing'. On the agreement that those things happened, Doris had the teams with her when the temporary move happened.

Then the decision on what was to happen in the 'refurbishment' was also taken away from Doris. It was deemed to be 'capital planning' and the service manager no longer had control over this. How could she reward the people who had moved so co-operatively, other than by saying, rather unconvincingly, 'Well done'? Morale slumped further.

Doris continued to try to support staff on the wards by being seen, by meeting them, listening to them and talking to them. But her role took her further away, even from the place of patient care. She had to do that to stop things being taken away from the services and from patient care. Rather than improving things, stopping things getting worse had become the goal.

Managers were on call. To start with this rota was one in seven, because the service managers and the executive directors of the trust — the senior managers — shared it. Sometimes there was nothing, sometimes they were called six or seven times a night and at weekends. While on call, they had to carry a bleep and a mobile phone. When executive directors decided to take themselves off the on-call rota, four of them were left doing it one in four. They got no extra money for this, but they were busier.

The larger organisation

Doris believed that no amount of training could have prepared her for the politics of a large organisation. Fighting for budgets, putting her case, trying to improve services without more resources, battling with consultants and with other colleagues. And always wondering who would be next. Would it be her or would it be someone else? Doris gave me the story of the director of nursing as an example. This person was a couple of years younger than Doris and would have been called a matron in the old days. In the restructuring of the trust and its emphasis on management at the service manager level, with localities or units, the job of director of nursing was to disappear. She was told that there would be no post for her and she was made redundant. Staff gave her a leaving party and had a collection for a present, but she was offered no counselling for this sudden life change, and she went off to work as a staff nurse somewhere else.

When the trust merged with another, one of the service managers had to apply for his own job. He did not get it. He was told to clear his desk that day and to go. The head of a different department had gone under very similar circumstances. And they all knew of senior managers who went at a day's notice.

Doris felt that she was never on top of her job, and that she was rarely achieving the new demands being made. She felt that in those rare moments when she was on top of her work, no one was interested because she was almost immediately told to do something else.

She could never sit down to sort anything out. She was no longer part of a team. She worked longer hours. Her personal life was affected. At home, in the evening, and certainly almost every weekend, she felt that she could never get away from her work. This was especially so in January and February, preparing for the end of the financial year, and in April and May working on the new contracts and what staff levels could be afforded. She was irritable with friends and family, her energy was down, she was sleeping badly, waking in the night with sweats and panics over losing her keys or her briefcase. Her dreams were often repetitive and reminded her of countless 'must do better' dreams of her childhood and adolescence.

Organisational audit

The trust was forever calling in outside consultants. If there was a matter of how a clinical service should develop, they never asked the people doing the service, but would rather pay thousands of pounds to outside consultants for a study and a report. Often the report carried almost word for word what some of the leading clinical people had been saying already.

One of these consultations was on 'organisational audit', which bore little resemblance to 'clinical audit' described in the introduction to this book. They brought in enthusiastic consultants on the subject of the organisational change. It was part of the constant change that managers would always be living in. The consultants had a system. They had many forms, they went to the wards, they went to staff, they went to patients. They worked at setting aims which were agreed by all.

The next stage was to interview everybody again to find out how they thought they had been getting on with the aims. The final stage was to interview other people to see if they thought those people had achieved those aims and if what they said they had done, had been done.

Then they produced a report.

I was invited to guess how that had helped staff morale.

We had the Patient's Charter

The executive directors and the trust board wanted the service managers to set targets for each item of the charter. Then they were to work out how well they were approaching them. All of this was to be done with no extra resources, except forms.

There was special productivity in complaints. The Patient's Charter encourages complaints and so nowadays there are far more of them. Doris had to investigate each, very rapidly, and draft a response for the chief executive to sign.

The ending

Doris decided that she could not cope with the hard management role and certainly could not do so for another 20 years. She could not please everybody, nor even a bearable proportion of people. She did not have control over the resources she needed to be able to do her job; and the resources were removed whenever she conserved them. She thought that she would never go back to work again in an NHS hospital, even in a clinical role.

I pressed Doris further on the last point: why not even in a clinical role, because she had told me that she had really enjoyed her early 'hands-on' times as a nurse? It was, she told me, no one thing, but rather a great number of little things, each one of which reminded her too much of the distress of management and the persistent pressure on all the staff in the wards nowadays. The general public has been led to have absurdly unreal expectations, which are then put onto the senior management and staff, who are handling the very sick people rushing in and out of hospitals with high turnover. The ward manager's job, let alone the service manager's that Doris had been trying to do, had been changed beyond all recognition.

By leaving, Doris lost money (a few thousand pounds a year in salary and her performance related pay) and she lost a great deal of stress. I asked her what she had gained. She had gained time which she can measure. Peace and integrity which she cannot really quantify at all. But the thing that keeps on going back into her mind is made of words so strange that she would never have uttered them a few years ago. Indeed she would have said to anybody who used them, 'What do you mean by that?' I was told not to ask Doris for an explanation when she insisted on finishing her interview with me with the words, 'I feel that I have gained contact with my soul, after I had left the service which had lost its soul.'

Doris had gone to work for a voluntary organisation. I think I did understand her final words to me.

Dawn

As head of district nurses under the old regime of the NHS, Dawn had been recruited under the '**management initiative**' of the mid-1980s to become one of two locality managers for the community nursing service. Between them they managed over a hundred people, including midwives, staff at family planning clinics, district nurses, health visitors, occupational therapists and a few others. They split their patch geographically but still shared their exper tise to mutual advantage. Dawn was more familiar with occupational therapists and health visitors, and the other with midwives and district nurses.

With the appointment of the first shadow chief executive of the shadow trust and the taking on of fundholder status by some of the GPs, new problems of communications arose. Senior management and Dawn and her colleagues were having to take decisions on the run.

The first thing to startle Dawn and her colleague in those immediate pre trust days was that their community services manager, who had appointed them to the two locality management posts a couple of years before, was sacked. He had been with the organisation for some six years and he was well known to many of the managers even before that. There must have been many opportunities to assess him and to tell him to change anything that senior managers wanted him to change. And they could have warned him. As far as Dawn knew none of that had happened. One morning he was told to go.

Dawn met him twice afterwards: he was clearly furious and upset at what had happened, but would say nothing. Dawn and her colleague assumed that he had been instructed to remain silent and had agreed to abide by those instructions. He was not surprised when both of them said that they were considering applying for his post, but in sadness rather than in enthusiasm.

In one of the sherry and biscuit, self-congratulatory, all part of the excitement events around the preparations for the application for trust status, Dawn and her colleague mentioned to the shadow chief executive that they were considering applying for the community services manager post.

The response stuck fast in Dawn's mind: 'No, ladies, you may not', as he pressed a cream cake on each of them.

Later the same evening they learned that one of shadow executive directors had been headhunting and a successor had been found, so there would be no need for an advertisement or interviews. Dawn's colleague started to say something but was frozen by her look. She herself had already learned when not to say things. In her head, she was asking why they were not advertising the job and reminding the chief executive of equal opportunities and was repeating the 'wisdom' that wide advertising was the way to get the best person. But she said nothing.

Dawn felt particularly strongly because she had once sent some of her staff on prolonged training courses assuring them that their jobs were being kept open. On their return the senior managers had insisted that the posts be advertised. In other cases, where staff had been appointed to their unit of management they were not allowed to move them around later within that unit without further advertising.

'You can always find irregularities in any group of people if you look hard enough. This applies to my discipline as much as to any other. We fall short of best practice. When we read of yet another colleague, from whatever discipline, being suspended, we think it could happen to us. It encourages us to cover up.'

The new manager

As the new trust was born, the new community services manager came in with a flourish. She had been in a fairly high-profile job in another part of the old health authority, although on the same grade as Dawn. (Dawn smiled and said how bitchy she had become.) They had known each other for years. She did not like the structure which she had inherited and wished to expand nurse management. It seemed unwise to Dawn and her colleague and they thought that the new GP fundholders, who felt that they were paying directly for something like that, would not wear it. Other people, they heard, gave the same advice.

The management was duly expanded and restructured. The area of the old district was divided into three, each to have its own locality manager. A third locality manager was appointed to fit in with this, and each had a number of patch managers. Conflict was stirred up between everybody and clinical work was neglected as many with such skills were submerged in extra management tasks. True to Dawn's prediction, the GP fundholders were murmuring disquiet.

Soon after the third locality manager was appointed, there was a sudden summons for all the other staff to meet the community services manager and the executive director (no longer shadow), but with the three locality managers excluded. More friction and more tongue biting.

The GP fundholders wrote formally to complain that 'their' money was being put into management instead of into field staff. They wanted there to be more people who would do the hands-on work and they insisted that the process be reversed. It was not.

Another appointment, again not advertised, was made to the post of project manager and coordinator for the community services manager. That man was to do the project work such as Dawn and her one colleague had done previously. There would then be five people (one community services manager, one project manager and coordinator to the community services manager, three locality managers) instead of three (one community services manager and two locality managers) before the trust.

Meanwhile the chief executive of the trust suddenly needed the community services manager to be acting general manager. Dawn and her two locality manager colleagues offered to 'act up' (do the job of) the community services manager for three months at a time; and to cover each other's work while delegating to senior field staff as they needed. The answer to this offer was that the project manager and coordinator for the community services manager would act up as soon as he started work.

The plan of Dawn and her colleagues could have been cheaper, but they were told that it was not necessary and that the department could wait for the newcomer. With that background the new project manager and coordinator started work. Dawn and her colleagues tried to say 'Welcome, good luck, and we are sorry that we were not allowed to compete with you for your job.'

They tried to get on together.

Gradually the GP fundholders showed more of their muscle: 'We are paying for this and we do not wish it to continue'.

A new structure

Shortly after he started work and was acting up for the community services manager, the new project manager and coordinator arranged an appointment to see each of the three locality managers. One at a time. In fact each found on entering the room that alongside the manager was the personnel officer, by then renamed the director of human resources. He was silent throughout each meeting. The manager read from a script. It went something like this:

'The trust has decided that the three locality manager posts in the directorate are now redundant.'

The statement went on to tell Dawn and her friend that there would be no jobs for them in the new structure. The newest, least experienced of the locality managers (the cheapest) was offered a job.

Later all three locality managers went back together and asked if they might apply for the one post, but were told no.

Now this was all done by the man who was brought in as the project manager and coordinator for the community services manager; or at least the message was read by him. Why had the community services manager (acting general manager), who had known Dawn for years, not seen them? They were told that of course they could see the acting general manager. They could request an appointment if they wished to appeal against the decision and then it would be arranged. Dawn had failed in her resolution to hold her tongue.

At the end of their individual meetings Dawn and her friend had been given slips of paper which were photocopies of handwritten statements on redundancy entitlement. There were 40 redundancies made in that way and around that time, so the photocopies of the hand written slip of paper must have served many people.

They were expected to do three months' notice, but they made a fuss and asked for payment in lieu. Dawn and her friend left in a month.

The ending

The senior managers had built up this large structure against the advice of Dawn and her immediate colleague and the GP fundholders; and then they took it to bits with a great deal of pain. Not once had Dawn received any formal appraisal, so she kept on wondering how they could have known how well or badly she might have been performing.

The general manager (no longer 'acting') and Dawn did not meet again. She did not come to Dawn's brief, low key leaving event. She did however make a video tape for managers to show to their departments. It was of her and the executive directors telling them what was happening. Dawn was instructed to show it to her staff because it was in support of locality managers. She showed it to them before she left.

Donald

Exchange and exile

When I met him Donald was not working in the NHS but had done so once. Soon after the reforms had been announced, but well before the christening of the first trust was in sight, Donald had been encouraged by his general manager to participate in a job exchange with an Australian colleague. It was to be for nine months.

'We need as many ideas as we can get so sending you away to look at a place where they are doing things differently is a good investment for us. And we may get something from the woman who comes in your place.' Thus spoke the general manager. Donald was single, unattached and enthusiastic about work. He was assured of his job to return to. It was not to be a complete jump into the dark because he had visited Australia and had even made some of his own contacts with hospital management there. (He knew that his own general manager had contacts also and he suspected there might be a hidden agenda for the general manager to get something out of it later on.) Donald went.

As arranged he sent monthly reports to his general manager. In the third of these he reminded the manager that he had agreed to send Donald news of developments back home. It was at the time of very strong management initiatives. Resource allocation and resource planning were in full swing as Donald went and he was keen to know how that was going, let alone to find out if there was news of the 'short list' for the first shadow trusts before the trusts themselves came into being.

Donald got no answer.

He telephoned. He left a message. He received a message that the general manager would telephone him at a certain time and he made himself available. Eventually he did get through. He found his old boss affable, enthusiastic and brief. There was a lot happening. Many changes were exciting and they were all terribly busy. But Donald was not to worry. They would send him a list of all the jobs that there were going to be, and with that information in front of him, he could decide what to apply for. There was absolutely no doubt that there would be something for him when he got back.

He got no list.

Homecoming

Donald landed, when he did return, into what he described as the activity of a revolution. The maelstrom of a revolution. The organisation was in the status of 'shadow trust' and was behaving as if it were a trust, but it was not one yet. People were working very late. There seemed little boundary between work time and recreation time. They took so much work home and there were many late night and early morning telephone calls and extra meetings. Some people were appointed on contracts given without even the semblance of an interview process.

Four of these high-activity, high-performance, high-energy people were sleeping together, in two pairs.

The grasp on power of the general manager, now shadow chief executive of the shadow trust, was tight and central. He told everybody to get on with it and needed to know in detail what they were doing. He was constantly fine-tuning, or crude-tuning, in attempts to maintain what clumsy market forces and purchaser drives could otherwise destroy... 'until we have had time to educate them.'

Money was lashing around, but only for some things. There was money for new writing paper, money for the creation and production of the trust logo, money for equipment and the launch of new offices, money for information technology (computers etc. for creating and running the statistics). And such allocated money not spent on those things could not be spent otherwise. 'Therefore we've got to use it. We have got to be seen to be the most enthusiastic runners in these reforms.'

Donald was given a job. It was to produce and coordinate all the documents which were needed to review the configuration of the proposed trust. This was to be a configuration both of the geography and the proposed services of the trust. Questions for him to consider included: should the small enclave on the top of that hill, 'geographically' in a neighbouring trust, be serviced by theirs because all the people were on the GP list of what was very likely to be the first fundholding practice in the neighbourhood? (The population, and through them the GPs, might be worth wooing.) Should post-operative physiotherapy services be managed by the community and priority services trust, or by the acute trust? Donald was aware of the extreme political sensitivity of some of these matters, and that he would be judged by how he handled the petitions and protestations of certain vested interests. This task took nearly a year.

The executive director and the chairman (both shadow or designate and then later confirmed in post) were delighted because everything which Donald discovered or fitted into his documents supported the case that they had put forward. The proposals were accepted. The ex-general manager, ex-executive director, ex-shadow chief executive, became chief executive of the new trust. The shadow chairman became the chairman. Most of the shadow executive directors became executive directors.

In the excellent work he had done for the chief executive and chairman Donald had, unfortunately, upset too many people who were close to the ear, or the bed, of the top pair. He was seen as the one who had 'caused' the trouble by producing all the evidence that caused so major a disruption. He became a notable *persona non grata* and got no job. For a few weeks he was kept on, shunted between the remaining undesignated bits of the organisation before they were incorporated in the newly created trust structure. He undertook reviews of services he knew nothing about and he produced piles of paper. And he tried to speak to the chief executive and the chairman. His six weeks' grace were up and he left.

Chapter 4

'Three hours to clear your desk'

At 8.30 am they told him to clear his desk and to be off the premises by midday.

The newspapers reported that the trust gave the reason as failure to meet performance targets. The department of which he was clinical director had taken on an extra consultant within the last year and the level of GP referrals could not 'sustain' four posts. Therefore there had to be a redundancy.

The BMA (North Western Regional Consultants and Specialists Committee) did their own press release. They pointed out that in making contracts without consultation with the consultants themselves, the management had not realised the necessity for, at least, more operating time. They had created something that was unworkable.

By the end of the autumn the mayor was quoted in the local papers as saying that the chief executive had been nothing but trouble since she started and should be sent out of town. The trust had commissioned an independent inquiry into the events around that meeting: the inquiry had concluded that the suspension was totally unacceptable and it criticised the trust for not taking appropriate measures to ensure continued patient care. The trust accepted that there had been insufficient grounds to justify dismissing the consultant by reason of redundancy. The consultant, Ian Mahady, would be reinstated. Mr Gerald Malone, Minister of Health, responded to a question from the local MP in the House of Commons by speaking of the value of openness. Later, in a TV interview, Mr Malone reiterated his position:

'I like to think that we have a culture of openness within the NHS. Not only where it is appropriate do we encourage people to speak out. We actually, in our guidelines, say that they should. It is their responsibility to draw problems that they notice to the attention of management and to have them solved.'

That much was very public and was broadcast on television.

Despite the assurances of Mr Malone, staff at the centre of some of these disputes which have received such national attention have been reluctant to talk to me and have said that they have experienced a frosty reception to any attempts to criticise or disagree with management openly.

But information was available. There were reports in the local and national press. In this town the general hospital is very much part of the community. Approached from some sides, the hospital grounds are entered when a side street appears to merge with one of the roads of the hospital. Walking around, it was easy to pick things up.

Furthermore, in some sense I had been there myself. I had been a consultant in the health service and I had been a medical director of a trust. I knew something of how managers were sometimes advised and trained to deal with doctors: how to ignore 'professional conduct' but deal with 'personal conduct', how to confront and how to split them by finding allies or dissenters in their midst. It was not difficult for me to work out some of the script that was probably used.

How it might have been set up

It blew up around a Bank Holiday weekend. There would have been at least an informal discussion at which the chief executive and chairman had agreed that it was time for this particular consultant to go and, if necessary, to be got rid of. As clinical director in the obstetrics team he had more administration to do and therefore would have seen fewer patients: easy to pick him off for low productivity. There might have been allusions to a history of trouble making: 'not supportive to the trust...critical of innovation'. (He did say in one of the television interviews that, as a clinical director, he was not there to give financial or management opinion but to give a medical opinion. If something came up which he felt strongly should be pointed out to the management, he would mention it. If he felt that the management was not listening, he was the sort of person who would continue to say what he had to say until they did listen.)

At this and other meetings, formal or informal, there would have been comments on the need to curtail the power of doctors, and to show who was in charge. There might have been talk of subtle messages from politicians or the NHS executive to show that the reforms were working. Strong management was needed to control the medical profession which was the group that had done so much harm to the NHS in the past.

Some of the members of the board would have come from an industrial business background, and would be firmly supportive of the notion that if somebody has got to go, then the sooner the better. Only the trust's medical director would be there to advocate the importance of continuity of care, in of post-operative visits by the consultant. (As one of 'them' — or was it of 'us'? — he might have felt inhibited from putting forward so 'wet' a view.)

Ian Mahady would have been called to meet the chief executive (or chief executive's deputy) and the medical director before the Bank Holiday. Probably summoned from an outpatients clinic. He might have been slightly tetchy over this and requested clarification. Was he being summoned as clinical director of obstetrics and gynaecology or as a consultant? If it was to be as the latter, he most certainly would have wanted his BMA representative present. He would have been assured, if he had asked, that it was as clinical director.

On being asked straight away in the meeting if he was prepared to accept voluntary redundancy, he might have said, 'No, no, no more. This is not something for me to discuss without the BMA representative.' There would have been a haggle over fixing a time for another meeting because, remember, it was before a Bank Holiday weekend. I know that there was an NHS 'stat' day of extra leave for staff on the day after that Bank Holiday Monday and I expect the consultant and chief executive might have appeared to vie for the position of 'who is most important' so that he or she has to work on that holiday. And there would have been argument over the operating list already fixed for the first 'working' day after the Bank Holiday. The management position would have been that they would 'manage' this: the junior doctor who was there or a locum could be brought in. The consultant (is it because they are always covering themselves or do they sometimes really care?) might have argued for honouring what he had told patients that he would do: namely perform their operations himself. That was something which they might have been expecting. Anyway I know that the operating list did take place, done by Mr Mahady, the consultant, and that the meeting took place on the following morning.

The meeting itself

It would have started with the BMA representative introducing him or herself. The deputy chief executive (in the absence of the chief executive) would then have asked the BMA representative if Mr Mahady would accept voluntary redundancy. The BMA representative would have said 'No, he won't.'

There might have been some parrying remarks such as, 'Does he really mean this?' 'Does he recognise how serious this is?' But the BMA representative would have continued to say that the consultant would not accept voluntary redundancy. Soon there would be an adjournment, during which the deputy chief executive, the medical director and the BMA representative would have met privately for a few minutes.

On the meeting being reconvened the deputy chief executive would have spoken directly to Mr Mahady. It would have gone something like this:

'I am going to make this offer to you once more. Will you accept voluntary redundancy?'

'No. I won't.'

'This really is the last time you are going to be offered this.'

'No. I refuse to accept it.'

'In which case I am instructed by the trust board to inform you that you are made compulsorily redundant. You must leave the hospital by 12 noon today.'

Mr. Mahady might have said something like, 'And where may I go in those three hours?'

'You may go to your office and clear your desk. You may go nowhere else but the corridor between here and there, and between there and the car park.'

The BMA representative might then have intervened with:

'Why 12 noon?'

And the deputy chief executive would have responded, 'I am instructed by the trust board to inform Mr Mahady that he is made compulsorily redundant and must leave the hospital by 12 noon today.'

(It is quite common in these meetings for there to be a set sentence such as 'I am instructed by the trust board...' which is repeated several times.)

The medical director would then have been addressed by either the BMA representative or by Mr Mahady himself. (This is commonly part of the process too: whether as part of the fight for survival or as part of assessing the medical director's 'true colours'. For whatever reason an attempt could be made to appeal to medical loyalty, responsibility, ethics, standards.)

'But I operated on patients yesterday and I should see them in the ward in literally a few minutes' time. I should go to see that they are all right. I also have a clinic to take, and this includes new patients who have been referred because they have specially asked to see me. May I go and see these patients?'

The answer would have been something like, 'No, you may not. You have heard. You are not to go to the wards. Other arrangements will be made.'

'Who is making other arrangements?'

'I am making other arrangements. You are not to go to the wards.'

I do not know if they pursued things any further (some do and some don't), but it could have continued with:

'It is good clinical practice for patients who have been operated on to be seen by that surgeon the next day, and the Patient's Charter says that if somebody wishes to see a particular consultant they should be able to do so, and that new patients should be seen by consultants. Are you saying that you are not allowing me to do these parts of good practice?'

'I am saying that I have made other arrangements. You may go to your office and clear you desk and you may go along the corridor from here to there and from your office to the car park. You may not go to the wards.'

Another sentence was being repeated. Mr Mahady would have then gone to his office, where the other consultants would have met him to find out what had happened. They would not yet have been asked to cover for his work, but during the course of the day the medical director would have given instructions to them or to the registrar. The latter would also have been to see Mr Mahady and would have been advised that, in this baptism of fire, he should seek all the support he could from the other consultants and refuse to take on any responsibility for which he felt not fitted; and maybe he was also advised, if in any doubt, to get in touch with the BMA itself as soon as possible.

Some people I have spoken to who had been in this position have told me that they had been quite terrified of driving a car because they have felt so devastated and anxious. Others have sought help from their GPs or other friends. A number have been placed on tranquillisers. I do not know how Mr Mahady coped with the next few hours in his room and the next few days out of the hospital. He left the hospital by 11.30 am.

What happened to the patients?

What did happen to this consultant's work and the patients who were expecting to see him?

I know something of the process from my own experience and from other people when they have told me of what has happened when a consultant has suddenly disappeared by being suspended or 'going on leave'. Each individual will have been told that whatever happens next with regard to the work is not his or her responsibility:

'The trust will make arrangements.'

'We acknowledge that it is not ideal, but it is our responsibility and we will manage.'

If consultants protest that it is unsatisfactory for patients, the reply is fairly standard:

'Yes, we agree. But it is our responsibility now and we will manage it.'

The person goes. A few key people are told on the telephone and the grapevine does the rest. Sometimes a memo is sent around from the chief executive with a 'I have to inform you' theme and appreciation of the valued service and contribution over the years given by the departed. 'Arrangements will be made as soon as possible to find a replacement and carry on the clinical service.'

Then a manager summons the other relevant consultants.

'There is no need to explain why we are here. We all know that Dr So and So left yesterday, and of course I am sure you will appreciate that the discussions with him were confidential and I am not able to say anything of them.'

(Sometimes in such meetings it is a different manager who does not know what the other manager said and heard. The line then is, 'As you know, I was not there when X and Y met, and that meeting was confidential, between them. I do not know any more of what was said than you do.')

'But we do have to decide what to do next because there are the clinical services to be run and patients to be looked after. So how can you plan to cover this work?'

Hesitation on behalf of the consultants is met by more:

'What has happened, has happened. There is nothing that we in this room can do about that. The question now is: What are you going to do to help the patients? What is your offer to support the trust?'

The consultants are fairly tightly trapped. If they protest over what has happened they are told that it is confidential and cannot be discussed, but the managers will agree that it is unsatisfactory. If they say that they think it was a dreadful thing to have happened and a dreadful way for somebody's career to end, the managers will agree with that too. If they make no offer to do extra work, to cover clinics, see patients on the wards etc., they can be accused of being uncaring, irresponsible, uninvolved, unresponsive. Their professional commitment can be called into question. They do not know exactly what it was that led to their colleague leaving. They will want to keep their own jobs. They may well have strong loyalty to the clinical service and care for its reputation and for the patients, some of whom they may know. They usually come up with an offer.

Some background that I picked up

A full day and a bit in the public library examining every news page of a year's local papers (thank you, *Burnley Express* and *Burnley Citizen*) and a bit more besides, and some walking in and out of the hospital, yielded a lot.

Many of the NHS items in the papers were really very mundane. This even applied to some matters which aroused strong feeling and controversy — car parking, for example.

The papers also carried items on spending and fundraising. There had been an appeal which successfully raised a couple of hundred thousand pounds. This was spent on a piece of equipment which sounds good and looks good, but is in fact only used a few times each year. It is called a lithotrypter and is used for getting rid of unwanted stones in the urinary tract. Far greater expenditure than if arrangements had been made for the work to be done in other centres.

Trouble over three months' leave not taken

A third of the way through the year a 'TOP DOC GOES' type of headline appeared. This turned out to be a different consultant. He had gone, and then he hadn't. I found out some more on this story. It seems to have started with the fairly usual sort of muddle and wrangle of a bureaucracy. The sort of wrangle that can go on sometimes for years, until something or somebody 'snaps'. There was a snap here. It was over holidays. One of the consultants had worked with few holidays because he was doing the work of two. There was nothing secret about it. In his specialty he was effectively working single handed and was on call a substantial part of the time, and so for two years he took little leave and 12 weeks of it had accumulated. When the trust had arranged for more staff to be employed to end an arrangement which was considered unsatisfactory, it became possible to see how things could be sorted out. This is the sort of matter which a personnel department would look into and resolve. But the personnel department in a new trust would be inordinately busy with contracts, job plans, skill mix, disciplinary procedures, redundancies and even, sometimes, staff support. (And the personnel department itself is under pressure and scrutiny and may have to be devising its own business plan, targets, mission statement etc.) This personnel department was certain to be targeted in the trust's drive for loyalty. One of the stories going around was that a known dissenter to trust style, who had worked in that department, was there one day and gone the next.

Anyway, the personnel department said they would come up with a proposal but didn't. There were further discussions, again they said they would and again nothing happened. The chief executive herself had been said to have raised no objection to one of the proposals, namely paying the consultant for the three months' extra work that he had done. The matter appeared settled.

A sudden summons to a meeting with the senior managers. The three months' pay idea would set a precedent and it could not be afforded anyway. Take an extra month's paid leave each year over the next three years instead. But that would push the new consultant into a very similar position in three years' time. The new person would be having to work full time on call for an extra three months: how would that 'extra-contractual' work be paid for? No decision. No decision by midday the next day and that is when something snapped.

Resignation letter. Accusations of gross professional misconduct. Said he would work a few more days until the medical director had been able to arrange locum cover for his annual leave. More sudden meetings. Several medical staff saying that there really was a risk of the whole medical service falling to bits if the management's act was not pulled together. Sudden agreement to pay the three months' leave. Accepted. Resignation withdrawn.

But, strangely, the payment, at the insistence of the management, was said to be for 'time and a half'.

Why the 'precedent' argument did not wash with the staff

I found numerous, interesting, widely repeated rumours.

Trusts have the right to pay salaries that they decide and to negotiate with work groups for any scale. The professional groups have consistently opposed local pay bargaining. Yet individual members of professional groups have been free to accept whatever contract they might be offered. A group which has been most active, both collectively in opposing local pay bargaining and individually in accepting unique contracts, has been the doctors.

Thus it was widely believed that since the trust had come into being consultants had been appointed at the bottom and at the top of the national scale, and that some had started at the level of a 'C' or a 'B' merit award. Some were said to have been welcomed with a 'golden hello' of several thousand pounds removal expenses, and one with a six-year contract (all at merit award level) of which five were to be worked. Additionally the trust's medical director, who features prominently in this story, was widely said to have a 'million pound contract'. This phrase referred to a clause which committed the trust to pay £1 million compensation if it sacked him. Now £1 million was an eightieth of the total budget of the trust, and may be relevant to the long drawn ending of his tenure. More of this later.

Meanwhile, the managers' representation on the NHS distinction awards committee further fostered feelings of suspicion. Whom did the managers support? Those who were seen as open or critical; or suckers up? Since the inception of the NHS consultants, led by the BMA (I believe to its shame), have accepted the secret allocation of funds in the distinction awards system. This has led to bitter rivalries, suspicion, and resentment. There is I believe no credit to the medical profession in the BMA's acceptance and often vocal support of this system. That managers are now involved has complicated a messy business and, in this trust, increased the rumours.

And I unearthed reminders of the past, that little packet of history 'inherited' by administration and work force alike when the trust came into being.

Ian Mahady, whose dismissal had provoked this row, had been a consultant in Burnley for 15 years. When appointed, he was one of two consultant obstetricians and gynaecologists. They served a population of a quarter of a million. They did a one in two on-call rota and when one was on leave the other would cover every night and weekend. In 1984, the consultant establishment was expanded to three. When the first formal 'job plans' were drawn up in Burnley at the beginning of the 1990s, they included the recognition that the number of obstetricians and gynaecologists was less than both the regional health authority and the Royal College of Obstetricians and Gynaecologists recommended. The job plans committed the management to endeavouring to improve upon this. Ian Mahady proposed not only a fourth consultant, but also an 'associate specialist' to concentrate particularly on family planning and termination of pregnancies. In principle this was accepted by the trust and the purchasers agreed to fund it. Arrangements were so advanced that by September 1993 a locum consultant community obstetrician and gynaecologist was in post.

The obstetrics department had links with the teaching hospital so medical students were regularly on placement there. It was also the first department in the trust to conform to the government's fixed level of hours for junior doctors.

The trust and contracts

The movement for trust status in Burnley had been management-led. (Lots in the previous year's local papers on that.) This had been so in most of the country, but the vote here of over 80% against trust status amongst the medical staff was one of the highest. The trust management which emerged was vigorous and confrontational. Loyalty appeared to be expected and demanded. People left quickly.

The clinical directorship system was introduced but the clinical directors were not involved in negotiating contracts with purchasers. They had to work to contracts that others had negotiated. (The degree to which clinical directors were involved in discussions over contracts varied greatly across the country. As other stories testify, some have appeared to have been ruthlessly, or ignorantly, excluded from the process. In other cases the managers openly involved the clinicians as much as they wished.) For whatever reason, little consultation took place in the Burnley trust. The first suspicions among clinical staff over the function of the clinical directors had been that they were to split the profession. Now they were seen more as buffers between the clinical teams and the increasingly distant, but threatening, managers.

How to spend £10 million

All the consultants were invited to a special meeting to discuss the next phase of the redevelopment programme. £10 million had been awarded from central funds for this. The managers' proposal was presented. The doctors pointed out some risks which the managers had not realised. The managers understood the objections and also the objections to yet another proposal which they put forward. It was a considerable reassurance for the consultants to witness managers listening and accepting that things had to be changed. (There are sound reasons for thinking about which departments to have as neighbours to psychiatry and for a children's ward not to be near the top of a building.) The managers then went on to say that they would still put in the proposal to the regional health authority for the original project because that was what was agreed. When they got the money they would do something else with it. The consultants were told that it was important that there should be no 'leak' of this discussion of objections to the proposal or of the plan to use the money differently when received. Managers were introducing consultants to another 'rule' of the 'real world': You don't have to mean what you say. Rather threateningly, a manager added that, if there were any leaks of this discussion, they would know where they had come from. (If you wonder where I got the story from... well, I heard it a long time later and, from the number of times I heard it, I think it became pretty common knowledge. Hospitals have good grapevines and they have been fertilised by many gagging injunctions.)

It did make me wonder whether governments also make similar statements in anticipation of possible leaks.

Nurses and doctors

G grade nurses (ward sisters and charge nurses) found that they were to be prevented by the trust from working weekends or Bank Holidays. In some cases this effectively reduced their annual income by £2,000.

The operating theatre teams built up over many years, were told that they would all have to work shifts and all would be doing, one month on nights. If they did not agree they would have to leave within 12 months. Now such teams would have developed over years and people in them would have built up their particular hours of work around family commitments. The NHS was dependent upon such arrangements. Sudden change in these requirements from management would have drastic effects on the private lives of members of staff and their families. Staff felt that what they said about these concerns, which in some cases extended to worry over whether somebody's health would stand the new arrangements, were disregarded.

In a strange way, medical staff and nursing staff were feeling closer, brought together through the way they experienced being treated by management and the way they were exploring and testing their powers to resist.

For a long time this story when the medical staff committee had a motion of no confidence in the medical director on its agenda. He always voted against it.

The Community Health Council

The CHC was often in the local papers and clearly represented a body of local public concern that felt shocked by what the trust was doing. It felt that it was made powerless by being kept in the dark. One headline was 'We've been snubbed'.

Over one matter, the trust was said to have communicated. The chairman of the CHC received a curious telephone call. The trust's chief executive suggested that it was irregular for the CHC to take on a particular person as a new member. This was because that person was closely related to an employee of the trust. The chairman of the CHC disagreed and the new member joined.

Other public matters

In a public statement in April 1994, the chief executive, worried over the performance and funding of 'problem' departments, referred to the possibility of 'downsizing', but was reported to be making strenuous appeals to the purchasers for special funding to be maintained.

On the other hand, at the beginning of May 1994, the trust proudly proclaimed that it had reached most of its targets and had, overall, balanced its books. And the figures were impressive: 95.5% of patients had their initial assessment within five minutes of arrival at the accident and emergency department and almost 85% of outpatients were seen within half an hour of their appointment time.

Matters and figures got even better. At the beginning of July 1994 the NHS league tables were published, giving Burnley trust top marks in 9 out of 23 areas, with the chief executive quoted by the *Burnley Express* as saying: 'We are shown to be one of the top trusts in the country. Very few have got such a large number of five-star awards'. And a week later, 99% of people questioned thought staff were excellent in the accident and emergency department and more than 90% praised the information they were given. That was made public in the same week that the chief executive of the NHS, Alan Langlands, visited the main hospital and told everyone that the NHS was in very good health.

The trust had tried mixed sex wards and heard, through the CHC this time, that they were not all that popular. Patients did have a choice and should be told of this when they arrived, the chief executive said. She added that the hospital had a protocol.

In response to a letter of criticism of her in the local paper, the chief executive wrote (*Burnley Express*, 5th August 1994): 'I operate an "open door" policy and I welcome constructive criticism on how we might improve our service for patients.'

Back to Ian Mahady, the clinical director who was suspended

Contracts drawn up without clinical participation can have interesting complications.

Targets for the directorate of obstetrics and gynaecology included a reduction in waiting time for outpatients, reduction in waiting time for inpatient treatment and an increase in day patient care. (The department was probably not worried over this and may have been eager to make such changes. I have come across countless consultants who were quite shocked when the reality of 'consumer neglect' came home to them. Increasing 'user friendliness' is something for which I found nothing but enthusiasm.)

Noting the extra consultant sessions being taken up, the new contract also required the consultants in the department, as a group, to be treating a greater number of extra cases within the year, and by a particular amount. This was to be one third up on the previous level.

There was a difference between the two sorts of requirements. The one, for changes in waiting times at clinics and for certain procedures, was clearly a matter over which the clinicians had some control and could act fairly quickly. The other, for changes in volume of work, was dependent on the relationship between this department's consultants and the referring, or potentially referring, GPs. And the relationship which these GPs had with other specialist teams was also important.

I was reminded of what I heard from GPs in Leicester, who were no sooner being told of a great service on offer from one trust, than they had an even 'harder sell' at greater length from another trust offering an identical service. I do not know who else, if anybody, was wooing or being told to woo these GPs in and around Burnley.

And how easy is it to increase work in gynaecology? Remember that this means doing consultations with, or operations on, people who would otherwise have gone elsewhere, or would have had no such consultations or operations. If you think that is strange, imagine the thinking if you are in an accident and emergency department and are trying to increase the volume of work.

(Interesting parallels in prostate cancer surgery were widely reported in the press in October and November 1995. Some surgeons had been advising men to have their prostates out in circumstances for which others had given the opposite advice. Drumming up business to bring in the money to pay for staff could have deadly consequences for some men who had not been fully informed of the side effects of the operation or of the consequences of not having the operation at all. Malcolm Dean wrote movingly and clearly in *The Guardian* of his own journey through the murky waters of ignorance among well meaning professionals spurred on to make the reforms work.)

Anyway, what had happened in Burnley was that the new consultant started work at the end of the calendar year 1993. At the end of the financial year that person had been in post for three months. Not much time to woo the extra cases, from whatever category or by whatever means. The target was not met. On the other hand, outpatient and inpatient treatment waiting times had gone down and more day treatment cases were being handled; these were matters more directly within the staff control.

Not getting their money's worth

The purchasers said that they were not getting value for money in obstetrics and gynaecology and Ian Mahady, as clinical director, was to give an account to a meeting of purchasers and trust managers.

Explanations of the length of time it takes to develop and expand clinical services, for new people coming into post to become known by general practitioners and other colleagues in the district, to develop and to take on a work load, were put to purchasers and trust managers, none of whom considered them satisfactory. The trust said that the figures would be reviewed monthly and that if there was no improvement by the end of the year one of the consultants would be made redundant.

'One of the consultants'? The trust had recently taken on a locum consultant with a month-by-month contract in the department: was ending that really in the management's mind? No, that was not considered an appropriate solution. There seemed to be bigger fish in mind.

Imagine Ian Mahady's position in being required to increase business. I did not pick up how much they were 'gagged' from talking to colleagues in other, neighbouring trusts, but I have come across reprimands in other places. Whatever they did or did not do or find out, the obstetrics and gynaecology team knew that it would take time to build up business. And they now knew the seriousness of the management's threat.

Meanwhile, in other parts of the trust, three of the clinical directors had resigned, but Ian Mahady resisted this temptation and stayed on.

He met the purchasers again, but near the end of the financial year. The clinicians had looked carefully at the contracts which had been negotiated without their participation, studied the figures and their implication (remember it could mean having to find women who might otherwise have no consultation or operation, and persuade them to have them) and concluded that they were too high to be realistic. This clinically based argument was not welcomed. The purchasers said that in future, rather than having a 'block contract' with the trust, they would pay case by case. Was the writing already on the wall? A target figure was easily arrived at by the trust managers.

A little later, in a meeting, the chief executive and the director of finance were able to show that only 90% of the target had been met. Referrals had increased by 10% over the year and, with the new staff taken on, were expected to continue to increase. Variations between consultants always existed. When one consultant took on the role of clinical director and gave up two sessions of clinical time, it was not surprising to find that he saw the lowest number of new referrals. The management made no response to these comments and arguments. They had to proceed with the redundancy, had already contacted the BMA and wished to know which consultant would accept it.

I expect that was another one of those short meetings.

The consultants also spoke to the BMA. None of them wanted voluntary redundancy and the BMA informed the trust on their behalf. The consultants could not find out what criteria were being used in making any redundancy decision, nor what the procedure was. When the BMA asked the trust for a sight of their redundancy policy the response was that the trust did not have one. The BMA industrial relations officer was then asked to assist the trust in preparing one. (One of my informants in Burnley suggested that if the trust had had such consultations before embarking on its efforts to get rid of Ian Mahady, at least they would have been able to have given a clear reason why he was being made redundant when he was, and the whole episode just might have been prevented. As it was it never seemed clear from the press releases or reports in the press why they had done it.)

What happened afterwards

The publicity took a long time to die down. Demands for both the medical director and the chief executive to go were vociferous. The chairman and chief executive were widely said to have been 'summoned' to the regional health authority, there to be told to sort their act out. Then they started to blame each other, the chief executive went off sick, and after a day's negotiations, a deal was struck. The chief executive, the chairman, and then, after many weeks of public acrimony, the medical director, all resigned. Maybe he stayed on longest because the £1 million tag to his contract inhibited the trust board and whatever management was still there from giving a bigger push.

The chief executive's deal included a payment of £$^1/_4$ million but this figure only came out after questions in parliament. (£245,000 was the gross cost to the trust of which she received £135,750 net, see *Hansard*, 28th November 1994.) The Burnley Health Care trust serves populations from three parliamentary constituencies: from part of Pendle, part of Rossendale and Darwen and the whole of Burnley. MPs had tried asking oral and written questions, but it was in the end the device of an adjournment debate obtained by Burnley's MP, Peter Pike, that elicited the information.

The independent inquiry into the affair concluded that the compulsory redundancy had been an error and that the consultant should be reinstated. He returned in February 1995: his secretary had been transferred to another department, some specialised computer equipment he had been using had been returned to the manufacturer and his office was now a store room.

Cost in money terms? At least the £$^1/_4$ million paid for the chief executive, plus all the salary they had to pay to Ian Mahady while his appeal and the inquiry were going on and the extra sessions paid to the other consultants to deal with Mr Mahady's waiting list in his absence. (The last was 'waiting list initiative' money which I have referred to in my introduction. When that budget was created I am sure it was not in the imagination of the most adventurous bureaucrat that it might be used to deal with the waiting list of somebody that the trust had already suspended but was continuing to pay.) As to the human cost, who can say?

The medical director

No answer was received to the question the MPs asked about the 'million pound contract' for the medical director. When his resignation was announced, the chairman of the medical staff committee said on the radio that his consultant colleagues would welcome the ex-medical director back, as a clinical colleague. A statesman-like remark, but it left me awed by the potential re-entry and reintegration problem. Here was a person so identified with a management that had fled, who had been the lone voter against repeated motions of no confidence in himself, whose own clinical work load had reduced to two sessions, who had been doing no on-call duties, whose contact with referring GPs had been greatly reduced and changed in nature. How was the work to fund his salary going to be earned from GPs and other purchasers?

No story really has an ending and in this one my telling of it finishes as two consultants were to return: the one who had been suspended and reinstated and the other who had been medical director until he resigned from the role.

I wonder what happened afterwards.

Chapter 5

The rheumatologist: Mary's story

I found this one of the most remarkable stories of bureaucratic and managerial ineptitude. I went back over it several times, I corresponded with my informant, yet it is still quite extraordinary.

Joint medicine is a specialty where the team is likely to be small. This is the story of a consultant rheumatologist, that is a joint specialist, whom I have called Mary and who, before the reforms, had a half time contract with a district health authority.

With the introduction of the reforms, the purchasers asked the GPs what services they wanted to be improved. One of the items on their 'shopping list' was the waiting time to see the rheumatologist. It was then at the national average, but the GPs considered that this was too long. The purchasers went on to ask their public health department to study the problem. They reported that the department was seeing more than the national average number of patients and therefore needed one more consultant and a few designated beds in order to be able to meet the reasonable demands of the GPs.

Meanwhile the purchasers and the trust which ran the hospital in which Mary had her sessions started to negotiate the contracts: rheumatology was priced separately from the others so it stood alone. She did not understand the significance of this but the chief executive told her that she might come to appreciate it later. It would enable her and her managers to see exactly the value of her service and for rheumatology to use any of its own gains or savings. The purchasers said that they accepted the need for an extra consultant and that they had the money available for this.

There were two meetings at which some of the purchasers' managers met Mary. In these creative meetings many an idea was floated for an ideal service but there was no proper discussion of what might, in real terms, be practical.

The first contract

One day Mary was presented with a contract written by one of the trust's managers. This manager had not been to any of the meetings with the purchasers that she had attended. The contract included the provision of a particular technique which, although it promised well, was still at an experimental stage at one teaching hospital. Mary pointed this out and was reassured that the document was a draft. A few weeks later, another draft contract was presented; the problem this time was that it made no mention of the beds which had been recommended in the report by the purchasers' public health department. Mary felt that the manager scoffed at her as he tried to reassure her. He told her not to worry about the beds, which could be included later, urged her not to delay and added, 'Let's get on with it.' Later, Mary learned that this was the first contract that this manager had written.

Six months later a colleague in the medical directorate happened to see a letter from the purchasers stating that the rheumatology contract was unacceptable and that the purchasers would therefore be putting it out to tender with no further discussion with the trust. The senior manager of the medical directorate thought that one reason why the rheumatology contract had been ignored for so long was that there were no beds involved in it: it was less costly and less complicated, and therefore had occupied the attention of all the managers less. Mary realised that this did not mean that the managers, from either the trust or the purchasers, were less interested. She decided to telephone the purchasers' manager to protest that she had not been told that the rheumatology contract was unacceptable. He said, 'Why should I tell you?'

(Much later on Mary realised that he was, technically speaking, correct. It was not the purchasers' job to inform individual consultants. That was the job of the trust. At the time it all seemed very confusing in this new world where talking to the person on the other side was not allowed or, at best, was highly controlled. From the way managers behaved later, it may have been confusing for them too.)

In discussing this incident with another colleague, Mary was reminded of the drawbacks of being part time: 'If you were full time you would have heard by now that the trust and the purchasers were not speaking to each other.'

Some GPs who were well known to Mary were telephoned to tell them what was happening and they made their protests. Although most of the GPs were not fundholders, they were very keen to have an influential voice in the shape of the new services.

But the process was not stopped. Six months later the contracts did go out for tender and there were half a dozen applicants. By now it was common knowledge in her hospital that their trust and the purchasers were not on speaking terms. In addition, there were strong rumours that the purchasers were on good speaking terms with the King John's trust a few miles away. (King John's is a fictitious name I have given to the teaching hospital concerned.) Links were developing between them already.

Consultant and purchasers meet

Mary was invited to a meeting between the purchasers and her trust's managers to discuss the tender. At it, the purchasers' manager said that it might be helpful to mention some of the features that counted against the service offered by the trust. These included that they did no joint aspirations or injections and that there was no associated physiotherapy. As both of these statements were not true Mary said she wondered how the purchasers had come to that conclusion. The purchasers' manager said he had visited the rheumatology clinic at … (he named one of the subsidiary hospitals of the trust) and was told that they did not do these procedures there. Mary took a deep breath to restrain herself, and explained that this was because they were done at another clinic within the trust.

It was now clearer to Mary how the purchasers got the sort of impression they did. It also seemed that they thought there were no beds and that the department did not see any specialist inpatient cases. She could in fact use beds at any time on the medical wards, and she regularly saw patients from other specialties if they had joint problems while inpatients on the wards. Again they had not asked. Clearly the trust and purchasers were not talking. How could a half time consultant influence that?

Mary decided that all she could do was to try and influence her own immediate management colleagues in her own trust. After the meeting, she therefore offered to redraft the proposal for a rheumatology service and present it to her manager at the beginning of the next week. The manager accepted this offer with enthusiasm: 'Now we are working together.'

And Mary spent the weekend doing it.

She produced a glowing summary of the comprehensive rheumatology services offered. It covered the different sites at which clinics were held and specified clearly the variety of diagnostic and therapeutic procedures available. Mary surprised herself by how she could present the work in such positive terms, while feeling all the time that she was such a novice in the art of medical promotion. A presentable draft was on the manager's desk by early Monday afternoon, but the manager warned that rheumatology was not the only contract he had to work on that week. Nonetheless, he promised to have converted the document into the language of the contract world, and to have a costing, within three days. In fact he didn't, and at 6.00 pm on the day before the meeting at which the purchasers would make their decision, there was still no costing. The most threatening rival, the King John's trust, had already published a glossy brochure, with prices prominently, but tastefully, displayed.

Losing the contract

The contract was awarded to the King John's trust. Suddenly Mary's trust appeared to be embarrassed by what had happened and embarrassed by the presence of this part time person on their payroll. The chief executive started to attend meetings with Mary. He suggested that they try to get a contract for her to do her sessions at the King John's trust. Several months later an honorary contract was offered, but it would have meant Mary working in three different places in two and a half days: a recipe for more confusion and tension. She would be unable to function as a member of a team.

Half way through one of the meetings, the chief executive of Mary's trust walked out and resigned.

There was still other work to be done because, although the service contract had gone to King John's, it was for residents who lived in the borough in which Mary's hospital was sited. Nearly half the work of the department came from outside the borough.

Mary realised that if her sessions were transferred to King John's she would be able to work only with patients from within the borough and that all the staff in the department which she had built up would probably lose their jobs. If she stayed put, she would be able to work only with patients who came from outside the borough. But her colleagues would keep their jobs and, because they were reducing their waiting list, their service might attract more business and expand. Then she would start competing with the neighbouring rheumatologists to the south and west. That would radically alter her relationship with neighbouring colleagues, who would cease to be people with whom to discuss cases, but would become people to take cases from. (Certainly not colleagues with whom to discuss her current problem.) And in all this, how big a threat was King John's? How far afield would it go hunting for contracts or extra contractual referrals (ECRs)?

Despite all this Mary turned down the King John's contract and decided to stay put at the trust.

The GPs' position

The GPs were angry over the contract because, for many of them, King John's now became the sole provider of rheumatology services. This gave the GPs no choice of where to refer patients. What about the Patient's Charter? What about 'money following patients'?

The GPs were further incensed, and the rheumatology team further confused and thrown into despair, when they learned that the purchasers had given the money agreed long ago for the new consultant, not to Mary's trust hospital, but as part of the package of the new contract with King John's.

To make matters worse for the GPs, not only did the King John's trust waiting list now increase to a figure greater than that of the original local service (which was reducing its waiting list), but patients were often seen by non consultant staff. They were being seen by people whom the GPs did not know and to whom they were often unable to speak on the telephone.

The GPs met the purchasers and said they wanted the contract back with the local trust's hospital. Although most of them were not fundholders they were still trying to exert more pressure on the purchasers to get the contract which they thought was best for their patients. Two months later the GPs were assured that the purchasers had agreed to review the contract in the autumn. Two weeks later they were told this was a mistake. Following that, the purchasers wrote to the press saying that the contract with the King John's trust was working very well. The erroneous claim that the local department did not have all the facilities needed was repeated. There was another confrontation, more public this time; but still the managers had not visited the clinic to see for themselves what exactly went on.

Meanwhile, even more confusing

Mary sat in the trust's hospital in the borough that used to be coterminous with the NHS district, seeing no patients from the borough. They went to King John's clinics, some going to the King John's main teaching hospital and some to locality clinics within the borough.

If a consultant from Mary's own trust asked her to see his or her hospital patients, she could see them if they were inpatients, but could not see them again as outpatients for follow up; and she could not see them at all if they were outpatients referred from another clinic unless they came from outside the borough. Nor could she see patients from accident and emergency unless they came from outside the borough.

Mary also had to discharge all her local follow-up cases, many of whom she had known for years, but for a tiny few.

For a time a way round this appeared, at least in theory, to be the mechanism of the ECR. A GP working in the borough could refer a patient to Mary as an ECR, because it would be work outside the purchasers' contract which was with King John's. There were potentially so many of these ECRs, and for each one the purchasers would in effect be paying twice. It was soon found to be too expensive for the purchasers, so that avenue was blocked.

In order to survive, Mary worked even harder and managed to reduce the waiting list to a tenth of the national average. Her department attracted contracts with neighbouring purchasers and GP fundholders.

The manager who had worked with Mary on the failed bid for the contract left suddenly and was replaced by a new one, a woman, who appeared to be much in favour of rheumatology. Communication between consultant and manager improved.

The service became more community-based. Some of the fundholding GPs wanted, and were given, clinics in their surgeries. On those days she drove through heavy traffic and major roadworks, had less clinical time and so saw half the number of patients.

While Mary did the clinics in the fundholding GPs' surgeries, her hospital clinic was being done by a GP, employed for a session as a locum consultant. Thus the waiting list was kept down. The fact that a GP was seeing the GP referrals at a specialist clinic seemed not to have been noticed by the referring GPs, the purchasers or the patients.

Another change in quality of work was that Mary was less interrupted at the GP surgeries, because other colleagues did not come in to catch her between patients. But those encounters had enabled two-way consultations to take place: rheumatologist to other specialist and vice versa. These now either did not take place, or another time had to be found.

Once a month, at one of the smaller hospitals run by the trust, Mary ran a clinic for patients of fundholding GPs, while along the corridor King John's ran one for borough residents. Patients for Mary were seen within weeks, while those for King John's clinic waited months. In the shared waiting room some felt confused and some felt angry.

Where did the money go?

And so it went on. Mary asked for another clinical assistant session in order to improve the service. This would cost £1,500 per year. When told this was too much, she pointed out the money made by the ECRs. 'Oh no,' she was told, 'that money goes to the medical directorate as a whole.' The rheumatology department protested: *they* were making the money. They were challenged to prove it, but they did not have the figures because the figures had not yet been produced by the managers who were collecting the money and saying 'Prove it'...

When Mary had more energy, she tried again. The new manager, who did see potential in the rheumatology service, was prepared to put in a case for a new consultant since more work was coming in. At an informal meeting with the new chief executive she was told that the figures were not good enough.

How could the figures not be good enough when there were the contracts with the GP fundholders and the ECRs?

An embarrassed silence.

Mary had a sudden thought and asked: 'Are you sure they are being billed?' The managers had to admit they did not know.

Subsequently, the manager of one of the GP fundholding practices said that they were not being billed for rheumatology. It was later learned that in the past year no bill had been sent for £20,000 worth of work. This was work which the management had encouraged the department to take on in order to bring in more money. So much for the advantage of being priced separately as told to Mary by the first chief executive at a meeting that now seemed very long ago.

Driving, parking, planning, negotiating, chasing money, responding to revised managerial requirements — all this was now taking over so much of Mary's time that there was much less available for patients. Anxiety about making mistakes grew. She was even irritable with some patients, although for the most part she still enjoyed working with the NHS patients — when she got a chance to see them. She felt that the system was destroying her work and she was losing energy for going on fighting it. She had lost her self-esteem and much of her desire to practise. There was so much more to keep up with. She felt sometimes that if she blinked a clinic could be moved, a contract changed or money lost. Being part time had become a greater disadvantage than ever.

She often woke in the night gloomily thinking that it was all her fault, that she was no good at her work any more. She was often in tears. She hated going to work and could see no end to it all, wondering what new administrative problems the next day would bring. Some GPs who were friends told her of their sadness; they had been instructed not to send her cases unless they were fundholders.

Mary's professional association wrote about these problems to the Department of Health, who suggested it took the matter up with the local trust and purchasers. For one moment Mary suspected the professional association itself: whose side was it on and might its officers benefit from fresh contracts if her service folded? A fantasy of the internal market forces?

Would things get better or worse? Mary had heard that in another part of the country, purchasers gave a specialist contract to a trust hospital 200 miles away with the consequence that the local consultant and department colleagues lost their jobs. Could such a contract be kept going? Would the Community Health Council speak up effectively on behalf of patients?

Once in a while she imagined that 'they' might back off and say, 'Well, we made a mistake, we are sorry and let's start again.' But they will never do that. The purchasers' chief executive would not see the consultants any more, giving as explanation that communication must all be done through the trust managers. Her own chief executive, similarly, was refusing to see consultants except through the managers. When she got fed up with the managers, Mary tried to remember that times were sometimes difficult for them too. Some had been encouraged not to communicate too closely with doctors and nurses, and most of them were finding that the rules by which they had to function were being changed all too frequently.

Postscript

Three years later Mary and her colleagues were keeping their waiting list down to two weeks but were still not allowed to see any local people. They were seeing more patients than ever before and making money for the trust, which had agreed staff growth. More of the neighbouring GPs had become fundholders and were sending cases back to Mary rather than to the King John's clinic, which had won the contract for the locals, taken on extra staff, but still had a waiting list of over six months.

And so it goes on...

Chapter 6

The medical director

Tom and a number of his colleagues were in that minority of consultants who had supported the NHS reforms in their early days. When the management said that they wished to make a bid for trust status, they decided to support that too.

They had clinical directorates set up and running, mostly with doctors as clinical directors. The new **unit general manager**, whom Tom liked and supported, wanted to have a 'shadow' medical director ready for the start of the new trust in April. Tom was one of a small number of consultants who expressed interest in becoming this person. They knew it would be for two sessions a week, that duties would include some line management and budget holding, and that modifications would be made in their work to allow for the two sessions. They submitted their CVs and were interviewed informally. Tom said that none of them really knew how seriously to take it, but were somehow carried by the unit general manager's enthusiasm. He decided to treat it all as if it were serious by the time he had the formal interview with the chairman and chief executive to be. Tom was chosen and agreed to what he considered to be an interesting experiment.

Tom started the two sessions with a series of mornings 'shadowing' one executive director after another: the directors of marketing and contracts, finance, human resources (personnel), nurses and other clinical staff and the acting chief executive himself. Tom was impressed by them. Of course he realised that they were, quite rightly, trying to welcome him and help him feel at home, and that they did have a full time commitment in contrast to his paltry two sessions a week.

After a pause, Tom told me that a particular remark by one of the executive directors had made him very curious. I waited. He told me that he had been asked, 'Are you prepared to lie?' I said that it made me feel curious too, but added that I would not ask him how he had responded. I did not want to create the uncertainties in my own mind that arise when someone's integrity is questioned. Anyway, I had already heard of someone else being asked the same thing.

Phase 1

Immediately after that, Tom was thrown into intense work which included leading people in devising formal strategies for the different units. (Some of these were well advanced already, but some were barely started and would not have been ready on time for the final trust application if Tom had not done what he did).

The second area of immediate intense work was to do with the health of doctors. Some went off sick and Tom became intimately involved with the personnel department. He discovered that it had far less expertise than he had thought in the recruitment of doctors, especially how to 'trawl' for locums.

Tom found that his management work had mostly to be done between the hours of 9.00 and 5.00 because that was when his fellow managers were most accessible and when the secretarial staff were available. He was doing a great deal of paperwork and from very early on had to come in on Saturday mornings to catch up. He realised soon that his non-medical management colleagues, by working full time at management, were always crucially ahead of him in receiving, reading and understanding documents. He worried for his patients to whom he gave less time: 'We had not yet got somebody to take on some of my clinical load.' (I noticed how Tom was saying 'we', which might be a sign that he identified with management at this early part of his story.) The patients also got less quality: he had almost completely stopped supervising junior staff. (They risked losing Royal College accreditation for their training programme.) Patients to be seen by Tom, 'their' consultant, outside the rather cursory ward rounds, got him after 6.00 pm. 'How was that for quality of care?' Tom asked me.

Tom learned how difficult it could be for the full time managers, too. The introduction of trusts was supposed to push financial accountability downwards, permitting faster decisions and, by allowing savings to be carried forward for the next year, getting rid of the traditional rush to 'spend the budget' in March before the end of the financial year. But then the government and the Department of Health changed the rules so that trusts would not be allowed to carry savings over. That had the consequence of trust finance departments devoting much energy and their great expertise into beating the system (I think it was not unusual for a trust to have between half a dozen and a dozen systems going by which they could 'lose' money at strategic times, especially around the end of the financial year). The managers themselves, in apparent fear of reprimand and fear for their jobs, managed to create spending budget scrambles like never before

When Tom became medical director, senior managers and consultants were hardly talking to each other. Managers excluded consultants from their meetings and refused to attend those of consultants. The senior manager said to Tom that of course he would meet the consultants, but not on their terms.

Both sides agreed to attend a meeting if it 'belonged' to neither side and if Tom chaired it. Such a meeting happened, was repeated and seemed to work.

Was he having any effect?

In spite of everything he was doing, Tom thought he seemed to be having very little effect as medical adviser to the management. He gave me two examples:

First, a lock system was suddenly fitted to the panelling of some of the office doors. The consequence was that patients in the depths of sensitive interviews were being observed by other patients wandering about or looking for doctors, and such interviews were being interrupted by staff who seemed to have developed the reflex reaction that if they could see what was going on, it might be interrupted. Unauthorised entry into offices containing confidential material increased, and petty theft as well. Patients and relatives complained.

When Tom brought this up at a management meeting he was told that they did not seek him out for his opinion because he was always so busy. It was, Tom was advised, done in the interests of openness, had been done elsewhere (they kept on quoting other trusts) and anyway it had been decided at a meeting for which Tom was late because of a clinical emergency. So they agreed that Tom would always be consulted at the beginning and at the end of any discussion on a matter that might have clinical implications. Of course this did not happen either — because they, the full time managers, were also so busy.

The second example was when there was a rumour that the medical secretaries, who worked so closely alongside all the consultants and other senior clinical staff, were going to be moved into a central 'pool'. Tom told them that no such decision had been taken. The consultants were not reassured so Tom asked the manager himself, and at the next meeting with the consultants he confirmed that the story they had heard was not true. He told them, light-heartedly, not to be so paranoid. They trusted the medical director, sometimes.

Two weeks later the secretaries were moved. (Tom said he was furious too, but he did nothing, telling the consultants that his power was gone and that the trust board were likely to back the manager, whatever he did.)

The pressure was mounting up

By the end of the year Tom was working Monday to Friday from 8.30 to 6.30 and on Saturday morning. Every evening he was taking papers home and working on them. He was falling out with colleagues, rarely seeing friends. There was friction with his wife and his children. He was irritable with his secretary.

Tom knew that he was difficult to work with. Because he was taking so much work home, his hobbies had gone. Holidays were very difficult to plan and, when Tom managed a few days off, he could not get rid of thoughts of work. He slept badly and the one good thing to come out of this was that he would sometimes go jogging at 6.00 in the morning.

The introduction of the new management structure

It seemed that trusts were always refining their management structures. They were for ever having talks by experts, or seminars by consultants, or 'away days' for themselves. Each new idea on management and management structure had much to commend it. The full time managers became convincingly enthusiastic for each in turn. As soon as Tom had managed to catch up with a new idea and to understand it enough to start to pass some of it on to the medical staff, the trust's executive directors went on to the next.

Tom put a lot of energy into persuading his consultant colleagues to accept what was worked out during his time as medical director. Although the chief executive, very reasonably, warned them that whatever was decided upon that year would need to be changed in a few years' time, what was devised did indeed seem to be a fairly good plan. It was a plan of devolution and Tom persuaded consultants and some other clinicians to accept what was called 'locality management' for specialist teams and 'patches' for area teams. He worked on job descriptions for the lead clinicians who were to be paid one session per week for this. He explained again and again to these colleagues, some medical and some not, that his role was to be advisory. They were to manage and they were to handle the budgets.

Thus Tom was able to pass on at least a little of his enthusiasm for the new structure and for the birth of the trust. When he heard two of the new clinical directors talk with enthusiasm of handling budgets without, as one of them had once feared, having Tom breathing down her neck like an ogre, he felt excited.

It was to Tom's surprise, therefore, that on the first day of the trust there appeared on his desk the personal files of the specialist (non-medical) managers and lead clinicians. One of the executive directors of the trust said that Tom was to manage them all and that this had been agreed, although other directors said it had been decided as Tom had agreed that his relationship with the clinical directors was to be advisory.

To his further surprise, some of the clinicians were not too put out, but Tom soon realised that this was because they saw a chance for power without financial accountability. He, Tom, was going to be lumbered with the accountability (Tom had emotional, but not managerial, sympathy with them for that.)

The chief executive said that it had been decided as the executive director had said; the medical director would run the units and be responsible for the budgets, for moving money from one to another and dealing with all the interdirectorate financial problems which might arise. Tom felt, as he often did, that his protests were disregarded with the chief executive's cheerful, 'I know everything is terrible. It is for me too. Look on it as exciting.'

It was certainly a problem for Tom and more than he could possibly manage on two sessions a week.

But it helped him to reflect on how decisions were being made.

'We had to produce "action plans" to a particular formula and present them to a meeting of managers. The plans were always ones which were really impossible to carry out, but everyone seemed pleased that we had one and then produced the next one and the next one.
Bids for new equipment were researched from a therapeutic, financial and business point of view including a paragraph on a market survey. With management agreement we informed fundholding and non-fundholding GPs and tested the market at professional meetings. Senior management withdrew the agreement saying that the figures (which had been agreed with the finance department) did not tally and that it was the responsibility of the clinical director.'

Time and again Tom was reading the minutes of meetings which appeared to give a very different story from the one he remembered from being there. Whenever Tom challenged this, and however gently, sensitively or aggressively he did so, he was always told that 'It was what we agreed.' It was sometimes added, 'The policy is already made.'

And sometimes, someone would add the gentle afterthought: 'Have you got too much work to do?'

The appointment of staff

Appointing a consultant had been a long and difficult process which the reforms were to speed up. But in Tom's experience the very mechanisms introduced to streamline the process unleashed power into managers' hands in a way which was destructive.

As medical director, Tom had discussed the appointment of a new short term locum consultant with the manager and they had agreed to advertise. Tom asked the personnel department to send off the advertisement they had used last time. When he called in to the personnel department the following morning he was told that the manager had phoned to say not to advertise yet. The manager was not available that day and the people in the department would not dare to go against his word. Tom tried the following morning, but failed, so he asked his secretary (medical secretary, for Tom had no extra secretarial assistance as medical director) to help by phoning. Both Tom and the secretary were very busy that day with work immediately related to their current patients; they 'prioritised objectives' and were prepared to put off dealing with some of the letters to GPs. Later in the morning Tom tried twice to speak to the chief executive and got as far as leaving two messages with his secretary.

(When Tom did work with patients, he kept on having flashes of despair, confusion, or downright rage. He wondered how he could ever get the other consultants to feel any confidence when he said it was possible to work with management.)

Eventually, the personnel officer tried again and spoke to the manager's secretary who repeated that the locum consultant post must not be advertised and added that she had been told by another manager to say that.

Late in the afternoon, after two phone calls from the other consultants who were starting to harass him, Tom went over to see the personnel officer who seemed to be as fed up as he was. While they were discussing what to do, a secretary came in with a message from the second manager (the one who had confirmed the veto that morning): he had spoken to the chief executive (who had not returned Tom's calls), who said that the locum post could now be advertised.

This was not the first time that Tom had thought seriously that there might be a deliberate attempt to undermine doctors, but it was the first time he had felt that it was being directed at him in principle or in particular. Tom told me that he had nothing against the insistence that doctors should work through the management structure, but the management structure had to be working.

The first time Tom thought he was being lied to

Tom said that the first time he thought that people might be lying to him was when a manager asked him to give one of the consultants a message. The consultant in question had offered to work in a different place and have a different contract. This was, by any account, a generous offer. It helped management, clinicians and patients. But he did need a new contract and that was a wisdom managers had taught clinicians. The manager rang Tom. Please would he give a special message to the consultant (he used his first name) to say he was sorry not to have been able to give him the letter as promised before going on leave. The letter was drafted and needed one addition from one of the departments. He wished Tom to assure the consultant that he would deliver the letter with his own hand in six days' time.

Tom gave his colleague the message and he sounded reassured. A few days later, when he was down by the managers' offices, Tom thought he would drop in to look at the draft. The secretaries knew of no draft.

Ten days after the manager's return from leave Tom received a further phone call from him about the new contract for the consultant. 'I am concerned that he has not received his letter yet. It is much more complicated than it started out to be, and it is not ready yet.'

When disillusionment really set in

As Tom was lied to more often and came to realise that lying had become an acceptable strategy, he felt that he was sinking into disillusionment. Before that, Tom had tolerated quite a lot, perhaps because he was resistant to admitting he had been mistaken in going with the reforms. He had also decided that inconveniences had to be accepted for the hope of greater or longer-term good.

Before I had time to ask, Tom told me that he had often asked himself why he did not challenge what was being done far more often. He told me that when he had tried, in subtle or in direct ways, he did not seem to have any effect. Perhaps Tom was too tired to be effective. He was worn out with trying. Whenever he had raised this sort of conduct or the topic of staff morale with the chief executive, he was told that, even if Tom were right, it must be necessary to go through this phase. He had to put up with it. Tom should expect morale to be shaken or low when such a very good job was being done. 'The trust board is 120% behind the new managers,' Tom was told time and again.

And all the time Tom was trying to play his part in running a high-pressure clinical service, prevent staff from leaving in disgust and keep himself sleeping enough at night. Rightly or wrongly, Tom decided that more frequent confrontations would make things even worse and might lead to more trouble for his younger and more junior colleagues.

More, and one survival strategy

Tom continued to work with the managers and often to identify with them. Consultant posts were an example. Tom knew that these should be seen as one of many jobs in the trust, without necessarily special priority. And Tom accepted the managers' argument that each time someone was leaving a post, the job description should be looked at again. Each time there could be a further 'whittling away' at some of the older fashioned aspects of medical tradition.

Tom therefore had some sense of being useful and smoothing a process through in another meeting between managers and consultants (at which, mysteriously, the senior manager arrived late with neither explanation nor apology). He was explaining an apparent delay over another consultant post being advertised. Tom chose to raise this himself to prevent a confrontation between the two sides. First, he explained that the department of human resources had a list of vacancies and an order in which they should be dealt with. Second, he explained how every medical vacancy presented an opportunity to review a job description. He added that the senior manager and he had been discussing this and had agreed on the need for both. 'I did not say either of those things,' was the manager's forceful interjection. As a chairperson of the meeting Tom had the choice of saying, 'You're a liar,' or shrugging it off with a rather lame, 'Well, something is happening now and that job description should be going off to the regional health authority for approval by the end of the week.' Tom chose the second.

Of course, Tom was furious. It was a lie and a stupidly unnecessary one. But some good came out of it. Tom had to attend a two-hour meeting that same afternoon and, as it began, manager X walked in (late again) and sat down near Tom. Now Tom told me that he was usually quite good at controlling his anger, but that he was still so shocked and furious after the morning encounter that the arrival of X seemed more than he could manage. He said that if he had known he was coming to the meeting, he would have made some excuse and sent apologies to the chief executive. So how was he to survive two hours in the same room? Tom felt hopeless and helpless. Worse, self-criticism set in: a more mature person would put it all behind him; a better manager would ride it easily. Tom had to do something to be able to stay in the room. Suddenly, he remembered an article a relative had once shown him on the treatment of a gymnast who had developed a phobia of the apparatus. The gymnast was taught to imagine doing her routines and doing them well.

He could remember little more of the paper and how the treatment was set up, but did recall that it had been successful. He had no clinical psychologist beside him to be his therapist or coach What he did was, Tom told me, the result of the nearest to pure inspiration that he had ever had.

Tom absorbed himself with the recurrent, vivid fantasy that after the meeting X, then sitting two to his right, would request a few words with him and they would go into his office

'Thank you for sparing a few minutes, Tom, I want to apologise to you. First, I arrived 15 minutes late for the meeting which you chaired this morning and I know that you had started it 15 minutes earlier than usual at my request, and I made no acknowledgement of my lateness. Second, in that meeting I lied to you twice. I lied to the meeting and I dug myself deeper and deeper into two holes of my own making. I apologise.'

The enjoyment of that fantasy made it possible for Tom to smile when X smiled, to be puzzled when X appeared puzzled; to listen attentively to what other people were saying and to make a few constructive comments himself.

Tom said that if there was one thing he could insist that I used from what he was telling me, it would be that strategy. It continued to give him pleasure when he looked back on it and he hoped other people might also find it useful.

Morale

Tom was not alone in his despair. None of the clinical staff seemed to be one bit pleased with anything the trust was doing, but all Tom heard at trust meetings was how good morale was. Even the non-executive directors said that anyone they met sounded enthusiastic. Against this tide of confidence, anything that Tom said was insignificant. Once, when his scepticism seemed to be noticed, one of the executive directors suggested a particular unit that Tom should visit, at least to satisfy himself.

Tom did make the visit. He got in touch first with the sector manager and second with the clinical manager. Willingly, they discussed times when a few of the trained clinical staff could be available. Tom drove there twice, in two separate weeks. He was told that staff had agreed to see him. On each visit Tom did the same: he went into a small side room with two or three staff and said that, as medical director, he was interested in staff morale, and that some of the other directors had suggested that he came to their department. Please would they tell him about morale? On each visit, the staff to whom Tom made that request responded in the same way. They cried.

When Tom mentioned this to one of his friends in the hospital and said how moved and surprised he had been, her response was, 'Moved, yes, but why surprised? They will talk to you, but with anyone else they use the safety rule and say they think the management's strategy is wonderful.'

The erosion of consultants managing

God knows, Tom said, he had worked hard at getting the consultants to take more managerial responsibility. Why did he say this so passionately? Because he was undermined again and again.

First, the medical secretaries, whom the new regime said should be managed by the consultants themselves. Tom pushed them to do this, but the consultants were reluctant to get more involved. Somehow they seemed not to believe that they were going to be allowed to manage 'their own' secretaries. Tom pushed them into believing that they would be supported if they did so, but as it turned out they were right and he was wrong.

Suddenly the rules were changed. The sector manager took overall managerial responsibility for the medical secretaries, appointed a secretarial manager (the number of managers up by another one) and, against the consultants' advice and against Tom's 'medical director' advice ('It's not really a medical matter, you know'), made change after change in their working arrangements.

Second, the junior doctors. Tom encouraged the consultants to become more involved in the management of their junior staff and he even ran a consultants' audit session on the management and supervision of juniors. The consultants became, gradually and slightly, more active and enthusiastic, but still remained wary. Tom thought real progress was being made. Then they had something more difficult to handle. A junior doctor who had been working with three separate consultants during the course of a rotation had been at the centre of a misunderstanding between two of the other departments. A complaint had been made. Tom was asked by the chief executive to sort it out and both of them thought that should be possible, by getting enough of the people concerned together.

First, Tom met the three consultants. They then interviewed the junior doctor, counselled her and drafted an interim report which they showed to Tom.

Second, he saw the junior doctor with the consultant who was currently supervising her. The consultant had checked with the two departments and heard that, when the doctor met them, all the remaining differences had been sorted out. Tom had also heard this and said so. They agreed that future supervision sessions between the junior and the consultant should include monitoring what happened when she visited those departments.

Third, the consultants produced a final report, which Tom approved of. With his agreement, they sent it to the management. The report noted what had happened, what they had done, how the difficulties had been resolved with the departments and how they were going to monitor the changes. They had managed something.

Ten days later, and without any consultation with any of the medical staff or with Tom, one of the senior managers wrote a remarkably inflammatory letter to the doctor and interviewed her himself. The doctor resigned immediately and they were back to the now familiar rush of looking around for a locum.

'But did you leave it at that?' I asked Tom. Not at all, he said, but when confronted, what did the manager say? 'You are quite right. We must improve our communications.'

At the end of the first year Tom told the chief executive that he could not continue. The experiment was unworkable and he wanted to resign. What would it take to make him stay? Tom had heard from fellow medical directors of all sorts of deals. Two extra sessions' pay, support for a distinction award. (Yes, Tom had now heard of several instances of the lure of management recommendation for lucrative distinction awards being used 'persuasively': 'We'll put your name forward,' or 'You realise that this may mean that we are unable to support any recommendation that may be made for you to receive a distinction award.') They talked of the possibility of really devolving management to the locality level, of paying him more, of fixing a date for starting extra increments.

The dates for 'changing his remuneration' were fixed and then changed and Tom kept on thinking, 'Could any money possibly make any difference?' That was how strong had become his wish to get out of being a medical director. The muddle continued. And meanwhile the problems with handling the clinical work, recruiting and keeping staff, got worse.

They did in fact recruit a new consultant, but last-minute changes appeared in the job description which Tom had not agreed to and which could cause no end of problems in the future if someone were to exploit them.

Then such a petty thing: a newcomer's relocation allowance, which had been agreed, was not forthcoming. More ill feeling and more murmuring that a medical director really worth his or her salt would look after the concerns of doctors better. Or was he imagining it? By that time, Tom was so near to breakdown that it was difficult to be sure which thought was whose.

They struggled on. Tom described it as stumbling on.

The last phase

His first 'proper' holiday was very early in the summer. Holidays had always been activity holidays, with travelling, touring, walking, exploring, visiting gardens, houses, museums. Tom would run or swim in the mornings. During these two weeks Tom left the package holiday hotel for two hours. Otherwise he sat indoors or in the garden by the pool and when he swam he swam lazily. Fortunately they had gone with friends and Tom's wife went out with them. They recognised that his apathy was symptomatic of his stressed state and they tolerated it. For Tom, it was the nearest he had ever been to a breakdown.

On his first day back at work, Tom got the news that the recruitment process for filling the remaining vacant medical positions had all gone wrong. Promising applicants had been lost. Tom had to do even more work with the department of human resources, which was by this time even busier with disciplinary hearings, counselling staff for their reallocations as the services changed, preparing their department's own business plan, fixing and meeting targets and looking after their own jobs and career prospects...

Tom had to get in locums very quickly. That first weekend he got a junior doctor in to start work, at 5.00 pm on a Friday. That was the nearest consultants had ever got to having to be in hospital, sleeping in themselves. All sorts of systems were clearly breaking down or very nearly so: prescription writing, medical supervision and so on. The hospital seemed to be on the edge of serious breaches of care and to be facing disasters, complaints, investigations. How could Tom and the other consultants adequately supervise the junior staff when they were running around so frantically completing forms, filling in returns, and rewriting business and management proposals, that even their own clinical work was skimped. Another thing Tom dreaded was that at the Royal College accreditation visit the genuinely neglected junior doctors would be honour-bound to report how little supervision they were getting.

When Tom went to see the chief executive to warn him of all this, he was passed a piece of paper with the statement, 'Sign this.' It was his revised job description. Tom said that he would look at it.

It was not right.

A week later the manager's secretary came to Tom's office with the same piece of paper, saying, 'Please sign it. I've been asked to get you to do it for the board meeting today.' Again Tom did not sign because it still was not as he believed they had agreed and, with all the other things crowding in on him,

he really felt it could wait. It was not something that was immediately jeopard-
ising patient care or risking bad practice.

At the board meeting some of the executive directors went over all the old
ground again. They complained that Tom did not drop in informally for a
chat often enough and, foolishly, Tom reminded them that previously they
had said they were too busy to receive such calls. Tom had provoked them
more. He was told that he had been offensive over the job description and that,
overall, his performance had been unsatisfactory and they had decided they
wanted him dismissed.

The chairman calmed everyone down with the suggestion that he and the
chief executive meet Tom at the end of the week. He had two days to prepare.

Tom had telephone consultations with colleagues who were medical directors nearby. They did not have any experience of the sort of line management
responsibility that Tom had found so difficult. His immediate colleagues were
very supportive, saying, 'Look, if you can't do it, then no one of us can.' The
BMA person, with whom Tom had a long telephone conversation, went
through all the 'options'. Tom checked his contract.

At the meeting with the chairman, Tom resigned and this was accepted. At
the start of the following week Tom learned that the extra two sessions pay
had started. 'Oh, we'll let it run,' the chief executive said, 'We may need to
call on you until we get someone else in and it will be easier to make that sort
of demand on you if we are paying you.'

On the next day the management cancelled one of the last things Tom had
set up. It had been an appointment committee to fill a consultant vacancy.

Vulnerability and internal conflict

Tom had too few sessions as medical director and this meant that he could
never keep up with the full time managers: they had more time to read the
circulars, to do all the other paperwork and to learn the language. They also
met each other frequently and were always several steps ahead of Tom.
Additionally, as a clinician with a leading role in a specialist team, Tom and
his close colleagues were managed by those managers: if they could not
control him, they would control his colleagues. Several times Tom had been
in a room with colleagues and a manager would enter, ignore the others and
address him; and if they, as a team, were to meet the manager, Tom alone
would be addressed by name. In these and other, even more subtle ways Tom
was given the message: he was to conform and help them to run the system
— including, if necessary, controlling the doctors. If he did not, they could
easily turn on those staff who were Tom's close colleagues. Tom felt depen-

dent on his clinical colleagues and he was fond of them, but as far as the managers were concerned, well, they did not even have to address them.

I pressed Tom further on the difficulty of being both manager and clinician. I remembered a meeting of medical directors I had attended at the BMA (see Chapter 23). When Sir Kenneth Calman, the Chief Medical Officer at the Department of Health, had addressed us, someone said to him that the most difficult part of being a medical director was the conflict between those two roles. How could one be a clinician, treating patients and working with clinical colleagues, but at the same time be a manager deciding the allocation of resources, working conditions and arrangements? Sir Kenneth gave his wry smile and said he knew what was meant. Tom had started as an enthusiast for the trust position and had worked hard to convince doctors to support it and to change the ways they thought and did things. In his later, disillusioned days he was increasingly taking the side of the clinicians and tried to protect doctors from management.

But he did have another story to tell. When he was at the point of arguing over his job description, one of the people he had met was a medical director from another part of the country. They had a 'worst moment' exchange. Tom had already told me his worst moment. His friend's experience was different.

In the other trust there had been a consultant of wide reputation who had run a professionally and financially successful department in his specialty. Anticipating his retirement, the consultant had negotiated with the medical director and with the trust's executive and chairman, and with the regional adviser in the specialty, for an advertisement to appear for his successor long before he left. They had agreed that it was important to prevent a gap with all the problems of searching for a locum and handling more uncertainty.

When a new manager came into post with the remit of revitalising all the clinical services, it no longer remained expedient to support the continuation of that particular department as it was. The argument was complicated. The new manager had to achieve a level of uniformity over a wide spread of services in order to promote the notion of corporateness. The manager had to be seen to be in charge and in control in order to carry things through. If one consultant was seen as being treated differently, a perilous precedent might be established.

The medical director, aware of the sweeping changes in practice that were going to have to be pushed through, and the difficulty of getting medical staff committee support for most of them, became convinced by the arguments. The problem was, how to make the change so late in the day?

Time was on the management's side, to a degree. The consultant's retirement was less than a year away and his power and influence were lessening almost daily. Delay, if sufficient and subtle enough, would suffice.

The medical director played for time, by meeting the consultant a few times and telling him that there were hitches with the purchasers, who had to be 'kept on board'. The purchasers must not get the impression that the trust was panicking because of a senior person reaching retirement age. The best way of reassuring the purchasers would be to have a review by the consultancy organisation they and the trust had been impressed by before. Then, whatever came out of that would have the backing of both purchasers and trust.

The consultant, as predicted, although wary of the argument, was far too preoccupied with his own imminent retirement, and worries for his health, to have the energy to try to tackle the purchasers himself. In fact he probably realised that even if he had tried, they would not have listened, for they on their part also wanted the trust to succeed in its general strategy. They would have feared upsetting the apple cart.

The 'review' by the consultancy bought time. The medical director easily persuaded the consultant not to be so provocative as to complain about either their credentials or manner of work.

The consultant left to a fanfare of applause from the trust and proclamations of commitment to continuing the service in a fine-tuned form.

The clinical service was suspended soon after the consultant left. The medical director let the trust give the standard explanation: something that was run successfully in the old days is often difficult to keep going in today's climate.

But what survived in that medical director was a feeling of heavy regret at having got caught up in such a degree of distortion of the truth and in misleading a colleague. His answer to the question, 'Are you prepared to lie?' was clear. And the price was, among other things, his 'worst moment'. A moment which lives on in his memory.

I thanked Tom for the story, but said that I could not publish it without hearing it from closer at hand. Tom arranged that. I am now satisfied that the story is true.

Why confrontation failed

Near the end of our meeting, it was almost as if he was reading my mind when Tom suddenly asked me if I thought he was a wimp. (I said 'reading my mind', because his story reminded me of several points in my own very brief medical director career when I had felt inadequate and guilty at not being made of sterner stuff.) I took the psychiatrist's way out by asking him what he thought.

Tom was sure that he had appeared a wimp and had often thought it. Some of his dreams had been of the executive directors taunting him for his weakness while the non-executive directors (the lay people) looked on from a balcony. He had often thought that a tougher man or woman in the post might have made a difference. But Tom was, in fact, no stranger to confrontation and had quite a reputation as someone capable of speaking out. (I checked on this and found it to be true.) Tom had after all tried some of this at the beginning but without success and he had seen the results of other people's attempts. Tom had, calculatedly, decided against this approach. Or maybe it was lack of energy.

But doubts of his own self-worth remained.

I pressed him further on what had happened when he had tried to be more confrontational. His reply was that nothing had happened except that he had come almost to admire the many ways which 'they' had of responding:

'It's better to say these things.'
'It's all right to get things off your chest.'
'I agree.'
'You're right, we must improve our communications.'

Additionally, every time there was a difference between a clinician and a manager in front of a more senior manager or executive, the manager's side was supported by that more senior person.

Tom had experienced this very vividly and painfully and had no doubt that it would continue. (Coming in on one powerful argument between a particular manager and him, when Tom was becoming furious with the manager's repeated lectures on management theory, the chief executive observed silently for a few minutes. Then he addressed Tom so calmly with:

'I know it's frustrating when you have worked to develop things in a way that was going well and when you are now being told it has to change, but remember that, from my more detached viewpoint, this is a "local difficulty". The total strategy is going well.'

That nearly started off another round of Tom thinking that if he had the energy or the will to have kept up the pressure harder and longer, it would have been ... but he stopped and smiled.

Tom had skills in which he had been trained for many years and he was good at using them. He did not want it to sound like sour grapes, but he did often find it hard when he was expected to learn a new set of skills to deal with a new management structure. He felt that he had been in no to cracking up much of the time. He had been working longer hours than ever before and nearly always taking work home. He was doing less clinical, face to face work than ever before: the least was one hour of clinical work in a week. He had been waking in the night most nights and was always waking early. He had been eating more to deal with an incipient duodenal ulcer (undoubtedly stress related) and had tension headaches. He had told his close colleagues and his wife that he might resign any day. Tom had indeed become vulnerable.

Now Tom no longer feels he has to act a mythology. He no longer takes masses of work home. He gives a better deal to his patients. He supervises the junior staff. His consultant colleagues at first gave him a mixed reaction, but on the whole they get on much better. Another person was brought in from outside as full time medical director (another one in the growth in managers). Tom gets on better with his wife and family and he is sleeping through the night.

Chapter 7

The GPs who were not fundholders

As I walked into the corridor which led to the small room where this interview was to take place, a telephone started to ring in another part of the building. It went on ringing and there must have been something in the expression on my face to prompt this story to start in the way it does…

'No, we are not answering it. That is the first difference that's noticed by somebody who has not been in the building for a few years: the telephones ring for longer. If you can hear our story out, we will get round to explaining why.'

The building, a 1970s or early 1980s health centre, housed GPs, health visitors, district nurses, a dental clinic and more besides. Over the years a lot of work had gone into all of them working together as well as with other professionals in the community who were not based in a building like theirs. They all had what was called 'coterminosity', with each professional group working the same geographical patch.

With the narrowing of tasks, budgets and targets and with them all competing with each other, all ideas of GPs working closely together with, for example, midwives seemed to have gone by the board.

The worship of information

Jean was a married woman, around forty with one teenage daughter; Andrew, the senior partner, was in his mid-fifties, married with grown up children. They started by talking of what they called the passion for data. Someone seemed to have realised that there was a great deal of 'information' somewhere out there in the community. And the most important thing seemed to be getting hold of it. As many professional groups were having to do audits by order of the government it did not take long for some to realise that one of the easiest ways of looking as if one is 'doing an audit' is to collect information. The GPs realised that this had little to do with 'indicator-based audit' which can sometimes have an almost immediate effect on improving clinical care, but it can make it look as if someone is doing it. (I knew of the positive effect of working out standards of 'good practice', and a simple way of checking how often that is achieved over a relatively short time.) The problem for the GPs was that it was they who got asked to help with everyone else's audit.

What is the number of patients you have seen with herpes in the last week?

What is the number of patients whose blood pressure you have taken during the last week?

Hardly a fortnight goes by without a questionnaire with items like those on it arriving through their letterbox.

More information is demanded directly by the Department of Health and, in part, GPs' income depends upon providing it.

They must record, and present annually, the screening advice they have given: the target, the numbers canvassed and the numbers advised.

I explained that the way they were going on sounded dangerously like a moan. Each gave me an example from work during the last week.

An almost constantly sad woman, whom Jean had known for years, came to see her. Throughout much of the 8 or 10 minutes of the interview, Jean kept on having the thought, 'I must get her to have a smear check. It will help to get to our target and then we get the money.' She hated having that thought and she did not in fact ask the patient to have a smear check, but she did not listen to her very carefully either. She did not help the patient.

A young mother with her severely handicapped epileptic son had come to see Andrew. Mother and son both had daunting problems. Both were on medication. Andrew said that a few years ago he would have known the other people involved in offering them help in the community and any one of them (GPs) would have offered to get in touch with the school on her behalf. What did this doctor do on this occasion? He found himself thumbing through the notes and the 'screening list'. What advice had she been given this year? Then he heard himself asking her if she smoked and advising her not to (government brownie point and money for the practice). The woman said that she knew that she should not smoke and that she would like not to smoke. 'But that's all you lot seem to be able to say now,' she added as she walked sadly out.

Andrew added a third case, 'Just someone I weighed unnecessarily.' So many women, and some men, are obsessed with their weight and, to be helpful, the last thing the GPs should be doing is weighing them regularly. But here again someone has got an idea of what makes people healthy and has decided that it is the same for everyone.

Not to smoke, not to drink and not to be overweight. And all the world must be measured.

Because part of the practice income depends on the count of activities to do with these ideals, they must get on with it. It erodes thinking about the patient and it erodes listening to what the patient wants. Andrew said that very often nowadays he says,

'I want you to realise that I am asking you these questions not for your benefit at all. It's so that we get paid.'

A lot of patients seem to understand.

Patient: I heard that my appointment with the specialist was cancelled by listening to the local radio. They did not give my name but they gave his name. Of course another appointment was sent later but it certainly was not an example of money following patients and I was not able to exercise my Charter choice of the specialist I wanted.

Choice

The Patient's Charter. A lot of that was supposed to be to do with choice. Ten years ago in this city practice the GPs could refer anybody to pretty well anywhere in the country. The reforms have narrowed this down and down until it is more difficult to refer anybody other than to the one hospital with which the purchaser has the contract. That is their local district general hospital (DGH).

A 60 year old woman who had suddenly started to pass blood in her urine came to see Jean. She had no other symptoms. Jean had to have several attempts at getting a department that would accept the referral for looking inside the patient's bladder by cystoscopy. The difficulty was, first, getting to understand which purchaser held the purchaser's contracts for where the lady lived (it was right on the border, in 'disputed' territory), for which sort of procedure, and then, with which provider hospital. The patient was seen as an outpatient and they admitted her for the cystoscopy as a day patient. She did the right fasting, was admitted to a bed, had the pre-medication and was waiting to go into the operating theatre when she was told that they had run out of operating time. They were sorry but she would have to go home. She went in a taxi. When Jean asked for another appointment for her, they said there had been a mistake and there was not a contract with the purchaser for where she lived, and would have to go elsewhere.

The department that did have the contract was a 'flagship' centre, the speciality and pride of its trust. It could not offer an appointment for four weeks. The consultant, whom Jean knew personally, said that he was very sorry but he was 'overwhelmed'. The patient was seen before the four weeks were up and that was to the credit of the people working in the department.

She was found to have a cancer which was then inoperable.

A bit on that flagship centre! It has wonderful productivity and turnover. Throughput is excellent. If performance related pay is brought in by the government, all the staff there will do well. They concentrate mostly on day care. The patients feel like they are on a conveyer belt and don't know who is dealing with them. And in some of the most sensitive parts of the body and mind. And who deals with all the complications after operations! Well, a lot of that now falls on the GPs.

Another two cases

A man in his thirties with an old shoulder injury had been to one of the London teaching hospitals for treatment. After some improvement over a few years, he had a relapse and was advised to have an operation. He agreed and was put on the waiting list. Then he was told that his operation was likely within the next four to six weeks. Suddenly a letter to say that there was no funding for the operation because the contract with the purchasers had been completed and the department could do it only as an ECR. Many more letters, furious telephone calls, transferral, the case accepted by another teaching hospital with which the purchaser did have a small contract. Onto another waiting list and eventually a very successful operation.

Result? The operation was done within the government's waiting list target time by the second hospital. Add the two hospitals together and you get two 'FCEs' (finished consultant episodes), thus enhancing one of the government's favourite indicators, the 'number of patients treated'. Look at the figures another way and you see that, if the waiting time for the whole thing, after the recommendation was first made at the first hospital, is put together, the wait is far greater than is acceptable. And if you think in human terms — which, Andrew added, he still managed to do sometimes — well, it all took so long that, by the end, the man lost his job.

And their local DGH itself used never to be full. Now it seems always to be full. If any of the partners telephones, he or she is now told by the admitting registrar, 'No, sorry, but we can accept admissions only through the EBS (Emergency Bed Service).' The GP then has to speak to the clerk at the EBS, answer a number of routine questions for unimportant information and write a very long letter because they do not know if the patient will go to the hospital which has the records and knows the patient or will go somewhere else, where no one will know him or her and all will seem strange. They no longer feel an affinity with their local hospital and their patients are being admitted there or elsewhere with no doctor-to-doctor talk beforehand.

> An alcoholic and schizophrenic man with a long history of difficulties, admissions to hospital and community support, lived in a small well run hostel. He and the staff at the hostel had really got to the end of their tether and Jean thought that it was cruel that he should not be admitted again to a psychiatric ward. The psychiatrist said that they could send him along but there would be a long wait and they would certainly not be able to admit him. They did send him along and he sat for 24 hours in the casualty department — which did nobody any good.

Both Andrew and Jean think that the staff running the psychiatric services are very good, but they have had their resources taken away. In this practice over the last year there have been three down-and-out men who suffer from chronic mental illness. When their illnesses were much worse, they were really disoriented and their perceptions very disordered. They were distressed and causing distress to others. They were seen by psychiatrists and they were admitted. I was invited to guess where: it was to single rooms in a private psychiatric hospital well away from where they lived, because they were no vacancies at the trust's psychiatric unit. How did I think that helped their sense of disorientation? And all at the expense of the purchaser, which means the taxpayer.

In vitro fertilisation (IVF)

Andrew and Jean said that they did not know my view on artificial or medical means of helping people to conceive, but asked me to bear in mind the Patient's Charter and what it said of patient's choice, as they told me this story.

The purchasers for the borough had no specific contract for IVF. Patients seeking IVF were being told to ring again in a month to find out if there was money available then.

The partners in the practice were 'neutral' about IVF and they would not mind very much if Britain followed the example of the state of Oregon in the USA where after wide public consultations it was decided what would and would not be paid for by state medicine. If the British government said no IVF on the NHS then that would be clear and they would get on with it. But the government does not want to be seen to be taking decisions like that. Instead it is passing them down to be made at a local level. So, through a process of local consultation with the community health council, user groups etc., the purchasers could make such a decision. They then described what was happening now to one such case.

> Serious appendicitis and peritonitis had rendered a young woman sterile. Both her fallopian tubes were severely damaged. The department of gynaecology at the teaching hospital where she went did many investigations and concluded that no benefit could come from surgery, but she and her partner could benefit from IVF. She was referred from the consultant at the gynaecological department to the consultant of the IVF and infertility clinic and an outpatient appointment was fixed. One week before the outpatient appointment, the patient received the following letter from the consultant:

>> 'Dear…
>> I am sorry to inform you that your local health authority is unable to offer funding for your outpatient appointment at this hospital at this time. I appreciate how disappointing this news at such short notice must be.
>> In some cases, depending on budget and financial planning, some health authorities may consider funding in a subsequent financial year, others have a definite policy not to fund any fertility treatment at all, others may not deal with certain hospitals or be selective of patients to whom they offer treatment. I suggest that you write to the Director of Purchasing at your local Health Authority and ask him or her to clarify the situation for you. The only way in which we could see you at the present time is, by you funding the outpatient and IVF charges yourself and I enclose a price list for your information.
>> You may also wish to discuss the matter with your GP so that you can discuss alternative ways of obtaining the treatment that you require.
>> Yours sincerely…
>> PS Your appointment has been cancelled. However if you choose to self-fund your appointment please telephone and we will be able to reinstate your appointment.'

Enclosed was a list of 14 services with prices which ranged from £50 (for an outpatient consultation) to over £1,500 (for MESA).

Andrew and Jean asked me if I knew what MESA was, let alone some of the other services on that list. I did not. 'What sense is a young woman with little education and on social security to make of a letter like that?' They doubt if the NHS will feel 'safe in our hands' to her.

(I give an example of how another specialist department dealt with this aspect of financing in a somewhat less clumsy manner in Chapter 20.)

Community care

An old woman who had suffered a stroke fell near a teaching hospital, to which she was then admitted. On recovery she was discharged from the teaching hospital and went home. But a few days later she fell again, injured her shoulder and knee and was unable to move. The teaching hospital said they would not readmit her because she was not from the area which had a contract with them. The local hospital said they would not admit her because she had just come out of the teaching hospital. Community care? She was stuck in her chair for two days pending 'fast track' into local authority accommodation.

For somebody to be considered for community care, they have to have three visits from a social worker and a 26-page booklet has to be filled in. There is therefore no emergency admission to part three accommodation and of course the hospitals dare not admit to one of their own beds in case it becomes blocked while the social services department struggles through the regulations.

Another system which has broken down.

ECRs — extra contractual referrals

Jean went to a three hour meeting at one of the specialist departments at the local hospital. It was plain very early on that the consultants were holding the meeting because the management wanted them to do a marketing exercise and the GPs were significant commissioners of the service. But rather than offering a package of the whole service for everybody living in the community, they were keen to promote the use of particular equipment bought for looking inside the bile duct from the gall bladder (bile duct endoscopy). They wished to create another 'flagship' to bring in money through ECRs from other districts and to use this equipment much more than would be possible serving the local population alone.

When Jean reported back to a staff meeting in the practice, it became clear to them that the lure of ECRs meant that the local hospital departments would never prioritise services for the local population.

Summing up!

So where do they go from here? Something like 95% of the practices in those two boroughs were not **fundholders** There are many stories of subtle differences in how the hospitals offer a different service for fundholding GP cases, especially those from other areas. Not a two tier system?

Andrew and Jean spend more time facing the computer and putting information in. They experience far more stress and they each have friends who have commented on how they appear. Particular worries lie in trying to get people into hospital or find other services for them in the community. The occupational therapists, the district nurses, the care attendants seem repeatedly to be 'closing their caseload' as the way of managing their services The funding of those services is special because it is strictly annual. This has the consequence that a new aspect of the service will be started and then stopped with the end of the financial year, sometimes not starting again. There is no sense that anyone has an overview for the community as a whole.

What the GPs are now expected to provide is so different from what they learned, developed and used to think was appreciated. Talking and sitting with a crying person is no longer valued. A doctor/manager asked:

'How do you know talking to your patients does any good?'

They fumble through the case notes and look at the computer when they are with patients. Expectations have been raised by government statements and they and their colleagues have less support than ever to see that these are met.

One of the GPs' central roles has been devalued and they have limited energy to fight for services and treatments for each of their patients. Their role is now the routine provision of valueless advice.

And they have become isolated. Andrew and Jean had promised to come back to the telephone that I heard unanswered at the beginning of our meeting. They told me that they used to share a lot of things in this building. If the family planning clinic did not have 'clini-sticks' for urine tests, they would come and use theirs. If they did not have any they would use some from that clinic. It was all part of the same NHS.

'Now we have separate budgets. *They* are "trust". *We* are GPs. We don't share things now. We used to run to answer each other's phones if we realised that colleagues were busy and the ringing went on. You see that we do not even do that now.'

Chapter 8

The fundholding GP: Philip's story

Like many of the smaller NHS buildings this one had started out as a substantial double-fronted family house with garden. It merged well with the grey urban desert near a large roundabout, but stood out by its bold fund-holding noticeboard displaying the practice logo.

It was a well established practice with five partners. Philip, whom I was meeting, had joined a few years before and, the way these things sometimes go, it was he, the newcomer, who became the doctor side of the fundholding business. There seemed to be a message in that.

Philip said that he had no doubt that fundholding improved communication at the hospitals and had made them more accountable. But he said that the benefit came only to some of the patients.

The doctor's role

Philip was asked to take on the fundholding management role in the practice because of his training in computers and interest in budgeting and data collection. It was agreed that he should have one half day each week plus two full days each month for it. The practice got money for one session of a locum doctor each week, but not for the other two days, so they were 'lost' to the practice. The practice also lost the extra time and energy which Philip put in.

Long before Philip's appointment, the practice already had a full time practice manager with a background in business. Determined that fundholding should be run as a 'real' business, the government allowed money for a fund-holding manager (sometimes called a business manager). The two had separate but overlapping functions. The practice manager focuses on the clinical side, including the clinical records and computer system, and manages the reception staff. The fundholding manager deals with the clinical contracts and liaises with the accountants and auditors.

The new fundholding manager was the person with whom Philip became most closely involved.

The preparatory year had been exciting enough with data gathering and the production of a business plan. Some practices had bought in the services of consultancy companies.

The practice

The total list of the practice was 11,000 people, which was a fairly common size. Fundholding was for permanent residents only and they had 9,500 of them. The 1,500 temporary residents were immigrants, refugees, vagrants, arrivals at the main line station and, sometimes, at the airport. These people will not appear on the 'official' list of the practice, so immunising them was not one of the targets which carried a financial reward.

Apart from being defined as above, what else was there about temporary residents? Most obvious, Philip said, was that they needed a lot of looking after. They were not comfortable, were not well, and did not have roots in the neighbourhood. They did not have networks for advice, support and recreation. They were at risk of more infections. They were the deprived and they needed a lot of looking after by GPs.

One third of the time and effort of the practice staff was going on that 15% of their population. Philip did not want to sound petty over not being financially rewarded for immunising immigrant children. He was talking of recognition. The system ignores work done with temporary residents. That work — which is most demanding, and some would say is of most preventive importance — is not noticed and certainly not valued.

The family health service authority (FHSA) tried to be helpful but did not have enough staff to deal with the demands of the fundholding practices and the trusts and the muddle that was created.

An overcharge

The practice had a block contract for outpatient services at what had been the local district general hospital, run by the acute services trust. Five days before the end of one financial year, neither the FHSA nor the trust knew the number of referrals from their practice to the hospital. Nor did the practice itself, which had not geared itself up to 'pull out' that information from the computers. Shortly into the next financial year came the figures from the trust and the FHSA. They covered 125 pages.

The bottom line was an overcharge of £30,000.

It took Philip and the fundholding manager three weeks to go through the figures and get some understanding of them. That three weeks included Philip taking a very large amount of the work home.

The year in which we were meeting had in fact started with monthly figures being supplied, but that level of efficiency was kept up for only a few months.

I tried to relate this to my personal experience. Philip came up with the idea of telephone bills. If I was sent accounts monthly for a while and then none at all until shortly after the end of the year when I got the whole bill, I would not be pleased. Of course, I could have worked it all out for myself by monitoring every call and recording destination, date, time, duration, price bracket. But then I probably would not be making very good phone calls.

The year's total figures

On a different occasion, in another year, both the FHSA and the practice thought that they were more or less breaking even. At least that was up to the eleventh month. In that last month the practice happened to spend less. Additionally they were given an extra £40,000 from central money for drugs for HIV positive people. They ended with £170,000 surplus for the whole year.

Their embarrassment (they had been saying they had to be careful and did not have the money for this or that) was very soon replaced by fear. If the fluctuation could go that far and that way, then another time it could go that far but the other way: they could have been £170,000 overspent.

Then they would have had to get rid of staff.

The size of their budget was controlled by the FHSA. Philip saw that much of the role of the practice in this 'equation' was as middle person between the FHSA and the provider. Over one year the FHSA cut its budget to the fundholding practice by 3% while one of the trusts put up many of its prices by 30%. The FHSA seemed not to challenge the trust but left that to the fundholders, who were expected to be tough.

At best, the figures are always at least one month behind. Between them all, they still seem unable to prevent the figures getting more and more behind as the year goes on.

Joining and computer costs

Philip's practice had gone into fundholding as a group decision, united in a strong determination to get on well and work together.

One of the GPs was very keen and said that fundholding was what he had been waiting for all his professional life. It gave power and influence to the GPs at last.

The second was neutral and, in a detached sort of way, curious. She voted to join for the money. There were bound to be benefits for fundholding practices: the government was determined to make it work and would throw money at it.

Two felt that it would be compulsory sooner or later, so better to join early, rather than be forced later. The sooner they did it, the greater was their chance of negotiating some of their own terms.

The fifth partner thought it was utterly iniquitous and would lead to a two tier system. He was prepared to support joining in order to get more benefits for the practice as a whole and for at least some of their patients.

Philip did not volunteer what his position would have been if he had been in the partnership at the time, and I did not ask him.

In choosing computers, they accepted the system recommended by the FHSA. Although some of them were sceptical, they did not want to start with an avoidable argument. The system cost thousands of pounds and, although not coming from their own practice funds, it was public money. They believed that the computer costs of fundholding itself would continue to be met from central sources. Soon they had to order extra software for the computer system which they had been assured would deal with everything; and then to order more several times.

In the year we met, the FHSA had stopped 10% of the current and future cost of computers. This meant that 10% had then to come out of the general expenses account of the practice, at the expense of the non-permanent resident patients not eligible for the benefits of fundholding.

It was then that they decided to make a fuss to the FHSA and that it was Philip's role to do so. To every question he asked, challenge or demand he made, he received the same response: 'That is our policy.'

The individuality of practices: and choice

First something on cost efficiency. The allowance was £34,000 to pay the fundholding manager's salary, secretarial assistance, and expenses. It was for negotiating the contracts for 9,000 patients. Philip was not convinced that there was all that much difference between the contracting requirements of the different practices, and the rhetoric had exaggerated what there might be. But of course the process justified itself. It was easy to fill the time and the computer space. The FHSA justified it, fundholding managers individually and collectively justified it. Some days, Philip said that he justified it. A disproportionate amount of money and professional energy goes in negotiating contracts for a few people. The private sector, with less costly overheads to carry, reaped some of the benefit.

Philip told me that, although one of their neighbouring fundholding practices often did refer to private services, his practice rarely did so. The prices in the private sector are nearly always lower, because they do not have the same management costs to cover, but Philip and his colleagues had less control over them. On the other hand patients, especially if they were insured, did sometimes ask. Philip smiled as he confessed their own inconsistency: they had a leaflet from one of the private health insurance companies on the noticeboard in their waiting room.

Philip expanded on his smile. He wanted me to remember that if the number of subscribers for private schemes went down, there would be a big effect on fundholding budgets. It was bad enough for any GP practice, for if fewer people were using the private clinics this would mean more work for the GPs in sorting through the NHS administration to get services. But for the fundholders, it meant their practice could save money. As fundholders they found themselves doubly pressured into encouraging people to use the private schemes.

Size of practice

Philip's is a relatively small fundholding practice, and they are trying hard to resist pressure to merge with others. They do not want to replace the old large system with a new large system. They are not interested in wielding great power (some fundholders have spoken of being able to destroy hospital departments they do not like). They want to continue their improved communication with providers.

At the moment it does not matter very much if they do 'suffer' a few extra hip replacements, at £5000 apiece. It will throw them over budget, but for something which is obviously clinically indicated, the authority will pay. With the amalgamation of the FHSA and the health authority into the new combined health authority, and together with expanding fundholding, such rescues will become impossible. It will be then that the pressure to combine with other fundholding practices may become overwhelming.

This led Philip to talk about choice. In most practices there is no real choice. In theory they can negotiate a contract with any trust anywhere and press for an individual patient to go there. But, except in a very few cases for second or third opinions, neither they nor their patients want it. GPs have less professional contact with the specialists at the other hospitals. The patients have a more difficult journey. 'Their' hospital is in their area. And, finally, to exercise this choice can mean very much more work. Cost effective?

Speed and waiting lists

But there isn't a limit: mean they can speed things up? Yes, Philip said, they can get things done more quickly, sometimes. They can phone around and find somewhere with the shortest waiting list for a hip operation. This may take several hours and it is usually Philip's time, though in some practices the fundholding manager does much of this. They do feel that they are under an obligation to get the 'best deal' for the practice and for the individual patients, but this is always at the 'expense' of the non-permanent residents who get, at each stage, relatively less of the GPs' time and thought.

Philip was amused by the effects of the fundholders' pressure on the providers to reduce their waiting lists. Their own practice had been well served by some of the initiatives. There seemed to be two ways for the trusts to reduce surgical waiting lists. One was to divert patients to a private ward. The other was to 'buy in' extra consultant sessions. In this case the consultants were paid an extra session to come in on Saturday mornings, but most of the other staff would have been there already and so did not have to be paid extra, only to work harder. Either way, the consultants got more money and it did not cost the NHS much. Philip said that the trusts did consult, or at least inform, the fundholders and this was part of their being better informed than before on what was going on in the local hospitals. Philip's concern was that money for surgeons was a factor in waiting lists and that there was a 'leakage' of NHS money into the private sector. Few managers seemed to mind this breakdown of the circular flow of the internal market.

Fundholders can play providers off against each other. Philip quoted one manager asking for the length of waiting lists for a procedure. In one trust the person he telephoned did not know, but when told that another had said four weeks, offered two.

What the pace is like for the GP

First Philip had enjoyed getting to grips with the business principles and details. He and his partners were convinced that it was important for a doctor to be involved in most of the contract negotiations, to stop clinical priorities and patient needs being forgotten. That having been done, he had hoped to extricate himself. Instead, he was still involved in the fine detail of contracts. While he and the fundholding manager agree over what he should be involved in, the telephone calls keep on coming in. 'It's a clinical issue,' they say to the receptionist who takes the call.

It is getting worse. Philip receives more telephone calls each day on the details of contracts or other aspects of the fundholding; he receives more memos telling him to be more innovative or cost effective, or more evaluating of the service; and he is invited, or called, to more meetings. Much as Philip would like to hand over most of this to the fundholding manager, they all agree it takes a medical person to appreciate the medical consequence of some of the decisions taken. It has become much more complicated than they ever imagined and they fear a disaster.

Philip knew that the fundholding manager was trying to make fundholding 'invisible' for the clinicians, by managing all the administrative side. When one of the GPs made a decision which required fundholding thinking, his or her task would end and the manager would 'make it happen'. In theory that might be possible, Philip said, but only up to a point. A clinician was still required to consider questions such as the importance of speed or the need for a particular refinement of procedure in certain cases. Anyway, Philip concluded, it was not happening invisibly, and he was still central to a great deal of decision making and discussion. To that he could see no end.

Now he is bored and frustrated with that part of the work, which is not what he was trained to do and not what he chose for a career. Instead of having worries and concerns over his patients, his worries are to do with the fundholding. Are they distributing the benefits equitably? Are they neglecting their non-fundholding, non-permanent residents? What are the figures going to look like? Are they breaking even? Is it immoral to make a profit? (On holiday he worries over fundholding problems, particularly the annual report and other reports that he has to make.)

For each of these questions Philip feels that he is the 'holder' of the worry for the partners. They support him well, because they share his conviction that a doctor should be involved, and because they do not want to have these worries themselves.

The money is not up for grabs and savings are not for free

Philip has to work out justifications for any savings they may have made. If the FHSA thought that they were 'gratuitous', rather than as a result of the GPs' careful planning, they would conclude that they gave the practice too much money in the first place and the budget would be cut. So far their own FHSA has not relieved them of any savings because it has accepted Philip's explanation for them. And they were not too big: if the practice had saved more, it would have required a lot of evidence to shake the belief that it must be a windfall, to be returned to the FHSA.

The practice always has a cash-flow problem. This is greatly compounded by the usual business phenomenon of having to wait months to be reimbursed for many things. And it is getting tougher. They have heard stories of GP fundholders who have been 'expelled' from the scheme after a couple of years' gross overspending.

I interrupted Philip here, and said that I had heard of some cases where the fundholding GPs had refused to return money. Philip acknowledged this but challenged me to work out the relationship between the practice and the authority after that. It was, he reminded me for at least the second time, 'paper money' which was being used to exercise control over the system. If the GPs refused to play the game, and refused to return the windfall, the FHSA would cut the budget next year. Nowadays it is called 'allowable' savings. And even the word 'savings' is used less as it is replaced by 'value for money'.

Yes, some GPs feared the FHSA would reduce their budgets next year. The annual business plan must include costings and savings. But this had not been required in the preparatory year of the first fundholding general practices and that was how some of those famous big sums got through.

The hospitals and the FHSA appear to be checking their data far more carefully and efficiently. In this way the 'pie' is being cut with increasing refinement and, while today's fundholding GPs may not have the same draconian power as the first ones, they continue to have more say in how their referrals are handled than in the days before the reforms.

As fundholding general practices increase and take control of relatively more of the overall budget, there will be less slack in the system to rescue any that err. Then there may be nothing to be done but stop particular procedures or remove the fundholder status of some general practices.

Personal capital

Some GPs have a financial stake in the capital value of their practice, where they are part owners of the premises. If fundholding savings put into benefit for patients increase the value of the building (repairs and extensions), then the absolute value of each GP's share will have increased. When an individual GP then leaves and 'sells on', she or he makes greater financial gain. Philip said that few doctors seem to feel very comfortable with this, but it is hard not to plan to partake in it. Another leakage of the public funds.

The relationship with the FHSA

The managers of the FHSA were very helpful when fundholding was started but they had become swamped by what they had been part of creating. At the time I met Philip, there was one person left on the staff of their FHSA who knew enough to be able to be of much help to them. Not surprisingly, she became inundated by questions from the other fundholders. Once there had been a queue of people waiting to speak to her: a waiting list for the manager.

Philip has been curious to observe how his feelings towards the people at the FHSA have changed. First he thought they were benign and neutral. Then he felt they were very helpful. Now he often has the fantasy that they are with-holding money, especially reimbursements due to the practice; and that they are doing this to deal with their own financial problems. They have their own books to balance. Philip was one of several of my informants to raise the ques-tion, 'Was he being paranoid?' Then he added that the FHSA people must have been preoccupied enough themselves when facing their own merger with the health authority.

A glimmer of light? 'Buying' district nurse and physiotherapist time

One trust's management did a skill mix and quality assessment of the district nurses. They gave them all psychometric testing. The one who got the 'lowest' score received her redundancy notice by letter. The GP fundholders withdrew their contract with the trust and employed district nurses them-selves. They kept the services of the colleague they valued so well, and had more control of the team.

In Philip's own practice, while not employing physiotherapists directly, they have direct access to them and consultants can no longer refuse their requests. It is not the command of the services that they have, but direct access (hitherto denied) to the physiotherapy department itself.

How much was this to do with fundholding and how much with GPs being more vocal? Philip agreed that this was not necessarily dependent upon fund-holding and that there were interesting examples of non-fundholders having a voice. He thought that it was easier for fundholders to become voting members of the commissioning group which dictates the purchasers' deci-sion. At least, it was easier if the majority of the practices were fundholding.

Auditors

FHSA internal auditors spent two whole days in the practice office and external auditors spent five days. Of course the practice manager and fund-holding manager had to be with them and the secretarial staff were heavily disrupted. Philip managed to hide much of the time.

Who paid? Philip explained that is all came out of FHSA, or central, funds. But accounting exercises cost money and he could not help wondering if less spent on checking the accounting of the GPs would have left their practice uncut by the last 3%. Or does it not work like that?

Where might it end?

Philip did not want to come across as all negative. Some of the work he found exciting and sometimes he was glad to be in it. But he often had the feeling that something unstoppable had been unleashed and that no one knew where it was going.

He wanted to talk to me more widely. Fundholding originally covered acute hospital services, inpatient and outpatient services, diagnostics, prescribing. Later community services were added. The exceptions, still funded centrally by the DHA, had been all accident and emergency admissions and subsequent activity, mental health inpatient services, all maternity services.

Mental health was hard. While inpatient services were excluded but community services included, it was expecting a lot of the GP fundholders to discriminate the right to fund community care. Such an observation seems to lie behind the often voiced grumble that the psychiatric hospitals are discharging their patients for the GPs to pick up the pieces and, if they are fundholders, the bill.

There was already talk of extending the scope to cover more elective surgery and outpatient work; and pilot schemes of 'total' fundholding practices.

The critical mass argument is that the ordinary fundholding practice is too small to be able to plan purchasing without shocks. It takes only half a dozen hip replacements one year to knock everything off balance. Merge half a dozen practices or bring them together as a consortium with a population of 100,000 people and you have stability. Accurate enough financial predictions can be made without any need for rescue by a parent body. It could be seen as a change from 'paper' to real money.

But as fundholding expands, with a greater absolute number of practices and more treatments under their purchasing, there will be less money for the health authorities to dispense. What price their 'purchaser role'? Their now substantial departments of public health carry out needs assessments of the community and link with wider academic epidemiological studies to work out priority of treatments. Some people speak of a time when the health authorities, with their highly sophisticated identifying tools for planning what should be purchased, have funds only for general medicine and emergencies. Or, if the pilot 'total purchasing' fundholders are a success, for nothing at all. They might disappear or, if they continued to merge with each other to get a wider and wider view, eventually they could become … well, you could call it a National Health Service (Purchaser).

Back to himself

As the managers become more fluent, they will do more, but it is difficult to see the system working without at least one doctor as involved as Philip is.

The practice had talked at one time of withdrawing from fundholding but dared not contemplate such a move because of the ill-will they would create within the FHSA and the providers. Philip, personally, would have felt that he was letting everybody down.

Now it is something that Philip no longer wishes to be spending his time on. As the other partners do not want to either, he remains saddled with it. They have agreed to discuss an 'internal contract' so that he can begin to think of an end to this role for himself. Then one of the others will take up what had become, if not a poisoned, at least a tarnished chalice

Chapter 9

The country doctors

Because I live in a city and had already met doctors from practices in two cities, I wanted to find some real country doctors. I looked at the map. There are several areas of the country where practices could be spread over what I call 'real' country, that is villages and farms and certainly no big towns. I made my enquiry.

As I fixed a time to meet a couple of the GPs in their country group practice, they told me that their productivity had gone up 10% a year for each of the last three. I wondered what that meant.

The village was almost deserted as the once-an-hour bus deposited me outside the pub. I thought it was like a mixture of a continental village at siesta time and a set for one of the old *Avengers* series on TV. But it was a pleasant village and I found a few small shops, a couple of churches, a hall and, to my great pleasure, a village cricket ground. There was a signpost indicating some industrial activity half a mile in the direction that the bus had taken. The surgery was past the shops, in a wood, brick and stone building, set amid shrubs and young trees. It had its own parking space and good disabled access.

I met two of the partners, Deirdre and Robert, who had both been in the practice for 15 years.

The practice serves around 15 parishes, with a total population of 7,000 people. The population is static and the practice list has been the same for many years. Yet this is the practice that has increased its 'productivity' by 10% a year. Yes, they assured me, 10% more patients have been seen each year for the last three years. That is, the number of patient-GP contacts has increased by 10% each year. How? I was told that it is the result of a combination of more check ups, more follow ups, better record keeping and different record keeping. More events are called 'patient contacts'. On the other hand, the hours taken on administration, the amount of paperwork taken home in the evenings, letters written and received on management itself, and meetings attended on management has, compared with the paltry increase of 10% in clinical activities, 'taken off'.

Deirdre and Robert were apologetic in admitting that none of the partners had made time to examine those different activities, as they would have liked to. They had been too busy doing practice reports, examining and reading documents, meeting purchasers and providers from the two lots of purchasers and two lots of trusts with whom they worked.

(As with the hospital figures of 'patients treated', no one really knew if the numbers quoted represented new or extra patients, or the same ones seen many times each. 'It is not really in anyone's interest to do that piece of research,' I had been told by someone else who had made a similar observation earlier in my enquiries. That person added, 'At least, not yet.')

All this activity was supposed to be geared towards improving the services, a direction in which these doctors were keen to go. But the result seemed to be that, frantically as they rushed, they were all standing still.

The figures required for the practice report were more demanding to produce each year. Items of terms of service had to be defined and counted. The banding of the figures was important and the higher the banding obtained the more money was brought in. But to achieve higher banding they needed more information.

They examine what is called their prescribing activity. (One of them rather ruefully drew my attention to the fact that they no longer prescribe: rather, they *do prescribing activity*.) This they do with the assistance of 'PACT', which stands for 'prescribing analyses and cost', and is in fact the Registered Trade Mark of the Prescribing Pricing Authority.

Their large folder of prescribing activity shows how monthly statements are assessed and commented on by the FHSA and are compared with the target budgets, the average for the particular authority, and with the average for the country as a whole. The FHSA adviser visits the practice regularly and the doctors are encouraged to reach a particular level in the proportion they prescribe of 'generic' as opposed to 'proprietary' preparations, particularly in certain groups of drugs. (Generic are the 'pure' chemical names — e.g. paracetamol — as opposed to proprietary names — e.g. Panadol. The wisdom of years of teaching has been to encourage the use of generic preparations, but recent research has shown a number of proprietary preparations to be superior in effectiveness. And some new drugs are available only in proprietary form.) The target for the generic preparations is pursued regardless of the clinical effectiveness of the one over the other in certain cases. The practice has to justify its prescribing performance in writing each year and for this purpose can have access to different levels or methods of analysis of the data.

They have been encouraged next year to create a 'practice charter' to be unique to them, but to go alongside the national Patient's Charter.

They are pressured to apply for fundholding status. It is rare for any subject to be raised in correspondence about contracts or the services provided by the hospitals without the suggestion being made that, whatever the particular difficulty is, it would be less likely to be a problem if they were fundholders. They are encouraged again to consider 'going fundholding'.

The county boundaries

Like several of the other rural practices that I investigated, this one had an area within more than one county. In the early days of the reforms Deirdre and Robert's anxiety over how this would be managed had been lessened on hearing from managers of both purchasing authorities and both trusts, who visited the practice and assured the partners that they would be able to continue to use the nearby hospital as they had done for years.

I questioned the words 'nearby hospital' because I thought that there would be two if there were two trusts. They explained that the two trusts did have two general hospitals but that historically patients from this practice had mostly gone to one hospital because of the distance. Under the old system this had worked extremely well. How would it work under the new?

Phrases used by the managers had included:

It will settle.

It's unlikely not to be sorted out (and even sometimes, Robert pointed out, with no double negatives, *It will be sorted out*).

Well, we'll wait and see.

One of the most confident statements was delivered by a 'shadow' chief executive who said he had put that question to one of the ministers from the Department of Health at a recent meeting in London. The minister assured the chief executive that provision would be made for that sort of geographical anomaly. And that shadow chief executive had certainly looked assured.

At other times managers had said that the contract would be set at a certain sum of money and that above that each case would be taken as an ECR.

The clinicians needed more reassurance. They emphasised that there were many good reasons for using only one of the hospitals in most cases. The public transport links were in its favour, the main roads were better and, for most of their area, the hospital of the one trust was, as the crow flew, nearer by far. In addition, the patients, their relatives and the practice staff had developed good links. The managers seemed to appreciate that and reassured the doctors who in turn reassured their anxious patients. Money was set aside for the minority of the patients who lived in one of the 'other' counties. Those people would be able to be referred to and to use the hospital they had always attended.

In the first year of the trusts the money ran out half way through, but very quickly the contract was extended and continued. A 'hiccup', they were told. It did seem like it, for the speed with which things were put right was such that hardly a patient noticed any delay or deviation in the service.

In the second year the money ran out half way through for the minority of the practice patients who lived in the 'other' county — and it took rather longer to sort out. Tolerance was less this time.

When, in the third year, it happened again, it did so with what the health service mandarins might have called interesting complications.

One week in the autumn seven referral letters were returned to the practice by the trust which managed the hospital they used the most. The trust's covering circular letter went over two pages and was headed, 'X District Health Authority' (one of the purchasers). It referred to the well known difficulty being experienced by that purchaser in providing funding to a level which would enable providers to be remunerated for the level of patient activity being commissioned by general practitioners. The purchaser had instructed the trust to return the referrals to the GPs. The GPs were to decide on whatever further action they might deem appropriate, in consultation with the purchaser. The letter expressed regret that delay would occur in dealing with patients' needs.

One of those referral letters had been with the trust for over two weeks. The referral was one which the GP and patient considered to be urgent, but the letter had not been seen by the consultant to whom it had been addressed, before it was returned by the trust.

The GPs had known that the purchaser was running into some sort of difficulty with funding and had been reassured that the administrative complications were being sorted out. They were therefore totally unprepared for a decision with such sudden and severe clinical implications.

The purchaser's letter was slightly different. It was dated a few days after the one from the trust. It acknowledged that the hospital had capacity to continue to do their work, but because the activity level which had been contracted was then 'forecast to over-perform', they did not have sufficient resources to continue to fund such activity. The purchaser had consulted the trust and had agreed to take certain actions. One such action was that all new referrals received later than a date which was in fact two weeks before that letter was written would be referred to them for authorisation. Such referrals would be handled as ECRs which would result in some referrals being returned to the referring doctors. They could then re-refer to other providers with whom the purchaser had a contract whose agreed contract level had not yet been reached.

Simple.

At the time I met Deirdre and Robert, they were having to ensure that each referral was accepted beforehand as 'urgent' by the consultant to whom it was going to be sent.

How the consultants made that particular assessment and how they did it without taking up more time which would otherwise be used for direct work with patients, and how they did it without causing more delay, Deirdre and Robert did not know. Another bit of increased productivity, perhaps.

To get consultants to assess referrals as they wanted, it was obvious that they had to put a great deal of thought into how to write the letters, whom to telephone, and which of them should sign the letters to which consultant. This was all in order to influence the system to get what they believed was best for their patients. It was taking up their time and that of the specialists, time which could otherwise be used in patient care. Furthermore it seemed obvious to them that if the purchaser was paying for these consultations as ECRs, there was money in the purchaser's purse anyway.

Why was it all getting so complicated and inefficient?

These doctors knew many of the managers at the trusts and at the purchasers. They were not stupid people. Yet they could not come up with a successful plan for the finances for this, the third year of the trusts. The conviction of all the staff in the practice centre was that the managers, trying to speed administrative processes, were repeatedly being tripped up by their complexities which were bureaucratic, time-consuming and, ultimately, delaying patient care.

'Money follows patients'?

The professional managers, they were told, had received a great deal of training and support. If they were finding it so hard to get it right, what chance did GPs have without the advantages of such training?

A new bureaucratic requirement

For a time there was another quite separate delay on some cases. Patients' addresses were being checked before referrals were accepted by the trust and this was causing even longer delays for residents with particular postcodes. It turned out that what had happened for several hundred people in this practice was that their postcodes made it look as if they came from a different county and so their hospital care should be contracted for by a different purchaser and different trust. These people were not to be confused, Robert explained, with the people from the practice who did live in the different county, did have that county's postcodes, but did, by the complicated aforesaid agreement with ministers and managers, have access to the hospital of the trust which served most of the patients of the practice and which was many miles nearer to them anyway. 'Or were they the same people?' wondered Deirdre. It was an anomaly of the postcode system found in several parts of the country which, as another minister had assured someone, was being carefully monitored. In this practice there was added delay for these patients too.

The director of public health had been very embarrassed: it was all an administrative error. One committee described it as a 'dreadful blunder' which should never have occurred. The managers said that, of course, it was something that the department concerned would in future sort out without clinicians knowing it had ever come up. 'Treat it as a teething trouble.'

And even the community health council, which had hitherto been neutral over fundholding, joined in suggesting it as the solution to the recurrent problems of over-contracting.

So more managers met the GPs and took more of each other's time, while the GPs wondered if they were going to have arrangements they had heard of from colleagues in other parts of the country, whereby there is an implicit preference for ECRs.

The area and the practice

And so it goes on. They showed me the map. Over 200 square miles, 15 parishes, individual villages, no obvious principal or capital village. It was easy to see that those few people living in the 'other' county, or with the anomalous postcodes, were for very obvious geographical reasons the more isolated. They were also, Deirdre and Robert said, the older members of the community and so had social reasons for isolation. They were the people whose urgent referrals were being delayed more and whose appointments were being postponed more. If it had not happened already it must inevitably mean that sometime, somebody would die unnecessarily. Lifesaving treatment will have been delayed in the name of the reforms.

This practice is one which has used computer technology for years. They have weekly practice meetings and meetings with other disciplines, negotiating packages of care, geographical areas of work, etc In these ways it runs and negotiates very much into a fundholding practice Relationships with the surrounding practices, all of which are fundholders, are cordial. The GPs in this practice are convinced that to convert to fundholding would not improve the service. It would certainly decrease the time the individual doctors spend on clinical work and increase the amount of time that has to be given to management More clerical staff would be required.

In a particular way, this practice, along with a very small number in the country, stands to lose if it does become fundholding, because that would entail a budget for prescribing. At the moment as a non-fundholding but dispensing practice they make a profit on their dispensing. This profit is sufficient to pay for the equivalent of a full time doctor. The 'market' works in mysterious ways.

But, ultimately, they do not want to be fundholders. They do not want to have the bother of it. They want to stop racing frantically to stand still. They are trained as doctors in doing medicine and allocating cases to other resources as required. They would like to continue to get on with it.

They expect that the pressures and the muddles will go on. Increasingly they are hearing of consultants and hospital managers murmuring, 'ECRs preferred.'

They showed me around their pleasing building. It still looked cared for. Highlighted on the calendar in the staff room were the birthdays of the members of staff. Deirdre and Robert said the partners were thinking of a five year calendar next, with their retirement dates.

Chapter 10

The general nurse

The managers realised how low morale had dropped. Eileen was invited, along with as many nurses as possible from her ward and some others, to a meeting. The clinical nurse manager complimented the seven of them who were there on tackling the changes made by the reforms as well as they had done. He spoke cheerfully of more improvements to come.

They were told, above all, to communicate and to let the manager know if there were worries or concerns about the changes, the work, or even management.

Furthermore they were told that if something had gone wrong, for goodness sake let the managers know straight away. The worst thing to start doing is to cover up.

'Managers and all the procedures are here to support you, so that if anybody does make a complaint, then management can support you.'

Really? Even small things? Eileen, who had been in her post for a month, asked this because she did not want to be pestering managers with petty detail. Yes, she was told, however small.

'That is the way you can learn. That is the way we can all learn.'

Eileen mentioned that earlier that day she had noticed something so trivial that she thought no more of it but now wondered if she should mention it.

She was encouraged to do so.

It was that the chart recording intravenous fluid and medication on a particular patient had not been filled in correctly, although the fluids and medication had been given correctly. Eileen was complimented on mentioning this, and the manager added that it was by bringing such things to their notice that they could all be sure that the people concerned could learn and keep to the procedures. 'And then we are all of us safer, including the patients,' he added.

The next day the nurse that had filled in the card erroneously was suspended.

The first things to learn

When I met her, Eileen had been back in this country for six months, working as what used to be called a staff nurse in a large hospital. After she had been qualified for six years, she had gone to work in Canada for two more, so was quite pleased to talk to me of her 'before and after' experiences.

The first thing she had learned after her return to the reformed NHS was not to be critical.

She had been asked at her first interview what she thought of the reforms in the health service and she was not enthusiastic. And the interviewing panel was not enthusiastic about her and she was not offered the job. 'Equal ops' (equal opportunities practice) dictated that she was given a reason. She was told that she had been unsuccessful because the other candidate had rather more relevant experience.

At the next interview she said that she was very excited by the reforms and thought that they offered a very interesting challenge. Her immediate future was ensured: she was offered the job.

On the ward, the first thing that Eileen noticed was how much time the nurses spent writing. I learned more of that later.

The 'named nurse' and multidisciplinary work

Within minutes of arrival on the ward Eileen had been photographed and two days later given a name badge. All the other staff appeared to be wearing these all the time. The obvious advantage — of people knowing who they were addressing and of the levelling of disciplines and hierarchies — was not lost on Eileen. She was enthusiastic. Soon, she realised that they were part of the 'named nurse' system and a new approach to responsibility for care. Each patient had a named nurse responsible for his or her nursing care. Being responsible meant also being answerable. If anything went wrong, it was the named nurse who had to answer.

Within three days Eileen had noticed how much general care had changed since she last worked in this country. Beyond her wildest imaginations, it had deteriorated. She was working on a 18-bed ward for women with severe heart problems. The patients, whom the managers called clients, were admitted in cardiac emergency, transferred after cardiac surgery or after other sorts of surgery but with cardiac complications, and some were admitted for investigations and were awaiting transfer elsewhere. Mostly, they were very ill and required a great deal of care.

Usually a nursing shift was two qualified staff with one unqualified care assistant. The second most common shift team was two qualified staff and two student nurses who were supposed to be 'super-numerary' (on the ward to learn and not to do the chores like student nurses used to).

In case that number of staff sounded all right to me, I was asked to think of what would happen if one patient developed a severe medical crisis. This would immediately take two nurses and could therefore leave one, unqualified, to care for all the other, up to 17, patients. What would happen if one of them needed help or observation from a qualified nurse? If a trained member of staff was off sick, it could mean that the shift comprised one qualified nurse, one care assistant and an agency nurse.

Eileen was thus liable to be not only the named nurse for her 'own' patients but also the person who had 'signed' responsibility for the agency nurse, was instructing the care assistant what to do, and was responsible for dealing with the transfers and admissions and all the paperwork.

The staff appeared to be gasping, and even the most experienced often looked distressed. They made mistakes in the paperwork, they often complained of feeling unwell and were off sick.

I asked for more on that word 'gasping' and Eileen explained to me some of the things that led her to use the expression...

Infectious diseases were not being handled in the approved manner. There is the well known, rarely seen and nastily dangerous MRSA (methicillin resistant staphylococcus aureus). Anybody in the hospital found to have this germ should be barrier nursed, that is kept in a separate room with special clothing worn by people going into that room which they then take off as they leave it. In the hospital where Eileen worked this had not been done because they did not have the staff and at one time the infection spread to as many as half a dozen people.

Sticking plaster and sellotape had been used to seal the door from one ward onto its patio because the night staff were so frightened of the ward being broken into again. One night staff person had to hand over the contents of her purse when confronted and attacked by an intruder. The broken lock on the patio door had still not been repaired over a year later.

Several times when critically ill people were admitted in emergency to this specialist ward, Eileen saw them and their relatives alarmed to find the neighbouring beds occupied by confused psycho-geriatric or psychiatric patients or, twice, by alcoholics being searched for dangerous objects. The relatives and patients were not reassured when they were told that they had to accept that there were not suitable facilities with qualified specialist nurses for those people.

What made them 'gasp' even more was the realisation that they were working in what seemed a 'good' hospital. It had done quite well in the league tables. Eileen wondered if having the appropriately trained staff was on the list of criteria.

Eileen, even at the time I met her, was still feeling very bad over the nurse who had been suspended. She had tried to speak to her colleague, whom she hardly knew, on the phone, but she had refused to speak to Eileen. The other staff on the ward told her to be cynical and to think that she had learned something about how the place was run. She would get to feel less bad in time. The nurse who had been suspended never came back to work because, before the formal investigation which had been set up was due to sit, she resigned and did not seek another job in the health service.

Manager to staff nurse: 'I am suspending you. I see you look upset. Do you want a lift home?'
Some weeks later the management presented 'no case' and the hearing reinstated the staff nurse with 'not a blot on your character'

Although this had been a nursing matter, everyone on the ward was affected. Eileen said that the doctors were particularly shocked because it was so different from how things would be handled in their discipline. If one of them had made such a mistake, they said, they would have been told off, and there might have been a big row, but no such shocking public ritual.

At interview Eileen had been told how the ward team worked in a multi-disciplinary way but in reality they found that often they had no qualified nurse from the trust's permanent staff able to go on medical ward rounds, so that communication between doctors and nurses was worse than she had ever come across.

Facing the budget

The three wards on their floor, they had been told, were £50,000 over budget. The managers cut £10,000 off the paper allocation and this seemed a good idea to all of them but, at the time I met Eileen, the staff were preparing to face £40,000 savings on staff. This might mean restricting over-time or sending some agency staff home at weekends if things were quiet.

Even the patients noticed how poorly staffed they were. They could tell when agency nurses were in because they were having to be told what to do and had not met the patients before. On the whole the patients tried very hard to support the staff and did not complain.

The staff were told how important it was for all of them to be aware of the budget figures and to think how they might make savings. But could they have a breakdown of the figures, the costs of all staff, training, food, cleaning, main-tenance, stationery, travel? Yes, of course they could, as soon as the finance department was able to finalise the figures for the whole trust. And remember, they were told, the finance department could not in all fairness (and it would not be politic) release one ward's figures until all of them were clear.

So, in effect, they were being asked to think of savings without knowing how much most things cost.

The paperwork

There were few things that were not to be documented. Even a telephone call to a social worker which lead to the revelation that the social worker was busy and not available, had to be recorded. Every patient had a care plan and assessment. Everybody in the whole place seemed terrified about lawsuits. Everybody was covering his or her back.

The care assistants and the agency nurses were fed up in a different way. They believed they were allowed to do less on their own than they used to; and they were reluctant to ask the trained staff for instructions lest they inter-rupt them too much. So sometimes they were frantically busy and sometimes they were idle and desperately bored. To be an idle qualified nurse in a busy hospital was a new frustration for some of those agency nurses.

But it was the named nurses, scattering mistakes in their frenzy, that were taking responsibility. Eileen and her colleagues asked themselves often if this new role of theirs was doing something for the government, like saving it from taking more responsibility itself.

(I checked out the experience of a few care assistants and agency nurses and was given a very similar picture from the one that Eileen had painted.)

Eileen was not against complaints and she said she had not come across people who, on principle, were opposed to the right to make a complaint. But she did say that if anything had not been 'worked through' before it was started, it was the encouragement given in the Patient's Charter and in other parts of government propaganda for people to make complaints. The trust where Eileen worked had, like most health service establishments nowadays, created a complaints procedure. There was a procedure for complainers to follow and a procedure for managers to follow in dealing with complaints. But nowhere in the procedure was there anything on how to deal with the work that clinical staff had to leave in order to handle the complaints. Sometimes it seemed to Eileen that all she or one or two of the other staff were doing was dealing with complaints. So clinical care got even worse. This weighed particularly heavily on the shoulders of the named nurse. The managers' immediate response to any complaint over a clinical event was to ask what the named nurse was doing. Responsibility is seen to lie with the named nurse, not with the hospital or trust.

Eileen quoted an example of a woman who had written complaining of the care her mother had been given when she was dying. Eileen had thought the complaint was very reasonable. She well remembered how rushed off their feet the staff were and how they had been unable to change this old lady's sheets as quickly as they had wanted to. The instant management response on receiving the letter was to call for reports and to look at the records and statements made at the time.

When was the first recording of the observation that the patient's sheet was soiled and needed changing? Had the named nurse signed? If the named nurse had signed this, and concluded that there was no member of the shift available to deal with the matter immediately, had they alerted the duty manager to this need (and potential complaint), and requested additional staff? If not why not, and was a record made of that?

Eileen was not telling me that the complaint was handled totally insensitively, nor that the management wrote an unnecessarily scapegoating or humble-pie letter to the complainers. Rather she was wanting me to realise that the intense bureaucratic machinery and its pressure to have the paperwork correct had in itself prevented the managers asking the ward staff a particularly important question on the experience of knowing that the lady's sheets were wet and that they had not been able to change them for an hour: what did it feel like for them? It prevented the managers from offering any support to the ward staff who had been looking after that dying person, and had tried to help her to die in peace and with dignity, when they were having to fill up all these other forms. Managers were unable to offer support to their staff who were sick to death of staying late, not getting their breaks during the shift and not having enough colleagues on the ward.

All that the managers seemed able to say was that the staff should manage better and prioritise their objectives more efficiently.

Some more senior nurses

Eileen had known some of the slightly older staff when she worked at the hospital before and had met up with a couple of them again. Both of them admitted that they had been openly critical of some of the ways in which the government and then the trust had introduced the reforms. They had not liked some of the decisions.

One of them, Jane, a senior nursing sister, had told Eileen that there were going to be changes in the ward that she was working on. She had told her that as part of carrying out their business plan, a 'skill mix' had been done. She had been quite sympathetic to the process of finding out everything that everyone did, how often they did it and determining which were the things that could be done by that person and by that person alone. What Jane had not liked was the way the 'skill mix' had ignored the question, 'What if two of a given procedure are required at the same time?' (I was reminded of what Eileen had said earlier of the position on the ward when a second patient needs immediate skilled nursing intervention and the qualified staff are occupied with someone who already does.)

Jane told Eileen that one day after the skill mix she was summoned to meet her own manager and the director of acute nursing services. They wished to discuss the redevelopment in the service and the redefinition of the goals. She was told that there were choices that she could consider. One was to take a lower grade job (but possibly at a protected salary for one year) in a day ward. The other was to leave. Jane took early retirement and the hospital lost a good and previously loyal person. Eileen said that managers were allowed to be critical of clinical staff in the interests of loyalty, so she did not think that Jane's criticism should be seen as disloyalty. As she left, she wrote a long letter on the changes and her reasons for leaving, but it did not make the pages of the trust's bulletin.

The other nurse who had been in charge of the nursing staff of a large acute department had been told her choice was a demotion to a lower grade post or to accept redundancy. She was still making up her mind.

Individual performance review and an old lady

If Eileen stays in the post the next thing in store for her is the new individual monitoring system of performance review. She will be invited to work out targets for her improvement (called professional development) over the next year and her manager will monitor it. She says it feels like offering coaching in swimming strokes to people who have been thrown into the water in a ferry disaster. They seemed to be so near to the edge of sheer malpractice much of the time. She quoted the following case to me.

An old woman had been in one of their beds for weeks. They could do nothing more for her heart and she was 'blocking' a bed. Everybody was saying that it was not his or her problem. The hospital managers were saying that she should be in social services accommodation. To get her there had been taking ages and the funding that social services had available was very limited. The old lady stayed and stayed. The consultant was troubled by the blocked bed and explained the dire financial implications of this: they could not admit an ECR from which they would earn extra money. Therefore the consultant said that she had to leave that week.

'Arrangements' were made. She was to go home on the Friday with 'support': meals on wheels and a home help for several hours a day. (There would be nobody with her in her flat overnight.)

During the Wednesday night, two nights before she was due to leave, she became confused and wandered out of the ward where she fell over. Eileen learned this when she came into work in the morning. She suggested to the consultant that she could not seriously be thinking of sending the old lady home in this condition: she could be seen not to be compos mentis by any 'person in the street', social services person, relative, coroner, or even purchaser. The consultant sagged her shoulders and hunched her back even more than usual and retorted that if she did not chuck her out, the social services, who had taken so long to organise care, would get a bill from the trust 'We are losing money and we are £50,000 over budget.' It was money.

Eileen won that argument: the old lady did stay longer and in fact died in the ward. But Eileen said that her mind was still reeling every time she thought of that morning and of the two of them being reduced to the level of having that sort of argument over a human being.

The story had another slight sting to its tail. A few weeks later Eileen met someone who had worked on the ward a year before. This ex-member of staff asked Eileen how things were. When he heard of the argument with the consultant, he said, 'You may not believe it, but that woman used to be able to show compassion.'

The use of the name badges

As we were parting Eileen remembered one last thing she wanted to tell me. She had spoken of having her photograph taken and what she called 'those lovely name badges' which all the hospital staff have with their photographs on. Did I realise, she asked, that the trust kept copies of the photographs? (I didn't say that of course they would so that they could replace the card if an employee lost one.) She went on to explain to me that when people were making complaints or the police were making enquiries, the management had been known to show the photographs to help get the identity of the person who was being complained of or was under investigation.

'How's that for staff support?' said Eileen. She added that she was absolutely certain that it did happen but had not heard of staff ever being told officially. She wondered if that was one of the uses that the government had in mind in drawing up that part of the Patient's Charter.

Chapter 11

Community care and the district nurse: Jane's story

'We have not had a restructuring of our management system for eight months at least. That's why I have time to talk to you.'

Jane explained her joke by telling me that in the last five years management had been restructured four times. Each new system had some good points and some bad points. When the things that are clearer are emphasised, the fuzzy bits round the edges do not get noticed so much. At each restructuring there have been some casualties: some take voluntary redundancy, some get promotion to a position in which they are very unhappy, some get pushed out.

In the first couple of restructurings there seemed to be more people who were optimistic and thought that it would make things better. One new manager was well remembered for having said, 'Come, on join us. We can make it fun.' The next day he disappeared.

Now there are not many people left who think these reorganisations are going to make things much better. The cynics are becoming the majority.

Even the managers are more cautious and herald change as something that has to be done or as a means to make the other changes that have taken place more workable.

The first old lady

A woman in her eighties, who had had a number of minor strokes, was well known to the district nurses. When she dislocated her hip she was admitted to the hospital.

On a Friday afternoon her son, with whom she lived, telephoned the district nurses because he had been told by the ward that his mother was going to be discharged on the following day. He was worried about the weekend.

The district nurse telephoned the ward and then rang the son back to reassure him that the staff were confident that his mother was now independent again and was walking with a zimmer frame. One of the district nurses would visit her at the beginning of the next week before reinstating a 'bath nurse'.

On the Tuesday of the following week Jane visited. She learned that shortly before midnight, ten hours before the discharge time, someone else from the ward had telephoned her son. His mother had had a fall but she was still coming home the next day.

The old lady was alert but distressed. In her room she had neither commode nor bedpan. There was a pad over her knee that had been fixed by the nurses in the ward but neither she nor her son had any instructions. She could not stand with the zimmer frame, let alone walk. Jane and the son together could not get her to walk (and the son could not wait, because he was fighting a redundancy threat at his own work). Jane telephoned the GP who visited shortly. He examined the old lady, found that she had a 'dropped foot', and on that ticket arranged for her to be readmitted to hospital.

Later in the week Jane was on the phone to one of her opposite numbers at the social services community care department and she mentioned this case. All the manager from the social service department replied to her was, 'Well, we had been told by the ward that she was fine.'

Where was the responsibility?

The old lady was discharged again a few weeks later but this time not on a Saturday morning and this time with a different sort of plan. She was discharged to social services department care.

Such cases, Jane assured me, were fairly typical. She reminded me of some of the features of the care in the community programme.

Ten years of changes

When Jane had been appointed ten years ago as a district nurse, she had to have at least two years' post-qualification experience and was expected to have varied experience in recognition of the isolation of the role of the district nurse, who had to be able to work independently and with no direct medical backup.

'Skill mixing' has changed most of this. So many actions of the district nurse do not require a nursing qualified person to be able to do them. This is why it has been possible for care in the community to be provided by social services, often by people without training. Even in the district nursing service itself, posts are advertised for less experienced staff with a position on the pay scale appropriate for the newly qualified. They can have had little experience of working alone.

How 'nursing care' is interpreted is crucial to the way the various roles involved in community care are allocated. The definitions of these roles seem to vary greatly from place to place.

Social workers used to see the district nurses as very 'medicalised' and these are the very aspects of the work that the managers on both sides are pushing so hard. The district nurse managers try to arrange things so that their staff do those activities, and those alone. The social services care staff manager aims to ensure that their staff do none of them. Both count the number of visits.

Thus trained nurses may sometimes be limiting their activities to 'skilled clinical nursing tasks' such as injection, continuous medication through 'syringe driver', wound and catheter care, and the management of diabetes.

'Personal care' and the use of skills of an interpersonal nature are not products that only the trained district nurse can market. Personal care is now part of social care. Anyone whose needs are social has to make a very great fuss and produce a few medical symptoms to get a district nurse through the door again.

Jane had always appreciated the relationship district nurses had with GPs, but told me of a change there as well. Some fundholding practices have 'bought in' an extra district nurse on a lower grade. She is not employed for her long experience or ability to make people feel cared for, but to do home visits on people discharged from hospital earlier than in the past, to give flu injections and to take blood samples, thus helping build up and maintain the numbers of 'itemisable' services performed by the practice. That means money.

The second old lady

Another woman in her mid eighties had been in hospital for nearly three months after fracturing her hip. No one could say that her discharge had not been carefully planned. There were meetings, case conferences and home visits.

This old lady was immobile in a wheelchair and there were very sound reasons for discharging her from hospital because she still had a chronic, discharging infection of the surgical wound in her thigh: much less chance of re-infection outside hospital.

Social services arranged for four visits per day to deal with feeding and domestic cleaning. The district nurse's role was to offer support and give supervision of her pressure points, to give continence care and to instruct and supervise the husband with the handling of the outer dressings of her wound, should they become moist between the district nurse's full redressings.

Day 1. No visit from the social services, nor news.

Telephone call to the district nurse from the daughter who had visited her parents.

Telephone call from district nurse to the social worker at the social services. Social worker not available.

Telephone call from the district nurse to the social services manager who said competently and in a reassuring manner, 'I will deal with it.'

Telephone call from district nurse to daughter.

Day 2. No news or visit.

Day 3. The carers started to arrive.

On the suggestion of one of the carers, the old lady's daughter telephoned the social services department herself. A social worker handling the allocation of the 'package of care' appeared unconcerned and said, 'I carried out my job. I did my paperwork. The manager must have delivered the package to the wrong department.'

Later in the week, when the district nurse and a social worker were speaking on the phone to each other, Jane said that she would like to try to find out what had gone wrong (in the past under the old system she or one of the other district nurses would have organised the whole package). Did they never check? She asked a social worker if she had found out what had gone wrong, or even if she had thought of checking that all the arrangements were in place before the lady was discharged. The social worker appeared very puzzled by these suggestions and repeated that she had done her paperwork. 'If they had a problem, they would have got back to me.'

Meanwhile, the old lady was admitted to a nursing home at the expense of social services. Husband and wife were separated again. This time over Christmas and New Year.

Three weeks later Jane heard that the old lady was to be discharged again and that all the social services arrangements were in hand. She telephoned the old lady's husband to discuss times when she might visit. He had not heard of his wife's imminent discharge. On the day before the planned discharge (a Friday again) Jane telephoned the social services department to double check on the arrangements. The social worker was not available. She telephoned the nursing home where the staff said they knew nothing of the arrangements. They were being handled by the social services care staff. The husband was not worried because within the last 24 hours he had been assured by the social workers that care had been arranged and would be 'delivered'.

On the Saturday she went home.

There were no visits.

On that day their daughter visited. She and her father together telephoned the duty social worker who said that he had not heard anything, but added that what they described sounded like a nursing problem.

Jane herself was telephoned at home at 10.30 pm by the husband. She was not on duty. She telephoned the duty social worker, not the one the husband and daughter had phoned earlier in the day. This social worker said she was sorry but no nursing visits had been arranged. The social worker said they would not be able to put any staff in that night because arrangements were more difficult to make. Eventually she did agree something for the next day. During the night, the duty district nurse visited and next morning the social services department care worker arrived. By the time that care worker visited the husband had already done his wife's incontinence care, cleaning and drying, so the care worker did no more than offer to give her a drink. In the afternoon when the carers arrived and heard again from the husband what he done in the night, they said he was managing and so did not return the following day.

At the beginning of the next week Jane rang the social worker in charge of the allocation of resources but he had no explanation for what had happened. He repeated that he had done his paperwork. When Jane suggested that they meet to try to sort out what had happened and to get their act of working together in better shape, he hung up.

The next day the social worker saw the husband and the husband saw the district nurse. By that time he believed it was all his fault because he had in effect sent the care workers away early on the Sunday morning after he had cleaned his wife himself.

Jane said to me that she could hardly bear it when he mumbled that it might have been better if he had left his wife lying in her own shit. He asked if he had done the wrong thing.

Training the aides

From Jane I learned that the district nurses have to train the social work aides in care tasks. First she reminded me that when she started as a district nurse she had had to have two years' experience after qualifying as a general nurse. The young people who are taken on as auxiliary carers are often people who walk off the street into the job centre. They are often employed through an agency. Vetting cannot be thorough.

There are so many skills for looking after dependent people that it is almost impossible for an aide to be trained in all of these before first working in someone's home. The skills required range from how to hold somebody's arms when they bruise very easily to how to work a hoist for lifting an immo-

one person from a bed. Jane told me that the sort of muddle described in those two cases was typical of her experience. It was also typical of what many of her friends, working in other departments had told her when they heard that she was coming to meet me.

She also described the confusion over the 'ownership' of cases. Patients could be transferred to social services care without the district nurse having been informed. When she had wanted to say goodbye to the patient and family, she had been told that this was not cost effective.

When they had taken these difficulties to their supervisors or managers, they got lectures in being more skilful in prioritising their cases and their tasks; and off-loading that which does not require a particular skill. Off-loading to whom? Another response which the managers have often given is that in these uncertain times the district nurses will have to carry on as they are. Meanwhile, the manager has to make preparations for the new reorganisation; or work on a paper which must be ready to be presented if the rumoured or threatened take-over from another trust, or merger with it, appears imminent.

The elderly man

He and his son were both widowers and lived together. He had a recurrence of abdominal pain at the start of the weekend and his son called their doctor. The GP, who knew him well, visited and agreed that he might have a recurrence of his ulcer. He arranged for admission to hospital.

The ward was run that weekend by agency nurses and locum doctors. They said that it was not his ulcer and he was discharged back into the community. Further investigations were said not to be justified. Four weeks later he was admitted again for the same complaint. This time he was seen by the permanent consultant who transferred him to an intensive therapy unit. He had a perforated ulcer and, despite the intensive treatment, he died.

The son told Jane, who had been visiting his father during those last four weeks at home, that he had no wish to make a formal complaint. He did wonder, if his father had not been seen by locum doctors and agency nurses, and not been discharged into community care immediately after the first weekend, and if further investigations had not been deemed to be unjustified, then what? Perhaps his father might have had early treatment and might still have been alive.

The middle-aged woman with terminal MS

For over ten years Jane has been a key person in the care of this woman.

For much of the time it has been complicated, using hoists to move her and careful supervision of pressure sore areas. Now she is back at home and wishes to stay there to die.

Care is being shared between the district nurse service, managed by the trust, and social services aide workers. All that Jane does is to try to supervise the care workers in the skills required for manipulating the hoist and helping her to monitor the pressure sores which are gradually getting worse. The care workers change often, so must be supervised often. There are more people doing the caring but, Jane fears, less caring is being done.

There seems to be no ownership of responsibility for providing the 'seamless' service.

Paperwork

Jane registers dependency levels of all her patients on a chart. She records tasks that she is doing, keeps a register and a diary and feeds information into a computerised system. The last three carry very much the same information. The computerised system has been running for over five years. It still fails more than once a year, and it is immensely time-consuming to keep up to date and to explain to the uninitiated. No one likes it. The senior managers find it useful. It was very expensive to set up, it is expensive to maintain and to train new staff to use. Therefore they cannot get rid of it.

Jane's travel expenses form is many times more elaborate and complicated than a few years ago. Gone are the days of referring to 'district visiting'. Even naming the street is inadequate; the postcode of the dwelling visited must be entered. The car mileometer figure at the beginning and the end of the day and at the beginning and the end of the month have also to be recorded. And all for 6p a mile.

One of the reasons for there being so many more forms to fill in and records to keep is that the legal side of the work has expanded. Anxiety over complaints and litigation has gone sky high. A few of the managers are really appreciative when compliments are received and they appear to go to great lengths to ensure that they get to the attention of higher management. But most often, when a complaint comes in, someone, somewhere in the department, is 'hung out to dry'. The staff at the trust say that the managers are 'going for the kill'.

When Jane wanted to attend a part time course and asked her manager for approval for her plan to work lunch hours to make up for the 2 $^1/_2$ hours per week, she was told, 'But district nurses work lunches anyway.'

Supervision sessions with the managers tend to be like a sophisticated game of picking and choosing. Difficult or unwanted cases are deemed more appropriate for social care. The intention is encourage the district nurses in this because, as they say, the social services department really has the upper hand: if the formula 'nursing care is required' is used, the case comes bouncing over. In practice this often means that the district nurses' case load is made up of those people with multiple health problems: strokes, diabetes and some of the more severe personality disorders. And then, when a district nurse appears to be keeping one of the cases for too long, or the visiting has become chronic, the manager is almost bound to say that she is spending too much time on social care: refer back to social services.

And so people's care is passed to and fro, from either side of the seamless scene.

Jane's way out

Jane is 47. She envies her friend who, being three years older, has been able to retire, frustrated and worn down by an increasingly managerial role and no more money.

But in her pre-retirement years, Jane is able to see a glimmer of some positives in what is happening. She described some of the fundholding general practices as being able to get in very good equipment and 'buy in' outreach clinics from specialists, so that their patients are seen quickly by the dermatologist or the rheumatologist. She notes, almost critically, how some of the fundholding practices have decided that they are a 'good' size and are desperately trying to remain that size. This means that they have to work very hard to resist the pressure to grow, to merge or to combine into another consortium. They keep having to plan strategies to stay the size they want to remain. But some of the fundholding practices are deemed by the others to be too choosy. They are said to avoid the difficult cases. And the district nurse, whose department's services are bought by several practices, is often the carrier of tension between them.

Jane said that she is swamped. She feels downtrodden, fearful and devalued. She reckons that her manager does too. Her hope is that she can last out the next three years.

Chapter 12

The health visitors

I met two health visitors who worked 200 miles apart. These are the stories told me by Margaret and Amanda...

Margaret's story

Margaret had spent 12 years as a health visitor and had worked in the borough in which we met for half of that time. With the reforms of the NHS in the last four years, while staying in the same job and working in the same geographical area, she had had three different managements. They were not a trust, they became a trust, then, with a merger, they became a different trust. There had been several smaller management changes between times and, at least four times, they had been given a great big 'family tree', showing the management structure of the whole organisation.

She used to love her work and to think she was good at it. She did not get into muddles. The adults and the children that she worked with seemed to find her useful and she got on well with the GPs, the district nurses and the others.

Now she feels that she does not really know what is happening and, worse, that no one can tell her. A couple of weeks before we met, on the Thursday afternoon, one of the senior managers in her friend's patch was told that his job was ending the next day. And he was gone. Someone said, 'It's the turn of the men in the grey suits now.' But that joke did not really help. It just made it more obvious that everybody seemed demoralised and to feel threatened.

In the bad old days of the old hospital hierarchy they all knew where they were. Then there was the 'democratic' phase when all staff were asked to give their opinions. Now, in the new phase, they are not asked for their opinions. Like in the old days, orders are being given but the big difference is that managers who are giving the orders do not seem to have a commitment to patients and do not even have any experience themselves of working with patients. Those old 'dragons' of ward sisters and matrons were very dedi-

onted. Margaret knew there was a lot of unnecessary anxiety for staff, but they did all realise that there was suffering going on. This was acknowledged by the managers. Now, tell the managers about a family in need and you get no human response. Instead, something to the effect of, 'Manage better.'

Managers used to give a lot of support. Now they give a lot of weight, and they throw it around. They do not seem to Margaret to be thinking of patients, or clients, or any word you want to put on those people they are all paid to care for. They seem to be thinking, 'How can you preserve me?' They want to spend as little time as possible near those people and to spend as little money as possible on them. Margaret and her friends talk of managers always having a very full agenda that always seems to have two things on it: to spend as little money as possible and to protect themselves from the person on their backs. The managers seem to many of the staff to be as frightened as the rest of them.

Chiropody was given as an example of what was happening to some of the local services. This had been a steady, well run service. They had very few 'DNAs' (did not attend) in chiropody. People want to have their feet dealt with. The department ran at 25 minutes for each appointment and that allowed time for them to fit in the emergencies that came up. Then someone higher up decreed that they could do a session in 20 minutes. So they now run on 20 minute appointments, which they find reduces the time they can 'juggle' to accommodate emergencies. Inevitably they expect quality to go down.

What is happening to district nurses worries Margaret and her health visitor colleagues. They see it at least as an indication of what might happen to them next. District nurses feel worried and saddened to see people they know well become so demoralised. The managers have told the health visitors that the district nurses are under the spotlight now because the purchasers have said that, 'On paper, it is a very expensive service.' So they have skill mixes, reorganisations, relocations and they are all having to apply for their own jobs or what is left of their own jobs. Rumours are rife, and not denied. They may be downgraded. Some of them may be paid 25% less. Some are leaving and are not being replaced, 'at least until the whole process of the review has been worked through fully and then no one is disappointed.' Of course their morale has gone right down. Might the health visitors be next? It seemed to Margaret that a number of preliminary shots had already been fired.

A few weeks ago Margaret was called out of a meeting with a GP and a social worker over a child on the at-risk register. It was a meeting that she had taken considerable trouble to set up. Conscientiously or foolishly (she did not know which) Margaret had left the direct line phone number on her diary sheet in the office. The manager was on the phone. An emergency referral had come in and Margaret had to do it. Margaret said that she would not because she could not walk out on the young mother, the GP and the social worker (and the child who was not present but whose needs were being considered). Margaret knew that there were colleagues in her own office, or who would be back there within half an hour. They would be able to handle the new referral and that was the procedure they always followed. Margaret continued in the meeting.

Early the next day Margaret was summoned to the manager's office and told that she should have gone to deal with the referral the day before. She and the manager, a young man, had previously seemed to get on quite well. 'He had his job to do and I had my job to do.' But this time he spoke very officiously to her when he repeated to her that she should have gone. Margaret did not argue, but the manager realised that she knew the case well, knew what her colleagues were doing at that time and knew that the one who did go out had handled the emergency well. Margaret said, 'Well we've got different views.' The manager did not keep her.

A couple of days later, one of Margaret's colleagues told her that she had seen her name on something being typed out in the secretary's office. Of course Margaret went to look herself. Among the piles of papers produced that day in the office was a report of her interview with the manager. He had said nothing to her of such a report being written. Where was the report going to next, or had it already gone? Was this a tactic on behalf of the young and inexperienced manager to cover himself, or was it more sinister in its implications for Margaret? She did not know, but was not going to ask.

By the time I met Margaret, that manager had — as managers do — left a long time ago. Margaret said that she had never found out where that piece of paper had come to rest. She had wondered if it had gone away with him or if it had gone into her 'personal file' and was kept in some management archive. But she did know that this was the day she had felt something die inside her.

From that day on, she got on much better with managers. She says 'fine' to nearly everything she is told.

I pressed Margaret further on that linguistic strategy. She acknowledged that she was not entirely consistent in the words she uses, but insisted that she was consistent in her behaviour. She never expresses her opinion unless it happens to coincide with the management line. She never does anything that by any stretch of imagination could be called arguing. When a manager criticises her for working late one evening and tells her that to work late means that she is being inefficient, she smiles slightly and says 'OK' or 'Fine'. When a manager spoke to them all about filling in their travel claim forms and then added, 'Do please be realistic,' she said, 'Time.' She realises that now she has joined that group of people whom managers talk of as being in favour of the changes.

And when she fills in her diary, forms and computer entries she may wonder if they look busy enough; and then she fills them in more.

Fortunately the clerks (the 'temps') remain very helpful and let them know if they are getting behind with their forms. They then spend an extra half an hour filling them in.

Nowadays they have new diary sheets to complete as well. This new large sheet includes space for the telephone number, address and postcode of the person being visited; and also which district the person is living in, because there may be a charge to be made for some services. There is also a space in which the health visitor is supposed to write an interpretation of needs.

When Paul went for his follow-up appointment all was well with the operation scar, but he wanted the consultant to see a new lesion that had appeared on his skin. It looked exactly like the small cancer six months before the operation. He asked the consultant for her opinion. 'Oh, please will you see your GP about that first?' She must have seen the look of disappointment and worry on Paul's face, because she quickly added, 'Don't worry, you know that we do see new patients quickly.'

It was as Paul was walking out of the hospital, that he realised the significance of her last remark. He was to become a 'new patient' again.

The computer system

I asked about their computer system. For every single clinical contact face to face with a client or on the telephone, the health visitors have to write on a piece of paper the address and postcode, the name of the GP and what the activity is. That is all. It used to be over 20 items. They have managed to have it reduced. They do that every time and it goes into the computer, whether it is an immunisation, developmental check, home contact, some other formal business, or a phone call of enquiry or for support.

There is also the main computer system where information on all the children is kept. This includes addresses, immunisation record, checks and meetings. It is a borough-wide record which means that Margaret can 'pull out' information on areas or patterns if she needs to. But it is two systems. Of course one system should inform the other and in theory that could be made to happen. But it does not. The managers did have a meeting on how to integrate the two systems when the new one was introduced. They said there would be more meetings and then further training, the cost of which, they were assured, would come out of 'central' development money rather than out of their own budget. But all that was over a year ago and nothing happened anyway. The managers seem to have other things on their minds now.

Meanwhile they continue to work the two systems very badly, terrified that they are going to be held to account for the next disaster. With a case load of around 300 for each health visitor, plus all the children they get directly or indirectly involved with, there are seemingly endless possibilities for muddle.

The reason for continuing in this way is the one they are given almost every time the managers have to make them do something without a great deal of logic to it. It is that 'the purchaser wants it'. 'Purchaser' has become such a rare sounding word, because hardly any of the health visitors or their other grass roots colleagues has ever *seen* one. Purchasers themselves keep on moving around between their jobs as they have their own reorganisations and when they do come and any of the health visitors do meet them, they seem to be most interested in the record system. They never seem to want to hear what the health visitors, or for that matter the district nurses or chiropodists, *do* in the time they spend between filling up forms or putting information into the computer. Margaret said it was as though they dare not take the risk of glimpsing pain.

The breadth of work that they in fact do is, of course, not reflected in either of these computer systems. As the purchasers never ask and their own managers do not tell, the health visitors are sure that much of the planning and contracting is done in ignorance of it.

From time to time Margaret and her colleagues feel guilty about this and think of trying to put their concerns more clearly to management. But they always come back to those 'personal' files and their worries for their jobs. They know that they could ask the managers if the rumour of the 'personal' files is true, but the managers keep on changing, seem unsure of their own futures and, anyway, no one seems to know whom to trust.

Most of their discussions on planning even the smallest detail of their work lives finish with someone asking, 'What's the point?'

Amanda's story

Amanda was hesitant to meet me because I had been a psychiatrist. She did not want to be diagnosed or interpreted to or advised, but when I promised to do none of those things, she agreed. I started by asking where health visitors got their support.

'Who compliments us? Who supports us?' she asked. First, the clients, those people who used to be called patients, give the health visitors a great deal of support. And colleagues do it for each other. Managers? Not now.

Clinical interest used to be encouraged a great deal, but it is so no longer. Amanda illustrated her point with a story.

One of her very old friends had a child who had always been a problem but in adolescence became very much more so. He was withdrawing into himself and was hardly looking at his parents, or at Amanda when she called round. He was saying some very strange things. Eventually he was diagnosed as being psychotic, put on medication and helped. Amanda became very interested and collected quite a number of press cuttings as well as information packs on psychosis. Her friend and her friend's son had found that both the information and the way it had been given were very helpful.

Later in an informal meeting at work, a colleague of Amanda's said that the older child of a family that she visited had been behaving very strangely and that the mother was taking her to see a child and adolescent psychiatrist. Amanda showed her the cuttings and the information packs. Her friend found the information helpful when her client brought the subject up again.

Sometime later when the matter came up in conversation with her manager, Amanda mentioned what she had loaned her colleague. She was told in a very firm and reprimanding voice that it had not been a relevant use of her time: handing over information packs on adolescent psychosis was not in her job description.

Muddles

Amanda said she could tell me so many stories of muddles. Vitamin K injections are given to babies after delivery to prevent haemorrhagic disease of the new born. Some have it in one dose and some have it in three doses. That is one of the pieces of information that the health visitors should have. When she was working with a young mother who spoke very little English and who was going into hospital again with her new baby, Amanda was keen that the hospital staff knew that the series of injections had not been finished. After several telephone calls, she got through to the ward, but found no one but 'bank' nurses to speak to. Later, she spoke to one of the locum doctors. Several faxes and telephone calls later, Amanda was fairly confident that the information was in the heads and notes of people who would be able to ensure that the series of injections was completed. But it was only a few days later that Amanda was certain ('Can you really be certain in the NHS?' she wondered) that it had been done.

Between them the locums, bank nurses and the health visitor (the GP was on study leave) got continuity of care ensured. I remembered all those forms that Margaret had described and asked Amanda if she had had to record each of the phone calls. With a smile, she said that there was a spin-off for the health visitors: she had completed an activity entry for every single phone call.

(Amanda was one of several to mention the confusion caused by the 'informality' of first names. Comforted, or confronted, by the charm of the speaker who answered the ward phone with first name or first and second names, it was not easy to ask with what authority he or she was speaking. Lack of differentiation between 'bank' care worker and doctor, or ward manager and student, could lead to information being taken too seriously, or not seriously enough.)

The leaflets

Amanda told me about some leaflets. The first were ones which the staff used to think were distributed to encourage complaints, rather like the advertisements that some solicitors have been known to place in local papers or on posters at airports or even, the rumour had it, in hospitals themselves. But they now realised that this was an unfair judgement. The leaflets were not to encourage complaints, but to encourage clients (note the word) to know how to make complaints if they wanted to. So some places, instead of having a suggestions box, started to have a suggestions box and a complaints box. They were both locked.

I asked how this was affecting a health visitor's working life. I was told that, apart from trying to cover up more than ever before, they now actively encourage people to put in writing anything good they may have said about the service. They have had some very funny looks. For years, health visitors have often had compliments from the mothers of the children they work with. Now, when mothers say they have been pleased with the service and are then asked by the health visitor to write to their manager, they really wonder what is going on.

The second leaflet I was told of was on research into 'client opinions'. Managers said that this was something the purchaser wanted. Purchasers wanted to find out what clients thought of the service and how they would like it to be developed. The health visitors knew that there was no money for developments so they saw this as another paper exercise which would increase the public's expectations and everyone's frustrations. They were given the task of randomly selecting a certain number of clients and, within two weeks, asking them if they would agree to fill out the form if they received it.

The health visitors immediately asked about interpreters and were told that of course the purchasers would make money available for interpreters to help ethnic minorities fill out the forms. That was not what the health visitors were asking. They were asking if there were interpreters to help them discuss filling up the form with the clients and to ask them for their permission. The health visitors did not see how they could get past the first hurdle, namely enabling the clients to become 'informed' enough to give 'informed consent' to receiving the forms to fill up. That the purchasers could be so unaware of the sort of the population they were buying services for was neatly demonstrated by that misunderstanding. The purchasers still think in terms of nearly everybody speaking English.

Forms in the dark

Amanda talked again about the forms. She thinks forms and she sees forms. When she goes home at night and she closes her eyes, one of those forms often flashes up as if it were right on the other side of her eye lids. She cannot get away from them. They are often there when she closes her eyes in bed before going to sleep.

Amanda ended by coming back to my having been a psychiatrist. She was worried that this interview may have sounded very negative or that I might even have thought that she could be depressed. 'I am not depressed,' she concluded, 'I do worthwhile jobs sometimes, but the soul has gone out of my work.'

Chapter 13

The unhappy dentists

Dentists elicit strong feelings and jokes. Some of their waiting rooms have dentist jokes on the wall. Greedy, selfish, disloyal, all accusations that have been levelled at dentists by some both outside and inside their battles with successive governments. The two that I met were well aware of these feelings and were not without self-doubt. Yet they agreed to see me and to share their story.

Part 1: What Anne and Douglas told me

It was in 1988 that Anne and Douglas had set up their practice together. The bank loan for the property and equipment at 7% interest was manageable. When the rates went up to 15% for a short time, they saw their income go down by thousands of pounds a year. To some extent, the high interest rates affected everyone in the country and they knew that we were meeting to discuss dentistry. But, they said, it set the background for their unhappy attempts to run an NHS dental practice.

In their late thirties, they were a very 'dental' couple. They had met in dental school and, of their four parents, three were dentists. They had a child within a couple of years of qualifying, but they had already taken the decision that they were going to do a job-share in running one practice together as soon as they could. They knew what the average dental income was and they set their sights on that. It was an income on which the two of them would live and they have managed to maintain it. They have avoided terrifying financial worries, and they have avoided the rat race of the highest earner category.

They had been dental students or dentists for as long as the present government had been in power. Two of their three dental parents had been in practice when the NHS had started in 1948. Since that time there had been 25 or so major changes in dental charges, eight of them in the seven years since Anne and Douglas had started their joint practice.

Dentists have been isolated as a profession and individual dentists have been isolated in their own practices. Their payment has always been arranged differently from that of others in the NHS, and it has not been the custom for dentists to attend as many postgraduate education events as for non-dental colleagues. Anne and Douglas were therefore unaware of the implication of the planned changes which were first being discussed in the late 1980s.

The government, they say, dreamed up one idea after another for dentistry and ploughed on regardless of what people working the system said. Sometimes Anne and Douglas have thought the same of the dental profession's negotiators. It seemed they did not listen to the rank and file either. A referendum of opinion within the profession as a whole, not the British Dental Association, had given a resounding 'no' to the proposals.

The pay structure

True, the previous pay structure was inequitable. There was no London weighting to compensate for the higher costs of property and rates for premises within the London area. This was so extreme a differential that it meant that dentists working out of London were significantly wealthier. The executive of the dental bodies negotiating team carried a preponderance of northerners.

The total money put into NHS dentistry has remained the same. But dentists must now fit more into it and there are many restrictions, for example on the frequency of certain procedures. Work on children is paid per capita: a capitation fee. Work on adults is paid per item. Both of those decisions are in keeping with the service being managed for cost rather than for quality.

A time restriction means that, for example, the calculation of fees and income are on the assumption of 17–18 minutes per NHS root filling. This is very little time for a well done job, except for very fast practitioners. This means risks are taken.

But the capitation fee had wider implications. Before the reforms, people did not have to register on the list of a dentist to get NHS treatment. Most people were not 'registered' in that way. Now they could do so: 10% of the money allocated by the government for dentists' pay went on the children's lists and 10% on registration fees for adults. Payment for items of service was for work on adults.

Dentists with large lists of children, with little to do on their teeth, did very well and those with children with high treatment needs lost out. Apart from increasing registrations, the way to get more money was to do a large number of items of service on adults. Thus dentists were encouraged to increase their rate of work by reducing the time spent on any item, and this encouraged them to cut corners.

The Patient's Charter and the demands which members of the public are now encouraged to make have also increased paperwork.

Their first reform

'Continuing care responsibility' was introduced with the 1990 contract. Fees paid for items of service given were reduced and 10% of the 'pool' of money paid to dentists went into a capitation fee for those registered. Smaller practices such as that of Anne and Douglas lost out.

To handle the management of registrations and collection of the fees they bought a computer for which no allowance was made. In itself this was not something to complain of, but GP friends were being offered thousands of pounds for technology associated with administration and audit. And similar windfalls of cash seemed to land on the desks of people working in those hospitals which were in the first wave of trusts.

They had to make their first choice. They could continue as an NHS practice which would entail having to explain its limitations and telling patients that some treatments could only be had privately. Or they could themselves go entirely private, but take on a vocational trainee to keep the NHS side of the practice going.

They started to become bogged down in administration and in having to explain to people again and again the complications and intricacies of the payment system. (They had to explain it to me again as our meeting went on.)

The government had a fixed 'pool' of money for treatment items and for these there were set fees. When the profession as a whole did more than the expected total number of items then the government called a stop. (Some called this crying 'Halt!' and others called it crying 'Foul!') There had been a miscalculation: the target for treatments done, and therefore the total sum going on dentist income, was exceeded. The government responded by cutting the fees by 7%. Anne and Douglas experienced this as a massive 'demotivator'. They felt they had been told to run a dental practice as a business in a commercial world, the rules of which the government kept on changing.

They already found the registration fee of 40p per patient per month to be disincentive enough. They knew of colleagues with 6,000 registered patients getting 6,000 times 40p (total £2,400) each month, for registration fees. Anne and Douglas' list was 1,500.

Six months into the new contract, in February 1992, the government said they had overpaid dentists and they must pay back £15,000 each. This meant for many of them a 30% reduction in profit. In the summer of 1992, more exits started from the NHS, some precipitated by bank managers' threats of fore-closure on overdrafts. (Dental business is one which carries a high overdraft.) Their closest friends left the NHS, but Anne and Douglas stayed on. They thought they could make it work.

At the very end of 1992 the Bloomfield Report was published. The House of Commons Select Committee took four months examining the proposals in this report and many a concern was registered over quality of service with no emphasis on prevention or health promotion. Anne and Douglas told me that the government clearly did not believe this Select Committee's report and went ahead with their own thing, *Improving NHS Dentistry*, in July 1994. There was an extensive consultation period, with much discussion. There was still the outstanding issue of every dentist owing them the princely £15,000. And a general assumption that something had to be done to reform the system for paying NHS dentists: no change at all was not an option. There was consid-eration of sessional payments for dentists or a purchaser-provider split as in the rest of the NHS. In early 1995, a decision was made that payment would continue largely by items of service but with the purchaser/provider model still on the cards.

Bureaucracy

The Dental Practice Board handles the money for dentists on behalf of the Department of Health. Its monitoring sub-section checks on dental practice. On its computer is recorded each item of dentistry done by NHS dentists, each of whom is given an annual profile. If the frequency of a particular procedure is greater than the local average, then the board may require that dentist to obtain prior approval before doing more of those procedures. The practice board can give a reprimand and require prior approval for a wider range of items.

Which procedures? The vary from conservative scaling and filling, to crowning and root canal work. Extractions are excluded because they are not a financial liability. An extracted tooth can cost no more to the exchequer while a filled tooth may require more treatment throughout that patient's life. Tooth pulling is NHS cost effectiveness par excellence.

The cost limit for items requiring prior approval by the board had been going down, from £500 in 1990 to £200 in 1992.

Anne and Douglas heard of all sorts of strategies to manage this increasing bureaucracy:

- doing more work on those people exempt from fees;
- doing that and treating privately all the 'payers', those who would have to pay a substantial amount anyway for NHS treatment;
- dragging out the completion of the work so that one half of it was done in one six-month period and the other half of it in another, allowing a total bill of more than £500;
- putting a bill for £1,000 worth of treatment in two lots.

Under the new system, a claim was put in individually for each item of service done and it was then paid in arrears.

But to complicate things further, each item of service had what was known as a 'fee narrative'. For example, treatment of gum disease was four visits to the dentist over three months, plus a follow up session three months later. There would be no payment for this treatment until it had all been done, so no payment for six months from the start. Nor was there any payment for minor parts of the treatment.

The market force pressure, and therefore the temptation, was to do a 'scale and polish' on everyone's teeth, if only because the dentist would be paid sooner. But then there was another trap, to catch the unscrupulous. There was a time bar of one year before certain forms of treatment could be repeated. And there was no mechanism of approval for exemptions. But more on gum treatment below.

Friends' tales of the simplicity of private practice accounting made them envious and furious. The NHS with its complicated methods of payment required more complicated bureaucracy and electronic links. Anne and Douglas did get a £900 grant to set up a new computer system with an electronic data link — but that was it. They referred again to friends in the NHS management whose computers are ordered with such nonchalance. One, an executive director of an acute hospital trust, was shocked to hear of their computer problems: she had received a new model every year for four years and when all the computers in the trust offices had been stolen, they did little more than shrug their shoulders.

Anne and Douglas and some of their contemporaries concluded that there were two possible outcomes. Those practices which invested least in equipment and least in cross-infection control (for example, equipment or procedures for sterilisation of instruments) would have their profits soar. Those practices which invested most in new equipment and premises and took concrete steps to meet the protocols for cross-infection control would have higher material costs. Their profits would go down.

The decisions were becoming ethical.

Number of patients seen and upper limits of cost

More was being said, among dentists themselves and in some of the documents from the General Dental Council, about standards. There was concern about over-prescribing, sub-standard work and the high numbers of patients being seen. Anne and Douglas had already worked out that in order to maintain their 'average' income they had to be seeing between 30 and 40 patients every day between them.

I had seen several newspaper reports on dentists' pace of work, from which it did seem that 35 or 40 patient visits a day was common.

They said they knew that their rate was common and but that for some it was nearer 60. They had heard of one dentist seeing 70 patients a day.

I worked some of that out in minutes per patient.

70 patients a day: 7 minutes each for an 8 hour day and 8 $1/2$ minutes each for a 10 hour day.

60 patients a day: 8 minutes each for an 8 hour day and 10 minutes each for a 10 hour day.

40 patients a day: 12 minutes each for an 8 hour day and 15 minutes each for a 10 hour day.

In all those calculations I assumed no breaks and no time spent on any other work, such as speaking on the telephone, meeting colleagues, reading or writing letters, dealing with suppliers, or studying professional journals. Anne and Douglas wanted me to put in such details to demonstrate the sort of calculations in their minds. I thought there might be something attractive in short visits to the dentist. Could that be good marketing and bad practice?

Anne and Douglas knew that they could press on doing what they thought was best for their patients and take whatever income they got from it. In their more idealistic discussions, that is what they thought. One of the troubles was that they were being very actively encouraged *not* to be idealistic, but to be realistic business people. And they were all too well aware that some of their colleagues were both realistic and successful business people. In a way, that was exactly what had gone wrong with the first reform, when total performance by the profession so exceeded expectation and the government ended up saying that each dentist owed them £15,000.

Gum treatment

Since I knew gum treatment to be so important and Anne and Douglas had said that it was hard to offer effective treatment on the NHS, I asked them to explain further.

Two visits are offered. This short term treatment is often not enough for dealing with any level of pronounced disease. What more can be provided under the NHS? A one visit 'scale and polish', for which the dentist is paid £7.40. The alternative is to say to the patient that he or she really needs an appointment with the hygienist; and that will cost them money.

They saw that I was bewildered but said that the public were even more bewildered. Anne and Douglas felt that having been determined to stick to the NHS, no matter what it was like, may even have been unhelpful for their cause. Or at least for the cause of their patients. It had become too complicated and then very hard to offer really good dentistry on the NHS. They had known many people try hard to find an NHS-only practice and, as dentists, to run one. They had failed; or had they been seduced?

Were they being greedy? This was where Anne and Douglas spoke most of their self-doubt. They wondered if I had written about the consultants who got others to lobby for them in the distinction awards committees, or published papers or sat on committees in order to be noticed by those who influenced decisions on the secret allocation of such money: were *they* being greedy?

They tried to put it another way. Some dentists had gone the whole hog and were rolling in the proceeds; some resolutely stuck with their beloved NHS and did not get rich. Anne and Douglas were in between (subject to market forces?) and tried to be ... well, 'reasonable'. That was when the forms and paperwork of the reforms got too much for them. They were relieved when I recalled all those forms I had filled in as an NHS patient, though I did them blindly and trusted the practice staff to complete them. But we agreed that this book was not on how the different professional groups have looked after themselves through the history of the NHS, although that has been influenced by the reforms. (I told them that I had mentioned extra pay for extra work by surgeons under the waiting list initiative and for the extra responsibilities of some clinical directors; and the grouse that everyone was working harder, but only some were getting more money.) One of the main differences with the dentists' story is that the reforms have been experienced as confronting them with more moral questions; and they have felt uncomfortable about it.

What about the figures that show more people using the NHS dental services? This is because the regulations allow an NHS register to be kept while much of the work is done privately. They also allow children to be kept on an NHS register while their families are treated privately. Thus more people 'use' the NHS (and inaccuracies in the collection of the figures gave over 100% of one county's children to be registered). Put another way, it is by virtue of being on the register that more people are said to use the NHS while more use private services by virtue of paying for them.

The private insurance systems? Close to 3 million people are now registered with them but over half are treated within the NHS as well.

Some of Anne and Douglas's patients tell them of friends who go to NHS dentists. Why can't they? Anne and Douglas must be wanting more money. They feel inhibited from putting forward the case that what they offer may be a better quality of service than it is now possible to provide under the NHS. It is often impossible to put over the argument. They have to explain that the paperwork for getting themselves paid got lost, and so on. They do not want to appear to run down the other dentists, or to be greedy. Put simply, what they offer is something which they found impossible to provide under the NHS. That is their belief.

Nonetheless their rivals appear to be more ethical, because they appear to be doing it all 'on the NHS'. So how can they do it? Anne and Douglas thought there were four ways. The first was to over prescribing (it does not take long to write a prescription). Second was to cut corners (take risks). Third was not to spend much on maintenance, servicing and replacement of equipment (take risks). Fourth was to be prepared not to make nearly as much money. Difficult to explain most of that to patients who desperately want treatment on the NHS, except perhaps the fourth point.

But had they got it across? Do they convince their enquiring patients? Do they convince me? Would I get it across to the people who read this book?

That was when they said that they could tell by the look on my face that I was unconvinced. They thought I might still be seeing dentists as no more than a money grabbing lot, having a whinge. They had acknowledged that the unscrupulous existed. What more did I want? They were not trying to put all the blame on the present government. Governments and the profession had, over the years, come up with a system which was grinding dentists out of the NHS. For Anne and Douglas, it had become intolerable. With a glance between them, Anne got up to present me with the last folder of papers which they had received from the Department of Health, the Dental Practice Board and the British Dental Association, before they finally left the NHS.

Part 2: How I became convinced

I had thought I was pretty hardened to bureaucracy and government papers, but I was surprised.

The Bloomfield Report (75 pages in a glossy green cover) reiterated the dangers of the 'treadmill effect', first eloquently defined in the Tattersall Report 30 years before. Given a limited sum to be divided among all the dentists according to fee for items of service, the argument goes something like this:

One dentist cannot be sure how fast everyone else is working. Alone, one dentist cannot, by going faster or slower, significantly influence the average rate. But if one dentist does fewer items of work his or her income will go down. Therefore each is likely to try to do more. More total items get done. There is a limited sum to be divided among them all, so the fee is reduced. Then... well, no one dentist can be sure how fast everyone else is working. Alone, one dentist... and so on.

Maybe that is how all those dentists came to be owing the government £15,000. Anyway, everyone wanted out of such a system.

The Bloomfield Report said the existing system was so complex that even those most affected often did not understand it. It was inequitable and could depress standards of care. The report called for views. Sir Kenneth Bloomfield had done as asked by the Minister of Health, Dr Brian Mawhinney, 'namely to identify a number of options for change, rather than a single recommendation...'

(It did end in a non-committal way, and the report itself started in a way which drew my attention. The first page was, as usual in these things, a letter from Sir Kenneth to Dr Mawhinney. It finished with: 'Dictated by Sir Kenneth but signed by his secretary in his absence.')

Next I looked at some responses in *Dental Practice*, the fortnightly news and views of the profession. Kevin Lewis has a regular column and I started by reading some of his usual pieces. A racy style, concise. Usually half a page, enough to fill one A4 sheet of paper. On the Bloomfield Report together with some general reports of meetings, he used up 16 pages (A3 size) over four issues.

What came out of it all? Next, I looked at *Improving NHS Dentistry*, published by HMSO in July 1994 for £7.10. It ran to 40 pages in a yellow buff cover and was called a 'Green Paper'. A clear historical summary and clear proposals for reform, consistent with the government's thinking on the NHS.

No change is not on. That is for certain. And forget pleasing everyone. There are so many different opinions that there will never be a system to satisfy everyone.

Because no one system could possibly fit every type of practice everywhere in the country, the working out of the details of the system should be pushed downwards to enable more sensitivity to local circumstances. So long as children have priority, the treadmill is removed and quality is supported. Dentists' incomes should then become more stable.

The Green Paper gave the government's intention for the introduction of purchaser and provider roles in general dental services and called for health authorities to volunteer to consult with their local dental professional groups with the aim of introducing pilot schemes

Then came the British Dental Association's 40-page response in October 1994. Lots of sub-organisations consulted, and motions from branches, but somewhere there is a plea (para 29) that if the Minister does decide to go ahead with purchaser/provider, please, please do a careful, evaluated pilot first.

In April 1995 there was a 'Dear Dentist' letter from Mr Gerald Malone, the Minister of Health. At least I was assured that it was from such a date, but the copy I was shown had '3/4' handwritten on the top and the year was missing It was a refreshingly unglossy letter, with even one misprint or typing error, and a definitely more conciliatory tone. The Minister is determined to move to having the local health authorities purchasing dental services for their own area, but over the vexed matter of that debt of £15,000, this is now labelled as an 'over payment' and the news is given that the government will not rule out waivers, on condition that progress in the fundamental review is made satisfactorily.

Next, the April 1996 *Statement of Dental Remuneration*. 89 pages. Even the Green Paper had warned me of its complexity, but clichés overpower me if I try to describe what I found among the 472 items which I counted. Here is an example:

SECTION IV — PERIODONTAL TREATMENT
NON-SURGICAL TREATMENT
Item 10:
Scaling, polishing and simple periodontal treatment, including oral hygiene instruction, normally only payable where at least 2 complete calendar months have elapsed since the last such treatment

	Dentist's fee	Patient's Charge
per course of treatment	£8.30	(£6.64)

[etc. etc.]
PROVISOS TO ITEM 10:
1. only 1 fee under any 1 of items 10(a), 10(b) or 10(c) shall be payable during the same course of treatment;
2. a fee under items 10(a) or 10(b) shall only be payable either in connec- tion with treatment under items 1(a), 1(b) or 1(c) (examination) or where a fee under items 1(a), 1(b) or 1(c) is payable or has been paid to the same dentist during the previous 11 complete calendar months;
3. no fee under items 10(b) or 10(c) shall be payable if a fee has been paid, or is payable, to the same dentist for treatment provided under items 10(b) or 10(c) during the previous 9 complete calendar months;
4. a fee under item 10(c) shall only be payable where the same dentist

has been paid, or is entitled to be paid, a fee for treatment provided
under item 1(c) (full case assessment) for that patient in the previous 23
complete calendar months;
5. a fee under item 10(c) shall only be payable where appropriate radi-
ographs are available.

When I put that down, I thought I understood why Anne and Douglas
used to be unhappy dentists.

Postscript

In June 1996 Mr Malone made another statement to Parliament. He
referred to the negotiations with the British Dental Association and he appreciated their co-operation. He was pushing forward with the purchaser/
provider split but gave a very firm government commitment to pilot and eval-
uate the system in several areas.

That £15,000 or more, once called a debt, was now very firmly called an
'over-payment' of which Mr Malone announced a total waiver (and said he
expected the calling off of the formal dispute started by the General Dental
Services Committee in 1992).

He did throw in (paragraph 8) proposals to set up new dental auxiliaries
and expand the range of work they can do, as if this had also been negotiated
and agreed with the dentists. In fact, it had not and the BDA put energy into
trying to have this pointed out as prominently as the government's statement.

I met Anne and Douglas once more. They acknowledged that there had
been a very significant switch. They had heard of the remark attributed to
Kenneth Clarke, when he had been asked why he had not authorised a pilot
study of the reforms ('The doctors would bugger it up') and I had heard it too.

'Yes, it does look as if the government may have learned something and
have become less confrontational, but unfortunately it is too late for us.'

Anne and Douglas thought the government and the British Dental
Association had been getting on better in serious negotiations. Could they
really manage to cut down on the complexity of it all? If the market forces and
the purchaser/provider split could release good, devolved local management,
why bother with trying to push through the proposals on dental auxiliaries at
a national level? Unless, of course, Douglas wondered, it was a strategic 'stick'
to get the pilot purchasing authorities to be strong and 'get on with it'.

Chapter 14

Mental health: hospital and community

To write on psychiatry has been the most difficult. The trouble was that I had been so immersed in it for years. I was a psychiatrist, albeit a sub-specialist in child and adolescent psychiatry. But I often mixed with general psychiatrists, both professionally and socially. It was important for me not to rewrite a story I already knew. I sought out other people, with whom I had not worked, in order to get their story. In all, I spoke to or met 15 people in eight places and I am convinced that the stories which follow are typical of much in the mental health field.

The consultant who got out: James' story

I started with a young and relatively recently appointed consultant psychiatrist. I expected to find somebody as energetic and enthusiastic as I had been 25 years ago, when I had my first consultant battles to fight.

James had been a consultant psychiatrist for four years. He thought he had received a good general psychiatric training. He had learned an approach which was called eclectic: it included giving medication, listening, talking, meeting relatives, working with a multidisciplinary team to bring in many skills and to help troubled people reconstitute their lives without dependency. In his last years as a senior registrar, 'care plans' had been introduced by the team within which he worked. He found them a sophisticated multidisciplinary way of bringing together the 'story so far' and treatment plans.

In the first two days of admission, people had to be met, investigations were to be done, programmes needed to be initiated and areas to be covered were written up, together with an outline timetable for the next three weeks which would probably include discharge.

What James had not been prepared for in his senior registrar training was the impact of the work load of some inner-city patches and the demands of the NHS reforms.

The community team which was 'his' had to take on something like 300 new patients per year, or up to 10 a week. It had been fairly newly set up: a social worker, two community psychiatric nurses, an occupational therapist, and part time, the most junior of doctors in psychiatry, a senior house officer (SHO). James himself was also part time. They seemed to have every potential for working well together, but because of management demands and everything in management never quite working out as it was supposed to, each team member felt that he or she was never quite up to date with anything. They always had that extra pressure of 'being behind'.

To make matters worse, they knew that their managers' main worry was not the patients, the relatives or the services provided, but money.

James had no objection to monetary restraint and had even done a small audit as a senior registrar, on cost accounting. He had no objection to being asked how much things would cost, nor how they were to be paid for. However, he very soon got the impression that something to do with money was in the first sentence of everything that came from management. It was so persistent that it stopped creative therapeutic thinking.

James' immediate medical colleague, the SHO, was on rotation from the local hospital. SHOs suffered terribly from the double pressure of the volume of work and the distress of patients and relatives. Half of the six SHOs who had worked with James since he had taken up his post seemed to be worn down and several of them complained of feeling severely depressed. Two had sought professional help. James felt powerless to help them to feel more optimistic, let alone to function as satisfactorily practising SHOs or be inspired towards psychiatry.

Directives without direction

In the last five years, James had been on courses, seminars and training days, all approved and paid for by management, on matters including:

Resource management
Clinical directorships
Business plans
Business cases
Audit
Indicator-based audit
Prioritising of objectives

James thought I might have seen him as brimming with management ideas and expertise. He said that the sheer number of new ideas on management, or the delivery of services, or the costing of services, which he had been obliged to study and try to understand, and the number of requirements which he was obliged to meet, had left him feeling. Management directives came with much frequency (and had been doing so for two years before James arrived) and with so many differences that the staff were experiencing directives without direction. He suspected that managers were on the receiving end of very similar things from the trust board or from the NHS management executive.

The first example he gave was a familiar one. Colleagues had been told that part of the service had to close. They resisted it, but were informed that it was the purchaser's directive and it had to be obeyed. It happened. Months later, after leaving a meeting on health authority premises, the consultant concerned bumped into one of the purchasers and they walked down the corridor together. The purchaser said very clearly that what had happened had *not* been at their insistence or suggestion.

Whenever staff collectively were having a problem and the manager tried to be supportive, all he could do was suggest they work a new direction. Never did he tell the staff to pause for a while, or to help them organise themselves into a time for reflection. It reminded James of an old record he had found among his parents' collection. In a satirical lullaby, there was a line encouraging the infant to be quiet because 'Daddy is reading another book'.

The 'lion's den' directive

James explained that there was nothing very surprising in a chronically psychotic person not keeping up maintenance medication and walking into a lion's den one winter's day in London Zoo. Equivalent behaviours had been happening for years in all the long term psychiatric institutions, but because of good staffing and supervision they had not had such dangerous, dramatic or public consequences. James saw the 'lion's den' directive — to create a list of people at risk — as little more than a cynical management manoeuvre to show that something had been done; and to create a queue of ready scapegoats.

In their district, the directive had led to a new policy. They had a list. The people on it frequently stopped taking their medication or having their injections and started comforting themselves with alcohol or illegal drugs; or the other way round. Any of these affected their perception and judgement. They wandered, so that they did not keep their appointments or attend the various support services which were set up for them.

And the response of professional carers in the community? Always the same thing. They called a meeting. Nothing was thought through, no arguments were put which were relevant to the immediate problems. But they kept minutes. 'Something' had been done.

The staff lived with the anxiety over what would happen if they appeared not to get it right. It was impossible for them to do all that was expected by the managers, referrers, relatives and patients, whose expectations had been so raised by government propaganda.

Within a few weeks of starting his job, James realised that he had a choice. One option was to practise mindless psychiatry in which care plans would become sophisticated drug prescription sheets. The other possibility was to have a breakdown.

He felt acutely de-skilled. All his knowledge of psychopathology, group or institutional dynamics, and leadership, was useless. He had to follow the rules.

James told me that everyone on the community team, including himself, was at times sobbing.

The ward and inpatients

Another duty James had was as consultant for a ward for those caught by the net outside, but not helped or supported enough to stay in the community.

Skill mix wisdom dictates that you do not need an RMN qualified nurse to sit with patients, observe or listen to them: unqualified people can practise those skills. The qualified nurse (there's always one on duty) receives reports from them, supervises and trains them, and is responsible for all the paperwork.

James' own clinical contact with the patients was channelled into tiny moments of the day. His inpatients were lucky to see anything of him outside formal 'ward rounds' which occupied half a day a week. In the ward round James saw each of the patients who were there that day and felt that all he did was to give some sort of a 'cursory blessing' to what other people were struggling to provide; and to give his name to the care plan which was often not even a clear summary of medication. In James' domain there were 14 beds. There were usually between 14 and 20 inpatients a week. James described the juggling with bed vacancies as a chronic nightmare.

There was a pre-discharge meeting at which relatives, carers, or workers in the community might be present, and at which the consultant should be in attendance. James rarely was.

On-call cover for the local district general hospital was provided by James for emergencies.

For half a day a week he worked at the day hospital with the community team itself, and they managed to spend some of the time in a meeting which was always too short.

He did domiciliary visits. Mostly he saw these as part of the job and did not bother to fill in the form which could have brought him in thousands of pounds extra per year. If the visits were before 8.30 in the morning or after 6.30 in the evening, he did fill up the form, a charge was made and he got extra payment for what he saw as unofficial overtime.

As part of his contribution to care in the community James went to the police station, where he would see floridly psychotic people who had been arrested. His main worry with these cases was always exactly the same: how could he avoid admitting this person, who had been wandering the streets, out of his or her mind and outside the law? Why was it so important to avoid admitting? Because they had no beds.

James gave outpatients very little time, with usually no more than ten minutes for a follow-up appointment. The patients seemed quite used to it and to expect it. Other staff got on with it and after a time in the job, James did too.

He would usually manage half an hour for lunch with sandwiches which he brought himself.

There was no space for 'let us all get off this roundabout for even a moment and look at what is going on'. They all stayed on and James stayed on too.

Audit

Did audit help? I had experienced such meetings as a time to get off the roundabout and look at what was happening.

The consultants had a monthly audit meeting and they kept minutes for the express purpose of being able to produce them if asked by the managers or the purchasers. Each month one of them raised something and they talked about it.

Audit, in the sense of examining how they were using their time or whether they were working within the criteria of good practice, did not happen.

So James had become a controller: of symptoms and of people. He was using more drugs and more ECT (electro-convulsive therapy) than he had ever done as a senior registrar or had ever seen other consultants use. He had stopped thinking about what he should do next by automatically doing something. He was fully aware that he did not do all that he should, in meeting relatives, friends and referrers, going into family backgrounds or personal histories. He said he was constantly aware that if he was caught out there would be hell to pay and that his position was indefensible.

He often felt that he should be trying harder and that he should have handled whatever it was better. In the evenings he usually got home late and miserable.

The managers

James had had a good experience of managers. There had been a complaint. The manager supported James and the other colleagues through the investigation and said that as far as they could see what had happened was not their fault. 'These things happen,' the manager often said, 'and we will see what we can learn from it.' But that was as far as it went. The managers did not help the clinical staff through any of the emotional debriefing which was a crucial part of getting out of the 'post-traumatic' stress which they were experiencing, and which they needed to get through in order to be able to think differently. James supposed that the cost effectiveness of emotional debriefing for staff had not been evaluated, and apologised to me for sounding so cynical.

James' general experience of managers was that they were a confused and frightened group of people. When they had ideas of their own they were countermanded by the people at the top. So much so that they rarely put any of their own ideas forward. When they were doing as they were told — acting as messengers — they were unconvincing, except as pointers to where the big stick was coming from.

They were patently instructed to recruit the user group, that is the patients and the carers and the relatives, as allies in the battle. I pressed James harder. He described how on 'stakeholders' days', when vociferous patients or relatives complained about psychiatric services, or said that they wanted many more small units, the managers nodded strongly in agreement and later quoted them. On the other hand, when long term patients or the elderly, or their carers, said they did not want to be moved, their statements were dismissed as evidence of neglect or indoctrination by old fashioned carers, and of bad treatment by psychiatrists in the past.

(There is more on stakeholders' days later in this chapter.)

If you can't stand the heat, get out

James had already resigned when I met him. He had resigned not in panic, nor in anger. He was going to work with an old friend in another part of the country where staff and managers seemed to be getting on together, people were not getting worn out and, perhaps most surprising of all, they appeared to have money.

So was it because he could not stand the heat? James said that it was, but went on to point out that very few people seemed to be able to stand it themselves.

One of the first things he realised on joining the ranks of consultants at the start of the reforms was the turnover of managers. There was internal turnover in which they went from one job to another as projects were initiated, developed and ended. There was promotion turnover, as they went on to higher things. There was private sector turnover, as managers went off to provide services in another sort of contribution to the nation's health. Finally, there was the chop. 'So-and-so does not work here any more.' One day's or one hour's notice. One manager 'took' voluntary redundancy two days after starting in their team.

What James could really not understand was how some of the staff survived in the other branches of the psychiatric services in the neighbourhood. (He faltered on the word 'neighbourhood' because geographical terms have become management terms, and he did not want to confuse me with the words 'district' or 'area'.) They seemed to have even worse things happening to them in their work, and yet they were putting up with it. Perhaps there was something connected to his age (James was 30) which had made him feel that he could still get out, whereas the others were awaiting retirement.

What were the other things that had happened? James told me two stories.

One consultant came back from two weeks' holiday to find that his office had been moved to a room with no curtains on its windows, paint on the carpet and on the telephone, and large prominent marks on the wall and on the filing cabinets where notices had been.

In another small trust unit, the clinical staff were told, 'You will now be working with a maximum of eight beds. That is a trust decision.'

Much protest was met with the line being repeated: 'You will now be working with a maximum of eight beds to be used. That is a trust decision.'

More protests were said to have reached the ears of the medical director.

Five days later: 'I think you misheard me. I said that we should try with eight beds to see how it went, and that was not a trust decision.'

James told me that the phrase 'I think you misheard me' was well known and carried much meaning.

The management team and deficit of care

'Young in years and young in experience' was how the ward staff spoke of the management team. They had been brought in by the new specialist services manager and senior management team. As individuals, they were given almost no autonomy, and had to take very nearly everything back to senior management and the specialist services manager for approval. This meant that they panicked at trivia.

A long term mental illness sufferer who had several prolonged admissions over a period of some 15 years was readmitted following a request by herself, a general practitioner and her carer. She was admitted in the evening and had her medical examination, which showed nothing untoward. She said that she had not been sleeping for many nights and had all the appearance of being tired but still very restless. She said she would stay up all night and the ward staff, in consultation with the night manager and the duty doctor, decided to respect this wish. They all remembered having been lectured by the senior managers on respecting the wishes of the users. 'Why should you not put up with somebody staying awake all night? That's what you are paid for,' they had been told. In the early hours of the morning the new patient said that she was feeling a bit sleepy and would sit in an easy chair. She still refused to go to bed, but sat quietly, was checked regularly and by 5.30 am appeared to be in a light sleep.

She appeared to be sleeping more soundly when the day staff came on at 7.00 am. When the ward manager came on duty at 9.00 am, heard the story and saw that the patient was still asleep in her chair, it was decided to move her to her bedroom. The staff could not rouse her. The duty doctor was called and saw her within a few minutes. She was transferred to the acute hospital where she died early the following day.

She died of natural causes. A cerebral thrombosis was found at post mortem examination, although no signs of this were obvious at the first medical examination, nor specific signs at the one in the acute hospital. The relatives expressed no concern over how she had been treated.

Some time later an inquiry was instituted into the level of care received by this patient in her fifteen hours in the hospital. Six months after the incident the nurse in charge of the ward that night, the night manager and the morning charge nurse and staff nurse were suspended.

The inquiry interviewed the staff suspended and they had to account for their actions and whereabouts, minute by minute, for the two hours preceding the transfer of the patient to the acute hospital on that morning six months before. They were criticised for not putting the patient to bed and for not changing the care plan overnight.

The inquiry team heard that the ward staff had been under strain, dealing with a racially abusive patient. They had to move black nurses off the shift and got white nurses in from other wards. (This was a common practice in the hospital and in several other places where I have enquired.) They heard that one of the ward staff had telephoned in to say that she was sick and the staff nurse had rung round other wards to get help.

The inquiry found that, while there had been a deficit of care, this made no difference to the outcome. The Inquiry further decided that the staff nurse in charge of the ward that night had shown a shortage of management skills, particularly for failing to telephone the 'bleep holder' to announce that one of the nurses was off sick. (It was acknowledged that he may not have telephoned the bleep holder because he may have been the bleep holder himself: no record was kept of this by the management.)

The staff nurse was given a final warning and was not to be allowed to manage staff or patients again. Downgraded with a loss of over £2,000, he was given learning objectives to be fulfilled within the next six months before review.

For the senior nurse who had been doubling up as night manager there was found no case to answer. Nor for the charge nurse and staff nurse suspended. They were reinstated.

As the new service developed and appointments were made, the senior nurse who had been the night manager did not get a job and later took early retirement. But meanwhile, because the management of the new programme was 12 months behind schedule, the staff were kept on, doing the same job in the same ward but for less money.

The specialist services manager was surprised to hear staff say that what had happened had a bad effect on them and that they were applying for other jobs. The manager reminded them that the senior management team had acted in 'the needs of the service'.

I came across five other suspensions in that place and all had ended in reinstatement.

The community care team: Bridget's story

Bridget had been manager of a community care unit supporting psychiatric patients living in a house in a residential street. The staff had been hand-picked for starting this project some years before and had been sent individually on courses in community work.

New management came in with new ideas and produced a strategy after a series of carefully managed stakeholders' days. James had already mentioned these events and I had a very slight experience of them myself, so I was glad when Bridget offered to expand.

Stakeholders' days: a definition

The organisers invited people deemed to have a 'stake' in the future service: nurses, psychiatrists, social workers, occupational therapists, GPs, probation officers, the community health council, users (who used to be called patients), carers, friends and relatives. A group of 50 or so gathered for a day in a building with large and smaller rooms. Presentations, small group discussions, plenaries and a 'Where do we go next?' final session.

'Everyone who has a stake in the services is represented here,' said the chairman in his opening address. Bridget said that nobody asked the silent or passive people who felt pushed aside by the change they did not want.

But Bridget's team was not worried. It had been in the forefront of development in mental health services in the district. Applauded by the Health Advisory Service on its last visit, it was one of the few teams which came in for positive acknowledgement or even praise from the new managers in their period of getting to know the staff and existing services. One of the psychiatrists was asked by the new senior manager, 'How can we get the rest of the staff to work like this?'

Nonetheless, the staff did consult their union on how to respond should management want changes in the service or in their contracts. Someone else advised them that if they approached the union they should also tell the personnel department, who raised no objection but added that they hoped they remembered that their department also offered staff support.

Three days later the new senior manager rang the unit directly. His very polite manner was reassuring at first. He said, 'I have to inform you…' and 'I have to pass this on to you…' The message was that they were not allowed by the trust, in work time, to see any union representative except the one acknowledged by the trust. The message was given in a clear, straightforward way, in a firm, quiet voice with an inflection on the concluding 'All right?' That 'All right?' was repeated twice.

Bridget's colleague who took the message was able to say, 'That is quite clear. Thank you for letting us know.'

Bridget and her colleagues had discovered a new role for the personnel department, namely to inform the managers.

The management decided that the unit's work was important and should eventually be incorporated as part of the trust's total mental health strategy. Meanwhile, until the total strategy for mental health services was worked out, this team's work should not come into it. That should wait until a new team had been instituted, as was happening elsewhere in the service. Therefore, the management said, referrals should stop. The staff who talked to me were not at all clear as to the reasoning put forward by the management, but were clear about the result.

Nonetheless their own immediate manager was extremely reassuring.

'You have nothing to worry about.' 'You've no need to worry over jobs.'

'People in your position will be wanted.' 'There will be new jobs in the community and people with your sort of training will be jumped upon.'

They missed the ambiguity of the last remark.

As the staff got really worried, they spoke more often to the manager and to the personnel department. After a time the latter said that as their own work was being amalgamated into a larger department of human resources, it was not really their business any more. Staff had better go to the managers.

Their manager continued to say that he really was trying to reassure them.

'We understand your anxiety.' 'We will keep you informed.' 'I will come to your business meeting every month.'

But he did not come.

The end and debriefing

When Bridget returned from her leave she found that of her team of seven, four had been encouraged to apply for other jobs or had been redeployed.

Of the three remaining, one was invited to work alongside the recreational activity officer with the elderly. There was no job description for this new post which carried a short term contract. What swayed her to take it on was not that she was told that it required someone with enterprise, or that the work had increased with the ward staff more busy with 'future planning' and skill mix assessment, but that she had the distinct impression that the alternative was redundancy.

Bridget herself was invited by her manager to a 'chat' about her future. She readily accepted but said that she did wish to be represented by a union official and the meeting was fixed for ten days' time.

Five days later she received a letter 'This is instructing you to attend a meeting tomorrow…'

Rapid consultations, and she decided to accept the instruction. She went to the meeting on the following day.

The manager confirmed that the team was ending. 'We are not downgrading you or regrading you, we are putting you in a job at a lower grade on protected pay and you will have a chance to apply for other jobs.'

Now the remaining staff had to apply for jobs. By this time vacancies in the units to be run on the lines they had been working on had already gone. They were advised to apply for work with long term support or on the still functioning acute admission wards. Some of Bridget's colleagues got jobs. Where they did not, the jobs were given to applicants without the community experience which their manager had said was their special feature.

Bridget and two of her colleagues went to lower grade jobs on protected salary. While it was not easy for them it was also not easy for their new colleagues to be in charge of people with greater experience.

Management arranged a 'debriefing experience', which turned out to be little more than a confirmation of the downgrading with protected salary. Some of the debriefing interviews had a member of the department of human resources present and some did not. They preferred it without them.

The last person on the team to be redeployed went into ward and outreach work.

The nurse who had been taken off the team to work with the recreational activity officer worked occasional 'banks' in the wards. While she was there two of the patients started to fight and one got a broken nose. The managers decided that although no blame was attributable to the nurse, she should be taken off the work with the recreational therapist, downgraded and placed in a long stay ward in which 'bank' sessions, if any, would also be done.

On arrival at her new acute ward Bridget found that there was a further unfilled vacancy for the same grade as one of her old colleagues, but she could get no explanation as to why she was the only one transferred there. That is, no explanation beyond the one in her own mind: that there was an intention that the old team be split up.

Bridget took out a grievance procedure. The letter ('You are instructed...') was attributed to a secretarial muddle (I noticed how secretaries remained the useful scapegoat for all) and it was acknowledged that what had happened was not fair. There should have been an offer of a higher grade post. It was not acknowledged that it could have been wasteful that she had been sent on a course for community psychiatry which had cost the trust £4,000, had been running a community psychiatry team — and had then been taken off it, downgraded and put into hospital ward work. The response was, 'Well you have still had valuable training. We don't know why you are complaining.' Worn out, she withdrew her grievance.

A reunion drink

Six months later, Bridget met a couple of the old team and they arranged to meet one evening. They had been told nothing of the plans the management might have for using their skills.

On the way to the small reunion (two or three others were to join them) Bridget remembered that when they had first started the community care team they had a wall poster of the 'charity' collect:

O Lord, who has taught us that all our doings without charity are nothing worth; send Thy Holy Ghost, and pour into our hearts that most excellent gift of charity, the very bond of peace and of all virtues, without which whosoever liveth is counted dead before Thee.

In the pub that evening they ended with raucous jokes and imagined what they could do to the managers. They talked of balaclava-clad attacks and vandalism to managers' cars. They wondered how they had become so dominated by aggressive, revengeful fantasies. How had they moved from charity to that?

Two years later none of the managers were in their old jobs. Those working were in junior positions in the private sector. Two had left locked in grievance procedures between themselves. The senior manager left at half past eight one morning. The building that Bridget and her team had worked in was being used for temporary staff accommodation and was in a bad state of repair. The group of patients living in the first of the trust's new community houses had to move twice because the managers had misunderstood the planning regulations and agreement.

Bridget still heard from some of her old team. Those who had jobs in the trust had become strategic. They had found that saying anything positive made managers smile. To say, 'This is exciting,' made them beam. They expressed enthusiasm for whatever strategy was in favour.

Moving out with the elderly

The nurses in an elderly patients section had an obligatory study day. Most of it was the same as the year before. Even the same hotel meal. The difference was in the final question and answer session. Hitherto, the manager's response to most questions was that they were on his list to do. But this was the year of their move. They wanted clarification and confirmation of certain matters. Many staff would have a considerable journey to work instead of the walk from home. Earlier, they had been reassured by being told that the transport arrangements would be exactly the same as for their colleagues who 'moved out' a year before (four years' travel allowance, as stated in the Whitley Council regulations, or the use of trust transport, available three times a day).

When they asked for confirmation of the transport arrangements, the manager said, 'Oh no. I don't know where you heard that.' When a more forceful nurse said, 'But three weeks ago you told me not to worry because there would be a bus available,' the manager replied 'Did I tell you that?' and turned away.

How it stopped in one place: Rita's story

How did such things happen in so many psychiatric places? It seemed unlikely that it was because psychiatry was in greater need of reform.

When I put that question to Rita, a young manager who had worked in two mental health units, she explained how psychiatry and mental health had more 'grey areas'. This made judgements more difficult to define and made it harder for staff to feel trusted and supported. For all the written policies and procedures there are many subtle variations of style which could be important. When staff made mistakes which, being human, they were bound to, they needed support. If they did not receive it, then in their vulnerability they became edgy and nervous, covering themselves.

The compliments and complaints procedure required that verbal complaints be taken as seriously as written ones. Rita told me that in a mental health unit she had known, the new management considered investigations to be evidence of how efficient they were. Staff, terrified of being investigated themselves, said how much better things were. Morale appeared high.

The trust senior managers told the purchaser of this rigorous pursuit of every complaint, to get its support.

Rita told me that the management kept the pressure up in many ways. The simplest was changing one detail after another of the old organisation. Advertisements for the replacement of secretaries and junior medical staff were delayed by repeated re-examination of job descriptions. Secretaries were moved. Offices (of consultants and others) were moved. Postal collection times were changed. Reports were demanded, and criticised when received. Instructions were changed.

The managers moved their offices three times and gained a receptionist, whose job description included making the tea.

The management stated that generic managers, not clinical specialists, were going to be leading community care. This would enable nurses to extend themselves with three year rolling contracts on a management grade. (The same money but without the security.) It was people who thought in terms of clinical specialty that held things up. A revolution was being driven.

But suddenly style appeared to change. Only later did Rita learn why.

The purchaser's money

In an informal meeting a purchaser raised with the trust executive directors concern over the number of staff (around one a month) suspended and, mostly, reinstated. None had been sacked. Over the year vacancies for trained staff ran at roughly twice the number of staff suspended. Now, the purchaser was paying for those who were suspended, and for those doing their work, as well as bank nurses for many of the unfilled vacancies. If the earlier suspensions had been to clean up the place, was it not taking a very long time?

And while the subject was being discussed, what of consultant and medical staff cover? Managers seemed to delay getting replacements while the purchasers paid for locums who gave little continuity.

There was talk of the purchaser not renewing the contract.

The executive director's daughter

The purchaser's tough talk was relayed to an informal meeting of the executive directors and prompted one of them to share with me stories she had heard from her daughter.

Awaiting a disciplinary hearing, but not suspended, one nurse was instructed by management not to take charge of any shift or ward. Managers forgot this several times and asked her to take charge. It was six weeks before she was cleared.

Five months after being told he was to be the subject of a disciplinary investigation, another nurse met the manager in the grounds and asked when his hearing would be. Appearing shocked, the manager gasped and apologised, saying, 'I forgot all about it.'

True or not, with stories like those, recruitment would not be easy.

The GPs find their voice

In their regular meetings with the chief executive, the GPs at last had something to say. They knew another consultant had resigned. In another psychiatric team, the decision to advertise for the replacement for a retiring consultant had been revoked. After the consultant retired that department was left with no consultant, no locum consultant, the withdrawal of the senior registrar (no supervision), no inpatients and very little income from purchasers.

'Get your act together.'

'Your manager is totally incompetent.'

'Where are the consultants?'

'Where is medical cover?'

'Does your management want to teach consultants a lesson and show them they are not needed? If it's a non-medical service you are creating, we could organise one much cheaper than what you are charging.'

'In fact we still want a medical service, with doctors. We want the opinion of psychiatrists. Are you interested in providing that service? If you are, get on with it.'

Why consultants and managers were so passive

I asked why the consultants and junior managers had not done something themselves. Rita told me that the chief executive refused to meet consultants without managers present. When any of the consultants did manage to meet the chief executive at some event or other she always said one of three things:

- 'The trust board are 100 % behind that manager.'
- 'Remember that I have to take a long term view. I know that you may see this as a crisis that needs major surgery, but I see it as only a hiccup.'
- 'Remember that things were so bad in the past, that they should be painful now.'

Try as they could, they could not get through.

As for the managers, Rita told me to remember that they were messengers: those who brought bad news back were 'killed'. 'Bad news?' Not of incompetent doctors, nurses, psychologists, art therapists, or any clinically involved person: such information only proved that clinicians were useless and that managers knew best. It gave someone to blame, something to clean up. Bad news was saying that the strategy was inconsistent or was not working: that GPs did not like the latest changes; that patients did not like being called 'clients'; that the junior managers were confused by their seniors' changes of mind, secrecy, and venomous criticism. For the carrying of messages like those, their jobs were put in peril; they would be the next ones for whom there was no new contract, or the next ones to leave suddenly.

And the senior management were stuck, painted into a corner. Perhaps washing some dirty linen had impressed the purchasers and showed that the management was getting to grips with things; but too much of it might suggest that things were still terrible. Or, could stopping it now suggest a cover up to keep contracts and to avoid compensation pay-outs; or that the earlier way been unnecessary and wrong?

Another doctor tendered his resignation and was immediately offered what James had told me right at the beginning the managers mentioned first: money. Did he want more money? No, it was 'respect'.

A key manager left. Quite suddenly, as they do.

Chapter 15

'To support you, I am suspending you'

'Suspension is not in itself a disciplinary action but is a neutral act taken to alleviate a situation and allow a full investigation of the facts to take place. I will keep you informed of any progress made in the investigation.' (Extract from a letter from a manager)

'I felt as if the floor and the furniture and the fields outside and all the people I knew or had ever known had disappeared. I should have been accelerating downwards faster and faster as I fell into a great hole, but I was not falling at all. I was standing still, so I felt unreal.' (Ward manager)

'For the first time in my career I experienced a sense of concern before I said anything at all. And when I had said something I started to worry what effect it might have on other people, or how it might be used or distorted.' (Consultant)

From the outside, the ward itself looked like many others in this fairly large and rambling, not untypical, district general hospital. The entrance looked different. Someone had taken trouble to put many old but bright posters on the walls of the entrance hall. These extended round corners to other rooms. Some of the furniture was non-standard and therefore non-institutional. It was apparent from these signs that, even before the era of clinical directorships and devolved budgets, people on this ward had somehow managed to use resources differently. They must have got money to buy the secondhand furniture or they must have been given it (perhaps by a relative) and had persuaded the managers that the items passed the latest and ever more stringent fire regulations.

It was the sort of unit that, at first impression, the critical visitor might think was approved of by the management. In the old days it had been one of the places of which the managers were undoubtedly proud: it was on the list that visitors were taken to see.

Staff had felt confident in their relationship with the new managers in the new NHS. They worked within their budget. Some of their extra spending had been possible because they had early on exploited the system of extra contractual referrals (ECRs) and had got in money over and above the budgets. It was not a very 'medical' ward. It had not been the first, but had been one of the first in the hospital, where staff did not wear traditional nursing uniforms. Rather, they wore simple overalls when carrying out certain procedures. The paperwork around admission and the way the case notes were written by all disciplines had for several years been done in a way that people would now recognise as 'care plans'. (The practices had included a form listing social and physical needs with spaces for staff who would pursue investigations, activity or training or treatment programmes and space for reviewing progress within days. At a glance, ward staff could see how much they had said they would do, and what was being done.)

Staff had close links with the community, especially with the patients' families, GPs and social workers. Many of their patients came for their brief stays from social services run, or social services inspected, establishments. For years the ward had a policy of short stay and shared care. Even assessments appeared to be shorter than anywhere else and the staff were always prepared to have people back as part of the process of providing respite for carers.

After the events related in this story, staff realised that they had a very prominent feature which was not doing them any good at all. They appeared to be doing their own thing. They appeared to be independent. They appeared to have taken great initiative without a new management structure. They appeared not to have the 'right attitude' to management.

The biggest difference between this ward and all the others in the hospital, was that when I conducted my interviews it had recently been closed.

The trust

This was one of the 'first wave' trusts in 1991. 1990 had been an energetic, exciting year of preparation and presentation of the bid.

Using part of the name of one of the hospitals and maintaining its high profile in the press, the trust established its identity and the management established its pattern.

In 1992 there was talk of a merger with a trust alongside. There was much energy put into presentations and considerations of this: surveying the strengths and weaknesses; the worst case scenario, and the best. The trust board 'bought in' consultants to help them consider the issues and the options and then to present the case.

In 1993 the merger took place and it became a different trust.

Late in 1993, concerns were circulating that the merger had not been as neat as it could have been: some refinements were needed 'at the edges' and in the size of the total organisation.

In 1994 it became yet a different trust and managers said that it was right.

These changes were not only in name but in management structure, geographical boundaries, and the way the different services were grouped together or managed. At each stage the jobs of the managers themselves were probably those most at stake. All managers must have feared for their survival.

For managers to embark on 'seeing through' difficult decisions, they had to be feeling secure. I do not know how long it would have taken to feel secure and confident of having colleagues constant enough for planning to be anything other than very short term. Meanwhile to manage their own survival, they needed to show they could manage their units. The easiest way of demonstrating that was to show that they could handle crises and deal with clinical staff who were not managing well.

Within days of the appointment of the new chief executive, rumours were circulating that he was openly boasting that he wanted to rid the trust of doctors' power. He would certainly have had strong support for this stand from at least two of the non-executive directors, who had been often heard to say that most of the trouble in the NHS had been caused by doctors. (It is not an uncommon remark.)

The warnings

The first encounters between the new management and the leaders of the ward were very friendly and they heard remarks such as, 'Why are other places not like this?' Nice to hear, but the interest was in the management and none was expressed in the clinical work or service. Later, they wondered if they should have seen that as a device to split them from colleagues.

Harriet, the service manager, had several groups or units within her domain. She was said by the secretaries to refer to this one as the 'playpen'. The ward staff never confronted her because they did not want to 'shop' their source of information in the secretaries' office.

Other colleagues told them that the managers would not be able to let them continue with the independence they had built up. They were warned that the managers would look for an excuse to intervene. 'And remember,' one colleague due to retire from another part of the trust said, 'these people are the government's adolescents: they have to stamp their mark.'

The event

Following prominent television coverage of an allegation of brutality towards old people in a local authority home in another part of the country, staff on the ward were not surprised that there was talk of disquieting rumours in their own area. A few days later, on a Monday afternoon, a social worker visiting the ward mentioned to one of the care staff that he had heard that a mutual ex-client had made a complaint about the ward. The name did not ring a bell but a colleague looked up the admissions book for the previous year and found it. It was somebody who had been in for a few weeks and a staff nurse remembered that the family had made two complaints about the consultant who was from another hospital. The social worker had not heard what the current complaint was, but appeared somewhat reassured that the ward staff said they were not really worried, beyond saying that obviously their ex-patient and the family were still having their difficulties. Many questions had concerned staff during the admission and they had shared these with the patient, the family and with the social services department. The patient had not been demented at the time of the admission.

On the next day the social worker rang to let the staff know he had heard that violence was alleged. This detail did not disturb them. They remembered more clearly the way in which the family had a go at the other consultant: like a dog worrying a bone, they would not let go for ages, then suddenly dropped it.

Alan, the ward manager, who had now heard of the social worker's conversations with the ward staff, mentioned them in passing to Harriet. A surprising response:

'Oh yes, I know. You must not talk to the social worker any more. Nobody should talk to the social worker about it again. It will all be handled through me.'

The staff on the ward heard no more from the social worker so wondered if he had been instructed similarly.

Early the next morning Alan, who could see that the continuing uncertainty was good for nobody on the ward staff, decided to ring his service manager again. Harriet did have more information. She had heard that the allegations were of violence and that the patients and family had named Alan himself. Alan was startled but also reassured. Startled, because he had expected it to be one of the junior and more vulnerable colleagues who had been accused, and reassured because he knew how he had behaved with patients and that nothing he had done with this man could remotely be construed as violence.

'Well, what is going to happen? Are you going to suspend me?'

He had said it light-heartedly. Harriet responded in a different tone and said she did not know if the allegations would lead to a suspension. 'I will let you know as soon as I do.'

Within two hours Alan had a message to go to Harriet's office immediately. It was a three or four minute walk and the office was on another floor. Harriet was there with one of the personnel officers.

'We wanted to let you know as quickly as possible that we are going to have to suspend you and we will do it this afternoon. Our advice to you is to get in touch with your union right away.'

Alan agreed to return at 2.15 pm.

On the walk back Alan was still not particularly worried. He knew he was 'clean'. They had had so many patients since this particular one and he would need to look at the notes to refresh his memory, but that was no big problem.

On return to the ward he told the charge nurse and the other staff and tried immediately to get in touch with his union. Meanwhile one of the other staff on the ward rang medical records, to request the notes.

Neither NUPE (National Union of Public Employees) nor the Royal College of Nursing could provide anyone to accompany Alan to the meeting that afternoon. They gave the same advice: say nothing.

Alan had no lunch.

All the ward staff were in a state of shock, but managed somehow to get on with their work. Some thought there would in the end be no suspension or, if there were, for a few days at most. They could hold their breath and get through that.

What else went on between the two meetings?

Alan wanted to rush to tell everybody. While he told immediate colleagues, he asked them to help him keep the right boundaries. They agreed and advised him to be terribly careful every minute while he was still on the premises. One of the youngest members of staff, a more militant union member, raised a finger at him and said very slowly:

'Don't give them anything else. Don't give them any excuse to write anything else down.'

One of the afternoon staff nurses phoned in and, hearing what had happened, came to work an hour early. She looked shocked and serious and said she was fearful. She said that the allegation itself did not worry her, because she remembered how the family had tried to 'get' people before and how the staff had discussed this with the relatives and the social services department. She also knew that Alan was extremely unlikely to have behaved as was alleged. What worried her was what lay behind the trust's handling of it. What was their hidden agenda?

At the 2.15 meeting Alan was again met by Harriet and a member of the personnel department. The former was in 'management mode'. She spoke formally:

'We all know what has been said, but I have formally to remind you that the trust has received a complaint from X and X's relatives that during X's admission you were violent towards him. The allegation is that X was hit by a member of staff and X has named you as the person who did it. Therefore, while the police and we are investigating this, to support you, I am suspending you.'

The personnel officer said Alan would be suspended on full pay, that a counsellor they had chosen was available if he wanted to see her, that a letter would follow and that meanwhile he was not to talk to anyone about the suspension. (The counsellor turned out to be another employee of the same trust, working on a different project. Alan did not see how he could talk usefully to another employee.) The personnel officer went on to add that she was terribly sorry that this was happening but that it really was the best way to support him.

He asked if the consultant of the ward knew, and was told that she did.

'And you would like to hear that she asked if there was any other way of handling the matter, but I explained to her why there was not.'

Alan told them that he had telephoned the Royal College of Nursing (he did not mention the other union) and would keep in touch with them. He added that in the ward they had asked for the records of the patient's admission because it was more than a year ago and, to refresh his memory, he would look at them before he left.

'Oh no. You are not to do that. And the notes are not to leave the medical records department.'

It had seemed so obvious a thing for him to do. Alan looked very puzzled, and spoke quietly:

'But why not?'

'In case you are guilty.'

The way home

The last remark had tipped the balance very suddenly for Alan. He had heard of this happening to other people. Was it now happening to himself? He felt more unreal than he had ever felt in all his life.

'I felt as if the floor and the furniture **and** the fields outside and all the people I knew or had ever known had disappeared, I should have been accelerating downwards faster and faster as I fell into a great hole, but I was not falling at all. I was standing still, so I felt unreal.'

The ward staff, upon whom he called briefly, were shocked that he had to go that minute and that he was not allowed to see the notes. Was that why medical records had not turned up the file as quickly as they usually did? Several of them thought they would get the notes for him later, but were not prepared to say so.

Men are not allowed to cry in the NHS, so he accepted the hugs, saw some of their tears, ignored a call from a patient outside the door (since when had ignoring a patient become part of his proper duty?) and left.

He described the journey home as a mixture of daze and thoughts rushing so fast that he could not catch them. Phrases and ideas went round and round again and again, but even, many months later, thoughts which took him a long time to share with me:

'What will the neighbours think if they hear that I have been suspended? Will they think that I am a murderer? Will they think that I have been killing patients? Will they speak to me or look at me? Are people looking at me already?'

He told me that 'pure' paranoia may be all right with the sense of certainty of persecution and being the centre of attention, but paranoia with doubt was terrible.

What to tell and to whom? Of course he told his partner and some very close friends. What to tell and to whom, never ceased to be a worry during this time. Relatives? Parents? Brother? Sister? Neighbours? How to account for being around so much? Should he hide? The postman? The milkman? The list of categories of people over whom this question was raised was endless.

It was a weekend of telephone calls from colleagues, but they could not help, because their distress fed his distress. Hearing them on the telephone reminded him of the difficulties that they must be facing in keeping the ward running. One member of staff was already on maternity leave and another had started two weeks' holiday.

The letter

On the second day of the next week the letter arrived. At least it was not by recorded delivery, but nonetheless, the very public nature of the postman delivering it through the door felt like further affront and humiliation. The letter itself was standard and formal enough:

Dear ...

Re: Suspension from Duty

I am writing to confirm that I am suspending you from duty on full pay with effect from (the letter gave the date of the previous Friday).

The reason for this suspension is to allow full and thorough investigation into the allegations of physical violence made by X.

I want to remind you that suspension is not in itself a disciplinary action. It is a neutral act. It alleviates an immediate situation and it makes it possible for a full investigation of the facts to occur.

While you are suspended you must not enter any property of the trust without prior permission. Furthermore, you must not discuss this matter with other colleagues, employees, clients or relatives of a client.

You must make yourself available between 9 am and 5 pm on Monday to Friday in order to be able to attend any meetings connected with this investigation.

You should sign and return one of the copies which I have attached to this letter. This is to confirm your receipt of the letter, and the other is for you if you wish to give one to your representative.

I will of course keep you informed of any progress made in the investigation but please do contact me without hesitation if you have any queries.

Yours sincerely,

The last paragraph was the straw at which to clutch. He decided to telephone Harriet.

The weekend had been terrible. He had hardly slept, and had episodes of palpitations and indigestion. He had felt restless but nervous of going out and had not left the house except in the dark. Friends had visited him and had offered to take him out and pressed much alcohol on him. He had drunk a little. They had encouraged him to contact his GP and he telephoned first thing Monday morning and fixed an appointment for later in the week.

Harriet was not available when he telephoned but he left a message. She did not ring back that morning so he tried again in the afternoon and this time got through. She had not received the message. The telephone call was warmer than the letter had been:

'We will be getting things moving as fast as we can, but we have to wait for the police to finish their investigation. I am sure you will be hearing from us very soon... Yes of course you can go away for a couple of days, but let me know and, if you have not seen them yet, let the police know.'

At the police station

The police said that they would not be able to interview him during that week, so they had no objections to him going away. He went to stay with his parents in the country for two days. It was a break. Neither of them was very well so he decided not to tell them what was on his mind. But he knew that they knew that there was something.

Returning to his own home there were several messages from colleagues. He first decided not to ring them back but changed his mind. He used their home numbers. They were very supportive, but they needed to talk about how difficult things were 'back at the ranch'. He wanted to hear, but he did not want to hear.

At the end of the first week he had heard from the police and fixed an interview with them for the beginning of the next week. He telephoned Harriet to let her know.

'Good. As soon as we hear from them and get clearance from them, we will get in touch with you.'

She added that the man and his relatives had been informed. Was there a slight cheerful lilt and very slight questioning in the voice when she added 'All right'? He realised that he had heard those two words often from managers in the last couple of years. He said nothing.

Alan's GP was sympathetic but said that he must know as well as she did what they had on offer. She could prescribe tranquillisers or hypnotics. They had a counsellor she could ask to see him. She offered him a prescription for tranquillisers which he accepted, but did not take to the chemist.

On the Tuesday after the second weekend, he went to the police. It was brief and surprisingly informal. The officer who conducted the interview gave nothing away and said very clearly what he had to do, and why; and then did it. One of the other officers, who was in the room for a few moments, said that if police were suspended every time there was an allegation of the strength of this one, then there would not be one of them left to do the job.

The police conclusion and the internal inquiry

The police's total investigation was finished two weeks to the day after the suspension. They concluded that there was no case to answer and that was the end of the matter as far as they were concerned. Alan was informed by Harriet at 9.45 that night. He was immensely relieved and immediately asked her when he could go back to work.

'Oh, it's not as simple as that. The trust will have to conduct its own investigation now. You will be informed when you are required. But we will get on to that first thing next week.'

He did not think until afterwards to question why he was being informed so late, and then the opportunity had gone. But later he learned that the consultant had been informed that afternoon, so Harriet must have known during office hours.

Over the weekend, more telephone calls. Some colleagues said Harriet told them that she was certain the story was a pack of lies and they had heard that other managers were also saying that the allegation was not true.

First thing next week? No news Monday morning. In the middle of the afternoon, unable to contain himself any longer, he telephoned Harriet.

'No news. You will be informed as soon as there is some. This may be the most important thing for you, but I am very busy today.'

Colleagues told him on the phone that Harriet and the clinical director had held a planning meeting and decided to interview other staff.

Now his palpitations and indigestion were returning. Headaches were starting. He asked his GP for more help.

The GP arranged the counselling and pressed him further to take at least one minor tranquilliser on going to bed, at least for three nights to break the pattern. Alan agreed. He told me that it was valuable to have been able to share with the GP his fear that he was having a breakdown. Her professional opinion was that he was experiencing understandable response to external events. Some people might call it a breakdown, but she was not one of them.

Three days later Harriet telephoned to say there was still no date for his interview, but that the internal inquiry was continuing and another member of staff had very firmly denied all supposed events. Had he heard of this formal 'internal inquiry' before, he wondered?

One week later he phoned again and was told by Harriet that the inquiry's final hearing would be in exactly two weeks' time. He was given the names of the people who would sit on the panel. Would he get an agenda? No, there was no agenda, but there was a procedure.

Alan's interview lasted two hours. He was accompanied by his union representative. The panel consisted of Harriet, a consultant from another part of the trust, the personnel officer who had been part of the initial suspension team, and one of the non-executive directors of the board. He was questioned mostly by the consultant and Harriet. He was asked questions far wider than what he thought was the subject of the allegations. He was questioned on consent and on hygiene. He did not understand why these questions were relevant to the inquiry into the allegation made towards him for specific behaviour and for which he had been suspended. He said so, but heard his union representative groan very slightly as he did. He answered the questions.

Afterwards the union representative said he knew he was intimidated by the questioning and the manner in which it was done. He assumed they were asking more widely because more than violence might have been raised in the minds of the senior managers as cause for concern. He was surprised that Alan had not been advised of this. Alan wondered if the ward staff had; he himself felt too confused to be sure of what he had been told. It was best to do as Alan had done in the end, which was to answer the questions. Otherwise, he explained, Alan would increase his reputation as a troublemaker.

A troublemaker? This was the first he had heard of that reputation.

The suspension was lifted and he was allowed back to work. By that time he had lost six kilos in weight, his indigestion was in a regular cycle and his GP had placed him on the first medication for a peptic ulcer. Apart from the three nights on the tranquilliser, his sleep was as bad as ever and his partner was on the point of leaving him ('I am sorry this is happening to you. I know it is not your responsibility. But I didn't live with you in order to have all this.') He was finding the counselling helpful. He had told the panel that he had been seeing his GP and he reminded Harriet that he had sent in a sick note.

Alan returned to work three weeks later.

He had received a formal letter reinstating him but not, as he had been promised, the minutes of the meeting. Back at work he visited Harriet. No, the minutes had not been done yet. It was because a number of people had been on leave and they had to collect information from others. He would get them as soon as they were done.

Two weeks later the minutes were being got ready for the executive meeting of the unit of management (a meeting that he himself was due to attend).

He asked if he might see the minutes before that meeting and received a nod. Three days later, the day before the meeting of the executive, he had still not received them. He telephoned Harriet.

'Yes, we agree we wish you to see these minutes. We suggest that you go to the secretary's office five minutes before the meeting tomorrow and see them then.'

Alan started to protest, was alarmed to hear a plaintiveness coming into his voice as he recalled her statement that she would support him. He heard her response clearly enough.

'Tough.'

In fact the secretaries were more helpful and he was able to see the minutes a couple of hours before the meeting. They were all right.

He left the trust four weeks later. During those four weeks he heard a great deal about the experiences of the other staff while he was away during the internal inquiry.

What other staff told him

He heard of staff being very anxious and frightened and then going off sick. There were as many as half a dozen different agency staff working on the ward within one week. Some of the staff felt that they were cut dead by Harriet when they met in the corridor. When they shared their worries with managers, they were told that their job was to manage the ward.

They were instructed to control admissions; to take admissions again; to offer a day service; then back to a 24 hour service.

There were frequent telephone calls for immediate information and whatever nursing procedures or clinical duties were under way had to be dropped:

'Would it be reasonable for a photocopier to be used in such and such a way?'

'Would it be possible for the nurse in charge of the ward, if it was a man, to be alone in the office when a female relative came in?'

When staff had been slow in coming up with answers, or sending reports, they felt threatened by being reminded that they themselves could be disciplined if they did not co-operate immediately with the investigating team.

Several were questioned over an alleged incident when there had been food on the floor beside a table: had a visitor been told that a patient had deliberately put it there? Were staff deliberately waiting before intervening? Had the patient been told to pick it up himself? If such an incident were to have happened, even hypothetically, what would be a reasonable time to wait before encouraging the client again, or picking it up themselves? What would be a reasonable thing to say to relatives?

Several staff were told that the trust had to go through the process of the internal inquiry because it was part of the business of looking after the staff. Although the police had said there was no case to answer the trust had to be whiter than white in making sure there was nothing which, although it might not be police business, was the business of the trust. Anything that might seem important to patients or to relatives and might lead to a complaint could be investigated.

Meanwhile it had been everybody's duty to go on managing the ward while they all went through the difficult process of their ward manager's suspension.

By the time Alan left, the internal inquiry into all the allegations had formally concluded that there had been no case to answer, the ward had been closed, and a review into the service had been started by the senior management team.

Staff were told later that if anyone heard of this complaint and made another one about a different member of staff, that person would be very grateful to the trust for having gone into things so carefully. It was all part of supporting staff. 'Pity that was not said at the beginning,' was the thought, but unspoken reply.

The consultant

When I met Patricia, formerly the ward consultant, now settled in her new post in another part of the country, she said that right from the start the management viewed the whole directorate as dysfunctional. She thought that, very early on, it was as though there was an inevitable process leading to the closure of something with some sort of endings of its own historical making. She remembered that I had said on the phone that I was particularly interested in hearing from her an account of how the unit was finally closed.

The management seemed to dislike people communicating except with themselves, but they actively engaged juniors in gossip over seniors. She gave the example of the letter which came proposing changes and the trimming ('downsizing'?) of a department. The consultant in this department, himself nearing retirement age, responded by writing to the chairman of the trust and to the chief executive, and sent a copy to a number of colleagues within the trust. By 'return' of internal post, most of the senior staff received a letter from the chief executive informing them that it was inappropriate for any member of staff to question decisions about the implementing of trust policy on size and configuration of services by writing directly to the chief executive or board. The next day, the consultant, mentioned in all but name in that circular, received his personal letter informing him that it was not expected that the board would hear that he had done such a thing again.

This public reprimand of a senior colleague was a clear and intimidating message to everyone else in the trust to keep silent. It was a turning point for staff relations and communications: loyalty to the trust was paramount.

For the first time in her career Patricia experienced a sense of concern before she said anything at all. And when she did say something she started to worry for the effect it might have on other people, or how it might be used or distorted.

The managers clearly saw every crisis as an opportunity to make changes. It was soon after the widely leaked 'We do no expect to hear that you have done this again' letter that the complaint against Alan arose.

Patricia had worked two sessions in the trust. She was not complaining of being kept in the dark over everything, because she knew how difficult it was to communicate with somebody who was there as little as she had been. But she did not like to be told that she had not been 'contactable' when she knew that the admin team, who knew exactly where she was, had insisted that no messages for her had come through.

What had been so alarming in this trust had been that the new style managers were suspending people almost as a reflex. At one point there were eight people suspended throughout the trust. For each one, they had what sounded a plausible justification, but the managers had not 'thought through' (language they use themselves) the effects of suspensions nor appreciated their impact. They responded to every hitch with the injunction, 'It has to be managed', and seemed totally unaware of the simplest requirements for the good functioning of a team. They confronted the staff as if they had no emotions or feelings.

Patricia was particularly strong in her comments on the misreading of the way a team would function when an investigation was under way. Many people have now worked with the process of investigation into child neglect and abuse. A family is never the same again once investigations have started: it becomes dysfunctional. Individual members find it difficult to relate to each other and to outside people. Often each person feels under suspicion from someone, and feels suspicious of someone. This wisdom has not yet penetrated managers' training. They still appear to jump to the conclusion that anyone who has complained, speaks the truth. And, of all unlikely things, they expect staff, working under the greatest professional strain of their lives, to be able to work well.

The staff felt battered by what had happened. First, the allegation of violence, the suspension and the police investigation. Then the internal inquiry for which there may well have been good reason, but for which there was never a good explanation given. Then the delay of that inquiry and the manner of all those telephone calls which felt so persecuting left the remaining staff feeling that the managers were looking to see how they could be tripped up. This eroded the ability of all the staff to make good judgements. It was very bad management, by people whose ignorance was most obvious in their focusing on 'incidents', which was how the unit was finally closed.

It was towards the end of the suspension period, after changing from a 24 hour service to a 9.00 to 5.00 one and back again, and when the telephone calls to the ward over fine detail of information to do with the inquiry were at their height (all the questioning on feeding routines, and some food on the floor seen by a visitor), that interest in 'incidents' started. 'Incident' is defined by a practice and a tool. It is the practice of writing incidents in the incident book. And it is clearly known what should be written.

Incidents might include daytime incontinence, shouting, falling, breaking substantial amounts of crockery or wandering away.

In short, staff write in the incident book anything about which they think someone else might say, 'Why was that not written in the incident book?' To have managers counting these, daily, raised anxiety even further. As Alan was preparing to leave, the trust decided that it would close the unit if there was another incident. It was therefore only a matter of time.

Postscript

I had one more question to put to Patricia. Did she have any comment on the position of the chief executive regarding doctors. She had an immediate response. she had heard him in an open meeting make the boast of ridding the trust of doctor power.

Patricia was in touch with me a year later to tell me, in the context of my final question to her, that three more consultants had left the trust very disheartened with the management style.

By then I had another question. How had the people who made the complaint, 18 months after the alleged offence, been able to identify by name so clearly a man they had hardly seen?

Patricia told me the managers had showed them the photographs of the staff.

Chapter 16

Work in the children's ward

Paediatrics is in a state of national crisis. In a recent year over 40% of the *BMJ* advertisements for consultant posts were re-advertisements. In an effort to find out why the specialty was so unpopular, surveys have been done of junior doctors. When asked why the path to paediatrics is so unpopular, they said: 'Look at the consultants: they work excessively long hours, have frantic on-call rotas and experiences, and they are at the sharp end of many life/death or medico/legal problems.' To find out how this was linked up with the NHS reforms, I met staff from several paediatric departments.

The much heralded reduction in junior doctors' hours has meant that in the relatively small specialties, like paediatrics, they become more isolated. I have found no one against a reduction in hours. But for a junior doctor to be on call for a wider range of specialties in a hospital would not be good practice, nor good training. Therefore, for their hours to be kept down to the required, agreed minimum, they have to have time off during the day. This means there is less time for juniors to meet day staff on the ward, other juniors and, of course, their consultants. Supervision and teaching are both interfered with.

Paediatrics is a specialty going in two important directions. The first is into community care, and paediatrics was probably the first specialty with high-profile publications on treating patients at home in the 1960s. The second is into 'high-tech', very staff-intensive work for relatively few severely ill children. Trusts and purchasers have handled this development in different ways. Some trusts have merged and, in so doing, have been able to provide, in one district, a single highly specialised paediatric ward with a manageable on-call rota for junior doctors and consultants. Other trusts have dealt with it by competing with each other. Both ways have meant extra administrative time for consultant paediatricians and other clinical staff.

In those trusts where mergers have taken place, one of the paediatricians has had to give up nearly all his or her time to clinical directorship. In those trusts which have not merged, several paediatricians have had to give up much time to the management.

No co-operation, please

One trust's consultant paediatrician was asked to produce a memorandum on the future of his specialty for the medical director. This was done over two weekends and a few evenings, and with several consultations with other staff. The finished memorandum drew upon many of the arguments put forward at national and international paediatric gatherings on the future of the specialty and concluded that it was probably very difficult for a paediatric service to survive in a single district trust, serving a population of 200,000–250,000. The paediatrician sent the document to the medical director who sent it to the chief executive, who immediately sent for the consultant and hauled him over the coals. The chief executive had been wanting advice on how the trust could keep contracts in paediatrics and was not at all interested in ideas of working in collaboration with other trusts. The brief interview ended with the words, 'And you'll meet the chairman next week.'

It was quite clear to the paediatrician, in subsequent attempts at discussion, that his work on the paper had been seen as an act of disloyalty. Co-operation with others in the interests of patients was not a matter to be discussed.

In another place, when the clinical team suggested that they merge with a neighbouring trust's department, they were accused of being disloyal and of not supporting their own trust. Even talking with colleagues in neighbouring hospitals had led to the criticism that they were naive.

One chief executive agreed in private that, 'The bottom line is what is best for the patients,' but added that they were a long way from that ideal. First, all the strategies for them to survive as a single trust had to be explored. A favourite phrase was that premature discussion of co-operation could get in the way of rational and tactical thought.

In another inner-city area, larger professional groups used to working without tight geographical boundaries in their societies and colleges told their managers of discussions on co-operation between several community departments. They ran into objections like:

'The purchaser wants to hear of beds being cut.'

'We cannot discuss community services until the inpatient services are rationalised.'

'You may be quite right that it would be rational to discuss co-operation with our neighbours, but I know that the senior management team won't consider transfer of resources to another trust because that is disloyal: it is not an option.'

'The trust board will not hear of the trust having no paediatrics.'

'The purchaser does not want to be dictated to by the providers.'

Meanwhile, the clinical staff were still being kept at arm's length from the purchaser which, in the absence of direct clinical advice, continued to produce papers which sounded good but were not specific.

The paediatricians and the medical staff committee meetings

The paediatricians in one trust said to me that there were two sorts of medical staff committee.

When there was both a manager and the medical director present (the latter a consultant herself and therefore a member of the medical staff committee) they had a pep talk. Half the time they were told how well the trust was doing and how a manager or the chief executive was pulling some coup over another trust or purchaser, and half the time they were encouraged to do better themselves. Dissent and pessimism were not allowed: enthusiasm and claims of increasing productivity were encouraged. (Several of the consultants said that it put them in mind of stories of the 'great leap forward' in communist China when officials joined the party hierarchy in boasting of unrealistic claims which could never be substantiated).

A middle manager was discussing with one of his teams the value of keeping each other informed. The consultant agreed and said she had been waiting to hear from the manager about the meeting currently going on in a neighbouring trust about a possible merger of the two services. She had been told about this a few weeks ago by her colleague in the other trust. The embarrassed manager could say nothing — but did take it up with his own manager at supervision the next week.
He was told he was quite right about the need to improve communications. But he must also remember that the trust's policy was for managers to manage, so not everything could be passed down the line all the time. And no, the senior manager did not know why the other trust was doing things differently.

When the medical director was there without a manager, things were little different. The medical director had told some of her colleagues that she had accepted the post because she liked power and kicking people around. She repeatedly reminded her colleagues that the world had changed and that they had to face reality.

With neither the manager nor the medical director present, the meetings took on a depressive and conspiratorial tone. They shared horror stories and complaints about the managers, the spurious data collection, the unrealistic and jargon-ridden business plans they were writing, and what they would 'really' say to the trust if they ever had the chance and the nerve. Those who were retiring were openly envied and everyone over the age of 50 could announce, often to the day, how much longer they had to go.

In medical staff committees, the paediatricians themselves found little support for their own preoccupations. Everyone seemed equally burdened by paperwork, targets, ECRs, quality standards. Some had the advantage of long waiting lists which seemed the easiest thing to change and even get money for doing so. Several were in larger groups, like the surgeons and physicians, who could make more noise. They could not remember a time when consultants were so united in their distress over what was happening to the NHS and the services they were running; but at the same time so riddled with rivalry, being suspicious of each other and unwilling to share plans. Old loyalties had gone.

How will the department develop?

Stephen, the youngest of the paediatricians in one trust, said that when he came there a few years ago people were proud of their local department. It was a good place to work in, hard work and fun. Now they were all just hanging on.

The junior doctors, training in the department for a year, met the consultants less. Even the ones on daytime duty had less time with the consultants because informal talking time over coffee or lunch was reduced.

As in other specialties, there are a number of paediatric practices which, if you are going to be any good at them, you must do at least a certain number of times each year. The same applies to teams which are carrying out certain procedures or running specialist services. Figures released during the reforms in late 1994 showed that where such procedures were done seldom, the death rate was higher. There was publicity on 'keyhole' surgery and the government department put out guidelines.

'Level 2' neo-natal intensive care is an example and to provide this, their trust had to make arrangements. Children could be transferred to another hospital, one of several, or the paediatric departments could have co-operated to share resources and create a joint unit. As co-operation with another trust was a subject that would not be discussed by management and as the paediatricians had their fingers burned too often to risk being dubbed 'disloyal' again, nothing was done. Stephen felt too worn down to press the case any more and so, here, crisis management would continue.

Shared care

Sharing care between tertiary centres and the local hospital enables children and their relatives to continue to be more confident of seeing the same person again and again (at their local hospital). Children with cystic fibrosis and some of those requiring particularly lengthy treatments for cancer are examples of the sorts of case in which this is particularly important.

Stephen was worried that this would not be allowed to continue as the contract system intensified. Will the children be allowed to attend two hospitals? What will the purchaser say? Cynically, one of the staff mentioned that someone should approve the idea because it would increase the 'number of patients treated' by having the children being counted at both trusts, as papers of 'finished consultant episodes' (FCEs) pile on top of each other.

Stephen told me of a physically abused child who had received severe brain damage from non-accidental injury. Stephen referred child and mother to a national centre whose report, which was illuminating, suggested referral and treatment at a further place. The suggestion made sense to Stephen, who then did whatever was necessary to approach the purchasers and the social services department for joint funding. After some time and no response from the purchaser, Stephen telephoned to find out what was happening. The purchaser had referred the family elsewhere for yet another opinion (the third). That specialist department, with a national reputation, took the case on for treatment and their treatment was cheaper than the other. After a time the treating specialists came to a further opinion themselves, and suggested a referral to the place recommended at the start of this story. This time the purchaser accepted the recommendation and some time later mother and child were seen and treatment started.

Stephen told this story to explain how hard it was to keep up to date with the rules. It was a story of 'money following patients', and one that showed some of the management procedures that have to be followed for that to happen. Stephen says that they will all try to remember that the purchasers may be referring agents themselves and that it is too much to expect the provider units to challenge their decisions because they want the money.

It had never occurred to Stephen and his colleagues that the purchaser might become a referrer itself. They were sure that no one had ever told them that when the reforms were being explained at those early meetings. Their managers had been sympathetic when hearing of their fury but said not to challenge them: we need their money too much.

Lifestyles

The paediatricians work longer hours than they used to and are interrupted at home more often. Out of hours calls are not only for clinical work. They are also for 'politics'. Senior colleagues telephone: 'I must catch you at home. It's too delicate to discuss at work....'

They spend hours producing papers for meetings. The time they spend with patients has gone down, as has the time spent with junior medical colleagues and those from other disciplines. They meet staff from other departments less and chatting or passing the time of day with anyone in the hospital has become a thing of the past.

And sleep? They knew that when they started in medicine their would be interrupted nights. But now Stephen has dreams of being ticked off by the chief executive, the medical director or the chairman. A colleague has dreamed of struggles in writing reports for the trust and of having them rubbished by managers. Every time one of them gets a summons to another meeting he or she sleeps badly and wakes early with worry. Stephen has found himself taking special routes through the hospital corridors to avoid meeting certain people. And feeling his heart sinking when he realised what he had done.

Working the system takes up so much of their time and they feel disloyal and troublemakers whenever they say so.

The neo-natal ward: Graham's story

I had heard so much about the small specialist units that I sought out Graham, a mature student whose training course required him to observe a small organisation at work. He had chosen a neo-natal ward of a general hospital run by a different trust. After some work by an intermediary, Graham agreed to meet me.

The first words he said to me as he sat down were, 'I am allowed to speak to you?' I thought those words could have many meanings, but what I did was to repeat what I had already put in my letter and on the phone about how I protected the identity of my informants. He explained to me that the trust for which he had been working was one in which to speak out was interpreted as an act of disloyalty. However, he decided to continue to talk to me.

Graham had met staff in groups and individually, and he had observed them at work.

Nurses, he said, are frightened for their jobs. They talk of being low paid, having too much work to do, being unable to fill posts so that much of the work is done by agency staff who have to be told what to do by permanent staff. Graham said that, compared with most other places in which he had worked, there is far less sense of 'community' because of the agency staff coming in and out. He was not being critical of the agency workers in themselves, but pointed out that they cannot know the children or the ways of working in the ward in the way that the permanent staff can. He had once met a plastic surgeon who told him that the only time a child had died in his care was on an occasion when there had been a change in the team. The management appear to think that it is satisfactory to slot people into shifts without knowing the people they are working with as colleagues or as patients.

The nurses talk of being low in supplies for even the most mundane items. They have to nag for them and they say that this is getting worse.

They find it increasingly difficult to get small amounts of money for simple equipment like the new gadgets for taking an infant's blood less painfully and more safely. So they are incensed to see a programme on television which shows a purchaser boasting how it is possible for them to contribute money for sending a child to the USA for a particular flamboyant form of treatment for cancer, which was available in this country all along.

They say they are no longer allowed to be flexible over babies and mothers who have come into their ward from areas served by other hospitals. Even if the mother becomes very attached to their unit she is transferred as soon as the managers can arrange it. They are very cynical of the early boast of 'money follows patients'. They see mothers and babies transferred with such rapidity and such frequency that they think the only gain must be statistical: a child being in more than one ward and under more than one consultant, and especially in more than one hospital, increases the figures for 'number of patients treated'. The NHS management and the government quote 'finished consultant episodes' as 'patients treated', so that it is quite possible for one illness to end up in the statistics as four patients treated.

Graham said that he had asked if they had ever challenged the managers on the point they were making, but they had laughed at him: 'Now that wouldn't be very loyal, would it?'

The junior doctors are very worried over beds being closed or, more accurately, unavailable because there are not enough nursing staff to maintain them. So when there is a very sick baby who should be admitted, they do not know where to send it. All they can be certain of is trouble whatever they do. They can: (1) admit to their ward, overwork the nurses and reduce the level of care for the other patients — and be told off by the managers; (2) admit (or try to) to another trust's ward — and be told off regarding costs and asked questions on who was going to pay; or (3) ring the on-call consultant when they know how tired they all are. And, the junior doctors added, if they do any of those things, they may be challenged by a manager to explain, yet again, why care in the community has not been tried when it is because it has been tried and has failed that the baby has had to be admitted.

The nurses have talked of their posts being downgraded. They describe their work in terms of endurance and something 'to be got through' It has become such a strained and unpleasant experience that they do not know how to integrate it into the rest of their lives: if they talk about it at all to their friends, they don't know when to stop, and that does not help either.

Because of the intense emotional experience of working with babies there is always a pressure to 'turn off' feelings about the work, especially when babies are very seriously ill or dying. This has become much stronger in the last two years. Furthermore the nurses feel they have to pretend to parents that the ward is safe, that things are all right and are being managed. To say anything else would be disloyal

There is no leeway if a nurse feels under the weather. They have to live a lie over safety and not talk to the relatives of staff numbers being reduced or the proportion of nurses who are agency staff

They describe staff meetings with the ward sister or a manager. These often start with shifty looks and bland statements of everything being fine. The conversation goes on as if staff or management are in control. But then, some days they will start to say, 'One day something will happen.'

Is no one allowed to make a mistake or have negative feelings?

Graham told me that, alongside the macho style of management, he saw an increasingly strong culture which seemed to embody the idea that one can work without making mistakes. Such an 'omnipotent' view suppressed honesty and supervision. Graham referred to some institutional papers he had read which described the negative feelings which staff had towards their patients or other people they were caring for. How could staff feel safe enough to talk of their angry or murderous feelings, their wish for some of these children to die; or to talk of their own distress? They did not dare own their own messy feelings.

Doctors seemed a bit more able to talk of their dreams and their nightmares about work. When Graham had asked a nurse if she had dreams of work, he saw a look of fear on her face. He smiled at her and asked what the look was for: did she think he would tell the manager? That had been exactly the fear that had come to the nurse's mind.

Talking to senior staff, Graham had realised that the country used to have a large network within which health professionals could share experiences and learn from each other. It had now become a country of competitors. For

the babies and parents in the hell of their pain, the staff are rarely in touch. If the staff do not feel cared for, how can they in turn give to those facing situations of life and death?

Everything had to be done for the show. Clean, looking right, better than the neighbours. Old colleagues had become competitors and sometimes they were no longer on speaking terms.

Junior doctors

The paediatric department was known to have fulfilled the government's targets for junior doctor hours so Graham was amazed to see how really shattered they looked. He tried to learn why. Had there been a 'hidden' cost to this apparent progressive change? They did have a shift system so they had time to recuperate after a stint on duty, but the time was enough for that and that alone. They seemed to have no time to have any other life. They had no time for relationships. The women were particularly hit by this because boyfriends would not tolerate their lack of availability. They appeared tired and lethargic all the time and they got through by telling themselves (and Graham) that it was for a short time and they were learning a lot. The senior doctors did not seem to be very sympathetic, saying that they had a far worse time and even longer hours when they were juniors.

But those senior doctors, the consultant paediatricians, appeared in themselves to be sensitive human beings, so Graham was still not satisfied. He probed further and learned of other changes, which had been more gradual but could have had far reaching influences.

Today's junior doctors have a room available for them to sleep in when they are on a night shift. But it is a room and nothing more than that. Their predecessors some 20 years ago had the 'doctors' mess' which for many was their home for six months or even for a few years. There they shared a somewhat communal life with other junior doctors. There was food and drink available all the time. They felt well looked after. The many arguments for closing down the 'doctors' mess' are compelling, especially those to do with egalitarianism and privilege. But the junior doctors have lost something that made them feel valued. Today's doctors do not have that when they are sleeping in. They have nobody to look after them and no particular place to call their own.

Graham finished by saying that one of the most shocking things for him, when he has asked himself why people are being treated in the ways he has observed, has been his own self-doubt. He is challenging himself with phrases like: 'Why are you making all this fuss? Why are you whingeing? Isn't this the way the world is?'

The children's nurse: Alison's story

A child was dying in the ward and both he and his family were very distressed. Alison, the nurse in charge of the ward, realised that they needed extra care but with the staff available on the shift it was impossible for her to arrange for them to have it and to provide the nursing care required for the other patients.

She rang the on-duty manager to explain the predicament and to ask for more staff. She was told, 'There are no more. You'll have to manage.'

It was said as boldly as that, with not even 'That must be very difficult' or 'I'm sorry', either of which would have made her feel better about the decision that the manager made.

As it was Alison said, 'All right. Well, so much can be done and no more.' She added that before she went off duty she would write in the notes of the patients who were not fed and not changed that it was because there was no nurse available to do it.

An hour later another nurse did come. She had been sent from a neighbouring ward which then became short staffed in its turn. Its staff blamed Alison for causing the problem by making the fuss. Her reputation as a troublemaker was established.

That was four years ago, at the start of the reforms.

Later that year, Alison moved to another hospital at the time the new chief executive was appointed. While she was working nights she attended a meeting which he addressed. She was impressed by him coming to such a thing at night. He appeared sincere in wishing to make himself available to staff. While there were no plans for them to become a trust, he said that they could still benefit from the reforms by getting more control over their money and deciding how to spend it because 'We, that is all of us in this room, and the other clinical staff in the hospital, are the ones who know where the needs are most.' She felt reassured and even felt some enthusiasm for the reforms.

Over the next few months she noticed subtle changes in language. Patients were becoming 'clients'. Admissions and discharges were becoming 'episodes'.

The second meeting with the chief executive was a year on from the first. The trust bid was now firmly in. Management was working hell for leather to get it.

At this meeting the benefits of trust status were praised. Alison asked a question. She accepted the arguments put so far but said that she was concerned over the effect of this on the other hospitals in the neighbourhood and on the services for people who lived nearer the other hospitals. Those concerns, she was reassured, were 'not an issue' and were not relevant.

Someone else said that he remembered a meeting a year before, when the chief executive had said that there were no plans for becoming a trust. What had happened?

'I know I said that then,' the chief executive agreed, but added that things had changed. 'Quite suddenly, it appeared to be the logical thing for us to do. It was inevitable really.'

He went on to say that they had been having consultations at that time and of course wanted to hear everybody's views. But with the possibility of putting in a bid this time round and the encouragement from the regional health authority, well there was simply no time for consultation at that stage.

'You used to complain that management never got things done. Well, some things have got to be grabbed and pursued very fast. This is one of them.'

They became a trust. They had directorates which seemed to be departments with clearer management lines and more teeth. Money and responsibility were devolved. Alison did realise that there was not endless money, but thought that there would be some advantages, especially from the devolution of management.

Have you got one? Yes or no?

One of the terminally ill children which Alison and her colleagues had been looking after was readmitted to die. As was usual, the child and the family were given a side room. The baby died before all the family were there and so they needed the room for longer.

Meanwhile, the parents of a child who was not seriously ill asked for a side room. Alison said that she was sorry but there was none available. When one did become available, they might be able to have it. They were told that the staff aim always to keep one side room free for support of the very ill children and their families who were coping in the community, in case they had to come back in an emergency.

Ten minutes later, the manager stormed in. The parents had been to see him.

'Have you got a side room?'

Alison started to explain, but was interrupted.

'Have you got one? Yes or no?' Then the question was repeated.

Alison said in an annoyed manner, 'No, because there is a dead baby and the family need more time.'

The manager stormed out.

Again, for Alison, some explanation might have helped. Why would a manager behave like that? Was it a particularly stressful day for him? Had something else happened that Alison did not know about?

Ruefully, Alison thought of that first meeting with the new chief executive when he had spoken so enthusiastically of getting away from allocation by the 'decibel' factor. 'It used to be he or she who shouts most, gets most,' he said. 'We will be able to make inroads into that because you and your voices will be heard.' This episode and a few other subsequent ones reinforced Alison's fear that under the new system, in fact, the eloquent parents and relatives of patients would be getting even more of a share of the cake than under the old.

Despite the threats to complain, those parents did not do so. Others did.

One of the complaints

When Alison was on night duty, one of the mothers who was sleeping in to be with her child asked for an early morning call. Alison said they would if they could. In fact it was a very busy night and Alison was five or ten minutes late in giving the call.

Two days later the child had recovered, and she and her mother went home.

Three weeks later the manager said that the trust had received a complaint from a mother regarding a night when Alison was on duty.

'What is the complaint?'

The manager said that the mother had asked for a 6.00 am call and while she did get it she was not given a cup of coffee or anything to eat which she needed because of the stress she was under. Alison felt flabbergasted and no doubt looked it. The manager said, 'Well, did you think of giving her a coffee and something to eat?'

Alison asked for a precise definition of what the complaint had been, and explained that it had been a very busy night. When they were not busy, she and colleagues would often make tea or toast and sit with the mothers. Alison said she was amazed that the manager was even investigating such a complaint. The manager said that the directorate's manager had wanted it investigated and asked her to look into it.

Again, Alison noted, nothing was said such as 'We support you' or 'I am sorry that this has come up'.

Division is power: the meeting for morale

As many people as could be spared from immediate ward duties attended the important meeting on morale. The directorate manager said that she did not wish to cut nursing numbers, but the directorate had to make 5% savings. This had been the instruction from the trust board.

One thing they were going to do immediately was to change the telephones to allow local calls only.

Someone said that he wanted to know how much saving was expected from that. What was the telephone bill? How many non-local calls were made? What would be the cost of the modifications to the telephone system? The directorate manager said she did not know the answer to the questions and please do not ask so many like this. 'You must realise that we have to be seen to be making cuts and here is one we can do.'

Realising that the exercise was largely 'being seen to be making cuts' helped many people at the meeting to feel more sympathetic. At least there was an explanation. But then the manager went on to say that there really was a big risk of the directorate losing one part of its contract. If that happened, then there would be much less money. 'So do not moan. I can do very little about these things and we have to cut.'

Many of the staff went into the meeting with low morale and came out in fear.

We shouldn't say we've not got enough, but we've not got enough

After the case of Beverley Allitt, a children's nurse who killed children, there have been very firm recommendations on the levels of trained staff that should be on a shift. In a children's ward there should be at least two specialist nurses per shift. In fact there are not enough specialist children's nurses working in this country to be able to achieve that. It will be some time before the ones who are being trained are qualified to make up the numbers. How soon there are enough will depend on how many of those who are already doing the job, stay.

Paediatrics is a relatively high-tech part of medicine. For example blood oxygen levels are measured by an oxygen saturation monitor. In Alison's trust nurses have sometimes had to take the monitor off one baby in order to use it on another who has recently been admitted and is even more ill. The monitoring of the baby without the oxygen saturation equipment may then be done by torchlight examination of the skin colour.

The treatment of cancer includes chemotherapy together with costly new drugs which stop children being sick when they are having it. These new drugs have sometimes been discouraged by managers and then started again after doctors have made a terrible fuss. Staff wondered if the management were worried that there might be a more public fuss if some of the more vocal parents got to hear of what was happening.

Many of the staff were quite sympathetic to the need to cut expenditure, but often thought that it would be more bearable if there did not still seem to be so many more managers.

Who meets the important visitors?

When needed, managers are often hard to find because they are in meetings or on 'away days', but have a visit by a VIP and there they are. When local sports people or politicians have been on a visit, staff have seen managers whose faces they did not recognise. It usually seemed to take five managers to welcome visitors. Nice children were found to be presented to them in neat and cheerful bays. No blood, no death, no staff in tears.

One nurse wondered if the politicians would spot the cosmetic cleanness and tidiness of the place and the controlled behaviour of the staff. He wondered if one day, one of the political visitors would do a 'walkabout' and really meet the staff. His friends thought him naïve.

Paperwork

As part of the processes of skill mix and work load monitoring, 'dependency forms' have been introduced into many hospitals. The idea is that the indices of dependency can be an indication of work load. Like all these forms, nurses filled them in, sometimes as best they could, and sometimes even better by making up figures. Starting levels were included in the forms so as to 'equate' needs with provision. In some children's wards and other high-dependency units, staff created an extra 'box' in the form and labelled it 'number of agency staff'.

Clinical staff have often insisted that agency staff were less effective than members of the regular team. 'Don't they have the same number of hands?' would be the manager's retort.

A friend of Alison in another trust had been filling in such forms ever since they were first introduced. Suddenly they were told that their use had been stopped. When asked about this in a directorate meeting, the manager said that the forms had not been filled out properly and so they could not be used. In fact, it was said that they have been done so badly that it had been a waste of time. Why this bit of paperwork had to be dropped became clearer later when a number of the staff were in a manager's office and saw all the forms there. Seeing them together, it was obvious that the dependency scores were so high as to indicate that six more nurses were needed, a figure that would never be achieved with the financial problems of the trust.

This time the staff really did understand why a management decision had been made.

Some more muddle and a complaint

On one occasion money was so short that they had all been told again that the budget would be cut if they did not make savings. For a time, even supplies of baby food were held up. Alison rubbed this point in: in yet another year in which more money, in real terms, was being spent on the NHS by the government, here they were worrying where the next jar of baby food was coming from.

Of course no one knew where the money came from or from which section of the budget. No one knew whose responsibility it was. Except that it was certainly not the mother's responsibility because the mothers were not allowed any responsibility. The parents were more than willing to bring in baby food themselves, but the managers would not allow it. Regulations to do with glass and tins being brought into the building were brought up. The nurses then had to deal with the parents, particularly the mothers, feeling 'disempowered'. (Alison glowed as she turned that piece of management speak against the reforms). The parents were allowed less and less responsibility, but when the nurses had asked the manager whose responsibility it was to have food for the babies, the manager had walked out of the ward.

Alison continued to live in fear of complaints. This was not because she felt she was a particularly culpable person or in danger of being disciplined, or worse. It was simply that, with the Patient's Charter and the initiative to hear the user's voice, far more complaints were coming through and every single one was taken up.

Another mother asked for a single room but was told that there was none available because one was being kept for use by a dying child who might be brought in.

The nurse thought no more of this, a relatively routine event.

A month later she was sent for by another night manager. In an aggressive manner, she was told that there had been a complaint that she had refused the single room. 'What happened?' Because the incident had been at least a month before, the nurse asked to see the notes to remind herself of what she had written. She was shown the letter only and realised that the mother had probably met the manager later that day and may even have been asked, 'Everything all right?'

It was not unusual for a manager to walk into the nurses' office, say 'There's another complaint,' leave a letter on the desk and walk out.

Carer power and market power

'Nurse, will you look after my baby while I go to the canteen?'

'Well no, I'm sorry. I can't do that. I will listen out for your baby but I can't be there all the time because I have got the other children to look after.'

'That's not good enough. You are the named nurse.'

A teaching hospital often takes private cases from other governments. They are a sort of 'international ECR'. They also take quite a lot of ECR cases from other parts of the UK. They are treated differently from other cases.

'I want you to do a CT scan on my child.'

'It's not necessary.'

'It may not be necessary but I want it done.'

Because they are paying cases or because they are ECRs so that the purchaser is paying money to the trust, such a demand is met — even though it is unnecessary, may have dangerous possible side effects and uses resources which would otherwise be part of 'spare capacity' available for the non-ECR cases. Thus a small but growing group is getting more of what it *wants*, but not of what it *needs* — at the expense of the majority who are getting less of what they want *and* less of what they need.

Sometimes they fear that things will go the way of one of the southern states in the USA, where a prestige private hospital had more CT scanners than the whole of Canada, while the state hospital next door had none.

Certain procedures called 'delivering treatments' may be done only by a registered sick children's nurse (RSCN). Examples include giving intravenous drugs, drugs into drips, and chemotherapy.

Because of the money from ECRs and private cases, many children requiring these treatments are admitted. Often there is one RSCN on the ward and therefore a big demand is placed upon that person's time. The procedures cannot all be done at the same time, so if there are more than a few, it is very difficult to keep them to a regular schedule. And they are not done as well as if there were fewer. Furthermore the RSCN is then not available for other cases where other special skills, such as support for the dying, are needed

Fear of discipline and punitive measures appears to lead all staff to be afraid of everybody else, and to live in fear of the hospital or trust being tarnished or of losing money.

So many things make Alison sad and angry, yet this very peculiar and special 'side effect' of the market forces is different. It arises not because of shortage of money or resources in the usual sense. It is more complicated and perhaps more subtle. Because the trust wants to get in as much money as possible it takes in the special cases that require the skills of the RSCN. The RSCN then becomes very busy and can no longer sit with the dying children when their relatives are away. They are sat with by the untrained staff, or left by themselves for their dying.

Chapter 17

That 'phone tap': what *did* happen?

When I was a consultant in the NHS and I was away from work, I always expected my colleagues to open my mail. At least it would reduce the pile to deal with when I came back. There might be urgent referrals, though this seemed unlikely because I reckoned that anybody with an urgent referral would telephone.

John Spencer, a consultant radiologist of nearly 50, might not have been ruffled to find his mail had been opened while he had been away, but he was surprised to find that each letter or circular had been stamped by the office of the chief executive of the trust.

Should this be ridden out as yet another example of the increasing bureaucracy and centralisation of the NHS reforms that he was becoming so familiar with? Or was it the last straw in an increasingly burdensome bombardment of regulations, resistance and refusal to listen to nearly anything that clinicians suggested?

He had a discussion with the BMA and they talked of the possibility of using grievance procedures, of which John Spencer probably had no experience at all.

But work continued. John Spencer was a consultant of a high-tech department and had been looking forward to the commissioning of the very expensive MRI scanner which had been installed shortly before he went away on his three weeks' leave (one week's study, two weeks' annual). The arrival of the scanner had been the culmination of years of negotiation which had required the utmost patience and tolerance of frustration, with submissions and petitions rewritten in whatever language or on whatever form was then currently being used in the NHS.

Back in his own office, something was not working quite right with his computer. I would have panicked and cried for help, but he was more than computer literate. He worked with electronic equipment. He checked the connections at the back of the computer and discovered a stranger: an extra wire had got around there, and it turned out to be coming from the socket of his telephone.

Well, strange things do happen in hospitals. There were enough stories of office furniture being removed, or the users of offices being allocated different ones while they were away on leave. And the days of the courteous, 'We have something to do in your office. Do you mind if we do it on such and such a date, or when you are away?' were long gone. Perhaps wondering about patients' rights to confidentiality when a technician worked in and around a consultant's desk, John Spencer unplugged the wire.

What you learn when you take a pee

Adjoining this consultant's office was a WC which he visited later. Maybe something had stimulated his critical powers of observation (some doctor training is very useful) for he noticed a new section of ducting, which he was sure had not been there before his leave. Again, nothing particularly strange, because it is not unusual in a hospital for building and maintenance work of one sort or another to be going on all the time. What was strange was that the panel covering the new section was fixed by only two screws. Fixtures on hospital walls are usually fitted with lots of screws. He was now feeling inquisitive. It was easy to remove the screws. There he found, underneath a notice saying 'Do not disturb', a tape recorder. Not much sophistication was needed to discover that the tape recorder had been connected to the telephone on his desk and not much ingenuity required to confirm that it was activated by the use of the telephone.

The BMA, an ever present help in time of trouble, suggested calling in the police. The police had not seen anything like this before and later in the afternoon wanted to take the equipment away with them, but could find no senior manager to authorise the removal.

The 'Do not disturb' was not being disturbed.

No real sense of clarity was achieved until in the last two minutes of the day when the telephone rang. The chief executive told John that he was suspended immediately.

The lull

It seems that in these things, like after many other crises, there is a period of numbness or quiet before acute reaction. First things went quiet. Then there was a curious, private, ritual. The man who had been personnel officer in the motor industry before starting his ten years as chairman, first of the district health authority and then of this acute services trust, did something: *he burned the tape.*

The storm

'Top Doc Bugged' ran the local paper headline.

From local press to local radio. Then to television and the national press.

You may well have noticed the Luton and Dunstable hospital if you have ever driven north along the M1 from London to Birmingham. It is easy to see. Furthermore you may have been observed from the hospital for the motorway has for years been one of the things gazed at by women passing long hours of waiting in the maternity ward. It was very easy for the media to pounce.

And it was very easy for me to visit and also to meet some people who had made their own visits over the months before.

The building itself is like that of many a sprawling modern hospital. 1960s rectangular style with lots of glass. Situated within good view of the country's main motorway and five miles from an international airport, the hospital is in a good position for picking up trauma work and was one of several sites chosen by the government for the influx of war wounded from the Gulf War, if they had come. It sports the usual corridors, lifts, stairs, notices and sign-posts. Outstanding good features to be noticed by the newcomer include the pleasant foyer with shop, cafeteria, enquiry desk and comfortable chairs; and it is generally well lit everywhere.

The staff

There were many accounts of an angry confrontational style among the senior management over the past few years. It was a hospital driven from the centre and by command. Tales of 'Right! What had we got here? Theft! Instant dismissal!' 'Theft again! Instant dismissal!' Tales of fingers being wagged in admonition. Of managers publicly embracing in jubilation on 'winning' a disciplinary hearing into somebody else's behaviour.

Senior staff shaking as they entered the hospital and looking over their shoulders as they walked the corridors. Several spoke to me of feeling what they thought it might have been like living in a totalitarian state: fear all the time and a fear of spies. They did not know whom they could trust and so they talked less to those who had been friends.

(The description reminded me of a change in my own behaviour in the two or three years before my retirement. For 20 years, whenever I had to go from one end of the hospital to the other, I would walk through the corridors hoping that I would meet people, at least to say hello. During the last two years given the same destination, I behaved differently, I would take an outdoor route, so as to reduce the chances of meeting particular people.)

And there were tales of obstruction to safe clinical practice. For example:

A routinely admitted patient became very ill and was found to have a rare bacterial infection resistant to all the usual antibiotics. Consultations took place between the clinicians on the ward and the staff in the pathology department with the conclusion that a small isolation unit would be necessary for there to be any confidence that the hospital could be reasonably safe again. The medical staff committee supported this. Nurses and doctors were in agreement, but found that the managers challenged every point of the recommendation and its argument, saying again and again that the ward and laboratory staff had to deal with the patient's condition within their own resources.

As predicted by the clinicians, the infection took a stronger hold on the original patient and spread to others. Not an isolation unit, but a whole isolation ward had to be created before the infection was got under control. This must have cost far more than the original proposal which had been derided by the managers. No one knew if the delay in getting the infection controlled had led to an increase in the pool of people harbouring the germs in the community.

Cynics have said that the last point was the least to worry managers: more deadly infections would mean more business. Worrying over public health was, after all, the responsibility of the purchaser, not of the trust.

There were also the all too common stories of reorganisation of the system of dealing with outpatients. Instead of working with the staff doing the job (see the 're-engineering' approach described in Chapter 18 following my visit to Leicester Royal Infirmary), at the Luton and Dunstable the managers reorganised the dedicated staff who had been running the appointments and outpatient systems not too badly over the years. They did this by central diktat. Some staff were made redundant and new staff were brought in to run the new service. Of course it settled down as most things do, but sometimes the trust was paying a consultant to do an outpatient clinic when no patients were there; or there would be the same number of consultants but double the number of patients; or the right number of consultants and the right patients and the right times, but no equipment. And then there was an attempt to return to the old system with some modifications.

Staff talked of the two years it had taken to change the hospital from being reasonably well known and competently run, with dedicated and enthusiastic staff, to being a place of high tension with fearful colleagues who were getting on badly with each other, wanting to get out and being afraid to talk. Several people told me that the most envied staff were the older ones, who were nearer to retirement. Staff did acknowledge that there had been a need to get into budget and that this had been done. Several people said they were worried about talking to me.

What else had the new managers done, with short term contracts, targets to meet, their own supervisors or managers making demands on them?

With the reforms came clinical directorships and then, as centralisation strengthened, a reduction in the number of clinical directorships. It became clear to the staff that the managers' intention was not that the clinical directors and the medical director of the trust should put a clinical view to the board, but rather that they were there to put trust policy to the clinical teams.

The new management appeared to understand well the value of splitting staff, if their intention was to cow them into submission. Several staff mentioned the terror of the splitting process: for example, if some people criticised the chief executive, others would jump to her defence, or try to make excuses for her. You never knew whose side it was best to be on.

Medical staff had to learn a new language: 'business plans'. They decided to co-operate with the reforms and so they learned this language and worked hard on the paperwork. They had joined the likes of all the people I was to meet in the new health service, people who were taking work home: papers and reports to read; memoranda to respond to; proposals and documents to work on; business plans to produce to a deadline.

The business plans were produced not in isolation, but in consultation with the managers and to formulae dictated by the 'new world'. But still this was not good enough and there were stories of the chief executive deriding the documents produced by junior managers and senior consultants as 'rubbish'.

(I came across this phenomenon in many other places and heard of it first from colleagues even before I retired. Several people, clinicians and managers whom I knew well, described hours of work on business plans, with outside consultants guiding the process. The finished product was then criticised by higher management as not being a business plan at all. I think now that those more senior managers were probably having the rules by which they were working changed under their feet as they went along. They took this out on those whom they could push around. It also reminded me of how I had come across managers understanding some aspects of the reforms differently.)

There had been attempts to challenge what was happening, but at the usual cost. One clinical director, struggling with the conflict of directing good clinical work and trying to support the trust line, was told in a meeting that a particular matter had never been raised. In desperation this consultant quoted the number of times that it had been discussed and put in writing.

I shall now reconstruct what I deduce happened a few days after that remark was made:

A friendly meeting started with concern. 'You are working hard…Are you working too hard?…Perhaps you are doing too much…Perhaps you should resign…You don't have to go on being clinical director for ever.'

But the clinical director wanted to continue.

'Right, I'm sacking you.'

A form of challenge which the medical staff did try was to pass a vote of 'no confidence'. They heard this had been done with the chief executive in a previous post. Sadly, they had not been trained in management techniques well enough by the managers or on the management courses that many of them had attended. They did not have the vote of 'no confidence' as an item on their meeting agenda, so the trust did not recognise it.

And several people told me that they had kept their heads down.

After the immediate publicity

John Spencer remained suspended. There followed secret meetings and what is known as a 'negotiated deal' of early retirement for somebody not yet 50. This happened quickly and the man was clearly shocked and distressed. He was the first of many consultants and senior managers I met who had seen their GP for stress and been prescribed tranquillisers or antidepressants.

Many remarks that were attributed to the chief executive during the furore of the next few days do not surprise me when I think of the tension there must have been. However, I was interested to hear that, during the weeks leading up to it all, some visitors were told by her, and with obvious pleasure, of her close relationship with consultants.

Both the chief executive and the personnel officer were suspended and then reinstated.

Later, with increasing pressure, this 'exceptional chief executive' who had been 'totally trustworthy and a first class employee', resigned.

The press release in November 1994

The chairman of the trust, who had himself destroyed some of the important evidence in this matter (the tape), commissioned an independent review of the phone tap. That review was conducted by the Anglia and Oxford regional office of the NHS executive. When their report was received by the chairman of the board, he issued his own report and a press release.

The confidential agreement for the early retirement of the consultant was within the authority of the trust, but one of the key comments of the report was that the chairman should have sought the views of the board. The confidentiality of the retirement agreement now prevented full discussion of the rationale for placing the tap on the phone. The board agreed that any future confidentiality clauses would be discussed by the board and reviewed by independent advisers before implementation.

Why John Spencer?

From what I could gather, he was a critic of the new management style and a persistent arguer for his own department, which he had built up to some level of prominence and success. The newspaper reports around the time suggested that the overt reasons for management concern and his suspension before midnight that day were to do with allegations that (1) he had been receiving sponsorship from an equipment manufacturer for attending a conference in Bali; (2) he had plans to set up a private ultrasound scanning service which would compete with the trust; and (3) a bank statement was found in the mail opened during his absence.

Disciplinary action for such matters seems strange in today's NHS where staff are encouraged to get sponsorship or money from whatever source possible. Being involved in private services or their setting up and development has, many would say, been actively encouraged by the government. Around the same time as this story was happening, Sir Duncan Nichol was leaving his job as chief executive of the NHS executive and was shortly to receive a post in the private sector. He had even been involved in the appointment of the senior managers for the eight regional authorities in England and Wales, and this only days before leaving his post. Was the thought of working in the private sector not there?

In the interests of open communication, it is a pity that, while the report recommended a confidential agreement should be avoided unless the matter concerned patient care and that the trust should 'establish clear criteria for confidentiality in trust affairs', it did not go on to recommend that whatever financial arrangements were agreed in his retirement deal should be honoured if John Spencer were now to say what happened. That is, there was no recommendation that the confidentiality clause should be removed.

John Spencer remained gagged.

Our meeting

I went to see John Spencer at his home.

'I will give you a cup of coffee and talk about the NHS if you like, but I won't discuss what happened to me.'

I agreed not to talk about it.

So we had a cup of coffee and discussed the NHS, but of this story I learned no more.

As I drove away I wondered if there would ever be some sort of 30 year rule for NHS documents, as there is for government papers.

Postscript: the Beverley Report

As I was editing this chapter I suddenly remembered something that had happened a couple of years before I retired. It had not been so public as the phone tap, but it certainly got out beyond Luton and Dunstable. The NHS management executive (East Outpost Team, Ongar Drive, Brentwood, Essex) was called in. Nigel Beverley was at that time executive director of the outpost.

The sacking of a member of staff who had fraudulently filled in a form for pathological services (at, I am confident, no risk to patients or anyone for whom the management had any clinical responsibility) and the handling of the outpatient services reorganisation had, I was told, been the matters which boiled over.

The visit was arranged in a typically centralised way. Nigel Beverley was given a list of names of people to see. The list, compiled by the management, did not include many of those who had spoken vociferously in meetings, but in fact Nigel Beverley was responsive when others asked to see him.

The Beverley Report was widely circulated, talked about and leaked in and after 1992. The management was recommended to improve communications and mutual trust between the board and the medical staff. The chief executive was encouraged to think how her management style was perceived. The board was encouraged to review the amount of control which the chief executive had and the amount of delegation allowed within the trust; and to consider the need for nursing leadership at board level.

The last requirement was most neatly met. It is a statutory rule for there to be nursing representation at board level. The chief executive had been a trained nurse and a matron before she was 30. Therefore there was nursing leadership at board level. It seemed to be thought by the board to be necessary to do no more. They had, after all, considered it.

Chapter 18

Leicester Royal Infirmary: a place that works?

In the year I retired, the 'Medical Manager of the Year' was Mr Nick Naftalin, a consultant gynaecologist and medical director of Leicester Royal Infirmary NHS trust (LRI). It seemed natural to contact him and he seemed ready to meet me.

Before the mid-1980s LRI functioned in the usual way. The people who shouted more, got more: the people who shouted less, got less. It took a long time. There were long waits, muddles and confusing bureaucracy. To get the approval for a new consultant required a dozen committees.

After the Griffiths Report in 1985, two hospitals were quick off the mark in appointing unit general managers (UGMs): Guy's Hospital in London and the LRI. One year later, the UGM in Leicester met consultants to discuss devolved budgets and more accountability. Staff in a number of departments were interested in clinical directorates. In obstetrics and gynaecology they wanted Nick Naftalin to be their clinical director and, after he had expressed willingness, he was duly appointed by the UGM. I noted that management made the appointment, but after finding out who had support.

In his new role, Nick Naftalin found that his department had no record of how much equipment it had, knowledge of its budget, or of the number of staff employed. For the first year and a bit he worked on data collection and in the second year could start the first business plan.

This was all happening already in LRI when the government launched the reforms in 1989. The ideas of purchaser/provider split with one group of people having responsibility for determining the health care needs for the population and another for providing services which could then be purchased by the first group fitted well with the way they were already thinking.

The trust is formed

One of the first things the trust needed was a medical director. It already had 14 clinical directors and they were all doctors. There were also half a dozen executive directors in other aspects of management. Nick Naftalin was asked to be medical director and he agreed.

One of the first things done by the new top team of chief executive, executive directors and medical director, was to reduce the number of clinical directorates from 14 to 8.

From starting with a deficit, the trust now balances its books. Its 'strategic direction' has some 70 strands, each the responsibility of one of the executive directors and each being tackled. The trust had spent more on new equipment in the last two years than the old management did in the previous ten years.

In four months, agreement was reached for a new oncology block, a combined obstetrics and gynaecology block, and the rehousing of ophthalmic services. A few years earlier, a change of comparable magnitude would have taken at least five years.

One surgeon became the 'Doctor of the Year' and another received the Moynihan Prize. The Hewlett Packard Management Development Prize (also national) was awarded for the 'single clinic visit outpatients system'. And the Medical Manager of the Year in 1994 was Nick Naftalin.

Re-engineering

Remember those ratings which the government introduced? LRI had been eleventh from bottom for having more than a 30 minute wait for an outpatient appointment; and in the bottom rank for those waiting for more than five minutes to be seen in accident and emergency.

But LRI was one of two hospitals which sent three of its most senior executives, including the medical director, to a three day re-engineering presentation by Michael Hammer in Boston.

LRI then applied to the NHS executive for funding and was successful, apparently the sole national site for a pilot of re-engineering in the NHS. At all levels of staff they held a large number of small group sessions with a dozen people in each. These were used to identify three or four dissatisfactions over the way they were delivering services. High on the list came outpatients. One detail of their discoveries: many X-ray films were never taken out of their envelopes. One of their 'laboratories' in phase 1 was to work out how to make their outpatient services more efficient. Half a dozen people worked on this full time for three or four months together with a couple of consultants giving one or two sessions per week with others available as ad hoc advisers. The laboratory produced ideas, a prototype, pilot study, test, revaluation, modification, re-piloting. By then they thought they had the methodology correct and disbanded the laboratory. The re-engineering team had the job of conveying what they had learned to the three hundred or more clinics in the hospital.

The result was a dramatic change in outpatient waiting times, efficiency in making appointments and getting letters out to GPs. Many of the clinics became single visit clinics, sweeping away much of the old waiting time (to see the consultant, for the tests and investigations, for the results of those, to see the consultant again; plus, often more waits for repeated or extra tests, and another for the consultant).

Everything now takes place in one visit, albeit a long one. Many of the tests, ordered by the GP, are done beforehand. Tests that are ordered on the day are done immediately and many of the results come back within one hour.

One particular well meant practice was discovered to disrupt the waiting times of some clinics. If an emergency patient was referred, the staff organising the clinic would slip the new person in at the beginning. This would make everybody else late. The consultant doing the clinic did not know, and of course the patients never complained.

In the accident and emergency department the re-engineering teams discovered that a person may go through over 70 'hand-offs' (e.g. porter to receptionist, receptionist to staff nurse, staff nurse to doctor, doctor to X-ray clerk, X-ray clerk to X-ray technician).

Seven people used to have a part in dealing with letters from GPs: opening, sorting, date stamping, transferring, putting them in consultants' pigeon holes. By the end of two weeks, the consultant would have seen them and be deciding what to do: offering urgent or non-urgent appointments, or writing a letter to the GP.

The result of the changes? Now 94% of outpatients are seen within 30 minutes. (If the fracture clinic is excluded from this, it is very nearly 100%.) 80% of investigations are received by the consultant within one hour of ordering them. In some clinics letters to the referring GP are dictated, typed and signed by the end of the day. The same number of patients is being seen, but the waiting rooms usually look nearly empty.

Re-engineering led to the appointment of a clinic co-ordinator to deal with all the letters. Now most replies are arranged within half a day. This made partially redundant six people, who were offered new work. Many investigations are now done by 'multi-skilled' people in 'near patient testing' (LRI jargon for doing tests in the vicinity of the patient): routine blood and biochemistry tests, ECGs and simple X-rays with a guarantee that the results will be back within the hour.

There were a hundred re-engineering projects, in various stages, at the time of my visit to Leicester. Leaving aside the jargon which seems to grow up around any new project and which I will not disclose, it's impressive.

Are the reforms all golden?

LRI is in the middle of an oval, ringed by good hospitals with whom there was a long history of cordial rather than predatory relationships. Where ECRs start to come into one of the LRI specialist departments, the management's response is to try to get contracts, so at least the predator role is not forced on the clinicians.

It continues to be easy to borrow almost as much capital as the trust wants, and LRI has been unable to prevent some spilling of capital before the end of some financial years. Some of this happens in the devolved directorates and some comes from higher up the hierarchy when the managers find spare and say, in effect, 'Look, there is more. Do you want some of it?' (In the financial year 1996/7 the capital available from the government is reduced by one-sixth but may be made up by the private finance initiative. The trouble is that the private finance initiative seems to be not quite as straightforward to manage as was first expected, like so much else.)

It was therefore easy to get more equipment or to put money into waiting list initiatives. Although the trust has created a dozen new consultant posts in its first two years, it is still trying to increase the number of intensive care beds and the services of vascular surgery.

The medical director's own work load? Nick Naftalin is half time medical director and half time consultant gynaecologist. He has given up obstetrics. He acknowledges that he takes an appalling amount of work home which invades his weekends and his family. He never reads a book. He is often far afield at 'away days' or weekend conferences. He cannot afford the time for a substantial private practice. Financially, in spite of performance related pay (PRP), he is markedly worse off.

By the end of 1996, he had done ten years in management. If he wishes to be a full time clinician again, who will succeed him?

I found other people to talk to

I got in touch with over a dozen people who worked at LRI and were prepared to see me. I met most of them. But first, let me describe the physical structure of this 1,000-bed hospital with eight clinical directorships.

Mostly neat, clean and tidy. It appeared busy. I found it to be no more difficult or easy to find my way around than most other hospitals. Some of it appeared startlingly good, such as a stained glass screen, commissioned ten years ago, along one corridor; a sign of care in the past. There were original paintings in many corridors and foyers.

Capital investment was obvious. The hospital is in good repair and appears well looked after. There were the usual major building works and on one site, among the skips and lorries, set in concrete and surrounded by used cigarette ends, I found a pleasant wrought iron bench. I sat on it in the sun.

Re-engineering again

Changing patterns of behaviour, structure and beliefs takes time. Some people have been taken away from their departments for weeks and other staff have had to be employed. Consultations and planning, not confrontation.

Re-engineering crosses discipline boundaries. The medication process as a whole was examined. Already a named pharmacist was attached to each clinical directorate and the part played by them and by physicians, nurses and others was scrutinised.

Flows through the hospital. There have been studies of the people walking around. (I was asked, very courteously, to answer a few questions and got away with saying that I had come to visit someone.) And on how information and objects move.

In pursuing the theme of the distribution of services, I learned that the pharmaceutical, pathological and radiological services had been 're-engineered' together deliberately, so that they simply had to co-operate across disciplines. Result: delivery of services from some of these departments can now be hourly.

Some enthusiasts told me that, within the last year, re-engineering had taken over the 'change energy' of the institution. It sounded better than looking at the possibilities of departments having individual contracts with other directorates. Now other staff are coming up with ideas and are themselves questioning what is happening in their work practice.

Some more history

Others too were enthusiastic about the story, confirming that clinical directorates and business managers started ten years ago. Pharmacy budgets were devolved to the directorates themselves. (I had come across a similar thing in London around that time, when resource management was first in vogue.)

When some of my informants started work at LRI it was a district general hospital (DGH) with a medical school attached. It had not been developed as a teaching hospital. Now it really is a teaching hospital with well integrated academic and clinical sides.

The long-standing clinical directorships and business managers made it possible for LRI to jump at the reforms and make the purchaser/provider split work for a shared care policy. In early discussion with GPs, purchaser and providers, it was agreed that the hospitals would provide the most expensive drugs. This required good communication between the GPs and the hospitals, with the pharmacists attending meetings.

Medical admissions go into one admission ward. The clinical firm 'on take' has this ward for 24 hours and must distribute all patients admitted within 6 hours. The patients must go home, to the acute ward or to rehabilitation. This has worked well and the stress of handling admissions has been reduced.

How was management seen?

I asked people for their views of the management. Several reminded me that LRI already had an advanced management style and structure before the current reforms got under way. The management is seen as up-front and honest, but trapped by having to obey the government and set the trust up against others when they all serve the same population.

When I pressed further on relationships between managers and medical staff I was again told that they were on the whole good. Recently there had been a meeting between managers and consultants at 8.30 on a Saturday morning. It was not a three line whip, yet 100 consultants turned up.

When management-led discussions on trust status started, the consultants felt that their agreement was required and their views were respected. Initially there was strong resistance from the consultants, concerned about the carefully developed complementarity of the three city hospitals, without duplication of the 'tertiary' specialities. It was only when there was a large body of consultants in favour of change, in the third year, that application was made.

Why so different from most places I had visited? My informants thought that it might be different personalities, or managers being more 'home grown'. Very few had been brought in from outside. They know what is going on and they have a non-confrontational style.

This pattern came nearest to being broken with the appointment of the chief executive. There was more than one interview with no appointment, before the internal candidate got the job. They appear to respect this person at LRI.

Unlike in many hospitals, the consultants have not felt the management has been looking over their shoulders all the time, controlling the minutiae of day to day work.

I asked if the reforms meant that fundholding GP cases were dealt with differently. Not exactly. Early on they were 'supposed' to call in a certain number of fundholding GP cases and these were identified by yellow stickers on the files. That pressure went very quickly when the rooms and files were flooded with yellow stickers. At one blow of inspired shopping in a nearby stationery shop, pressure to give preferential handling to fundholding cases was killed. And without, as far as I could make out, recrimination. Perhaps the management did listen.

There remains pressure for numbers. Clinical and commercial conflicts become a problem when winter medical emergencies occupy surgical beds, making it difficult for those directorates to meet their contracts. Towards the end of one year, management stopped teams that were ahead of target and 'transferred' operating theatre time to others. This created problems for the teams which had managed well (or struck lucky), together with jibes from some who said that others had got softer contracts and friction between the different clinical teams and between clinicians and management. There was much anger at having been told to be more efficient and then prevented from being efficient. Staff talked of the efficient being praised or penalised, and the inefficient being rewarded. That phase was now over. Contracts and efficiencies have to be worked on, but not in that way. Another sign of management learning.

How wards are managed: prepared to try and perhaps to learn

What is the role of the ward manager in this 1,000-bed teaching hospital, with its eight clinical directorates, each handling its own outpatient department as well as wards? Attending monthly clinical directorate meetings of ward managers, business managers, nurse manager and clinical director (between 12 and 20 people altogether), sometimes with a specialist nurse in attendance for a particular item; meeting the nurse manager (probably weekly); being nurse 'bleep holder' for the directorate (probably once a fortnight); doing the individual performance review (IPR) of each auxiliary nurse; reading, attending some consultant ward rounds to remain up to date and able to fulfil a leader role; handling routine management to do with sickness and sick notes; keeping a watching, and sometimes organising, eye on the training needs of staff and their personal and professional development.

The nurse manager of the directorate, with an individual office and direct line, is not a stranger to the wards, into which he or she will drop weekly and always go to the nurses' station first: they seem to know each other. The nurse manager does the IPR for the ward manager.

The auxiliary nurses sit in on the same hand-over as the trained staff. (Part of acknowledging that, although they are paid to do the donkey work, they are also valuable members of the team and that the patients will talk to them.)

Before admission to hospital, patients are asked to bring in their own drugs. This is partly so that the medical staff can see exactly what a patient was taking, and it was also for the implementation of a Leicester district wide drugs policy. 'Stock drugs' are returned to the patient immediately or kept in a cupboard, to be given back on discharge. Unusual drugs are dealt with differently and, at least in the first instance, the patient's own are used.

If someone comes up with an idea, it may be given a three month trial and then looked at again. Patient care plans on the wards were handwritten on two A4 pieces of paper before they were all computerised. There was a two inch wide margin for nursing evaluation. On one ward nurses suggested revisions. One suggested using one A4 piece of paper, portrait position (vertical); another, one A4 piece of paper, landscape (horizontal). The ward manager agreed to try both at the same time for three months, on alternate patients: then the nurses would decide which was best. The horizontally placed paper, with its longer line to write on, was favoured. The system worked well until the introduction of the present computerised standardised care plan.

Dealing with the job

The reforms and the media publicity have all raised expectations well beyond a point that can be matched by staff. Ward managers and clinical nurses, often unable to tell somebody exactly what is wrong, can at least be more clear than in the past about what is definitely not wrong. Increased openness is useful, but, as the public becomes more vociferous, some relatives have become more rude.

The ward managers often wear uniforms on clinical days but not for the non-clinical day, at least once a week. It was their decision to structure the week like this, with the non-clinical day being different each week.

The separation of clinical from non-clinical days frees those managers who do it to do hands-on work when they want. More than ward sisters ever used to. It has become part of monitoring standards. Patients may comment that something is being done differently: a flannel for wiping the hands after using the commode for example. On those days it is also possible to get a better awareness of the clinical work load of the nurses, to demonstrate and witness interpersonal skills with patients and relatives, and to notice how the other staff are handling the paperwork, assessment forms etc.

Other ways in which nursing has been driven by the reforms

The reduction in the junior doctor hours has expanded the role of nurses. Some have a certificate of advanced life support techniques. Nurses take blood samples, give intravenous drugs or defibrillate patients in cardiac arrest: no waiting for the doctor to put the equipment in place and press the magic button. Asthma nurse specialists see patients, prescribe inhalers and changes in therapeutic regimes.

At night, the nurse manager may certify some deaths and cannulate veins without calling on the doctor.

A positive skill mix

On one ward a late shift four years ago would have comprised one qualified nurse and three or four learners. When I visited, there were three qualified nurses and one auxiliary. All on a budget managed at ward level. The purchasers need 'quality' information so they need the correct skill mix. The staff have to monitor pressure sores, accidents, falls. The nursing dependency level for each patient is a measure of how much each requires and if this goes up for the ward as a whole to more than a certain number (it seemed to vary from four or six), they need more staff.

In negotiating changes the nurses, prepared with figures and proposals, are now better able to fight their corner. I saw it as an awareness of corporate risk and its management, with each discipline now more ready to compromise and listen to the others.

A twist in the tail? People seem to be joining the nursing profession because they like the buzz and are interested in getting a diploma or a degree. Patients are better informed regarding diagnoses and treatments and come with more sophisticated questions. The nurses must be more sophisticated in responding. Tender loving care (TLC) was sometimes what the nurses would put forward first as their special contribution. Now, far more, it is individual skills: a nurse may need some nurturing to be able to deliver TLC.

Junior doctors' hours

The gradual reduction of junior doctors' hours and payment for out of hours work has been a shared negotiation between the profession and the government. The government has been energetic on this. Some costing of activity has been a logical consequence, but the zeal for 'time/cost' has been a government initiative. I was therefore interested to find out how LRI had tackled it.

There, the house officers' right to a day off and precise limitations on hours was respected all through their training. In the relationship between junior doctors and hospital, every hour is counted and costed as never before. Continuity is reduced, and pressure on those on duty is increased: junior doctors are on call less, but cover more; and, on call, run far faster.

Three years before my visits, the coronary care unit was covered 24 hours a day by six doctors; now by nearly three times that number. Each of those doctors does one night in two weeks, but only one of them will be working in the coronary unit during the day, so only one is a 'culture carrier' and only one sees follow up for her or his decisions and actions. The others will not even be in the room for another fortnight.

I heard examples of surgeons doing lengthy emergency overnight operations 'talking' the junior doctor through stage by stage and spending time before and after the procedure to ensure the maximum training experience. Some consultants have then suggested going on to do a ward round together, to check on other patients operated on within the last 24 hours, only to be told by the junior doctor that it was not possible, because his or her off duty time had come. The consultants had a day's work ahead.

Here I did detect a feeling that management was not always understanding, or sympathetic. Talk of a memo instructing that work not finished by the house officer by 5.00 pm was for the consultant to complete. Talk of a junior doctors' forum at which one of them was noticed to be looking fed up. 'Yes,' was the reply, 'it had been a bad week, because for a couple of days work had to go on until 5.15 pm.' The manager said quite seriously that he was sure the consultant would look into that and turned in the direction of some of them. In an enterprise where managers and consultants are taking more work home than ever before, it was easy to understand how some consultants find it hard to see their trainees as people to be nurtured, because they cannot see them as successors.

What is going to happen with this generation of trainee doctors when they become consultants? They see less of consultants (and consultants of them) than their predecessors did. Apart from having less clinical training, one part of being a consultant of which the junior doctors have less experience is the assumption of overall awareness and responsibility (even planning a week). It is part of being a consultant, so far. (Some consultants I met in other places wondered if that role will be taken over by managers. It did seem to be in the mind of the trust chairman I mention at the end of the book.) At LRI I met consultants who were wondering if the new system will leave room for altruism.

What is happening to today's consultants is that they are working harder.

Consultants' work load and thoughts of retiring

The consultants are doing more clinical work as junior doctors do less and more paper and management work to meet the requirements of the reforms. $1^1/_2$ hours of paperwork each evening seemed to be the average for the consultants to be taking home, often around 7.00 pm.

Such a work load is impossible to maintain.

Two of the young consultants I met had started, against all their previous expectations, to take private patients and to make serious enquiries about retirement from the NHS at 50. (I met two consultants elsewhere, in their mid-thirties, who were talking of retirement.)

Concern for the district: duplication

I came across no one who was saying that the NHS was under-funded or was grumbling over money for the service. Some of the people I spoke to at Leicester said they were pleased that the government had questioned how money was spent and had forced efficiency into an area where there was little before. However, they thought that the purchaser looked for the lowest price, was not concerned about duplication and had little overall view of the city's needs. How had the city as a whole gained from competition between trusts? Defenders of the reforms said to wait a bit longer to see.

While communication with colleagues from other trusts was not encouraged, nobody seemed to have been reprimanded. It seemed to be outside the view of management, committed to the furtherance of the trust itself rather than service to the population.

Nearly three quarters of the coronary care in the city is done at the LRI and the bulk of the secondary referrals. But there was no cardiac catheterisation and no cardiac surgery when I was there. This is done at a tertiary specialist hospital, Glenfield, which draws its work from a very wide area. Trusts are encouraged to be self-sufficient and compete by providing specialist services. While this might make sense in business terms for the trust, it does not, I was told, make clinical or health resource sense for the city as a whole.

There is, therefore, some reluctance to incorporate in the LRI business plans all cardiac services on their own site, because it would mean a duplication of what is available at one of the other hospitals. Already some vascular surgery equipment is duplicated. I detected a horror that Leicester might become like some of the cities in the USA, which have several medical schools, each with most specialised equipment.

It is to the clinicians' immense relief that they are still able to talk to the trust management about retaining the complementarity between the hospitals in the district and they feel they are being listened to.

I made enquiries further afield to find out more on cross-district co-operation and duplication.

The therapeutic advisory group of LRI advises on drugs to be encouraged, discouraged, or not allowed without special approval. Such groups are part of good practice, cost saving and co-ordination. The ones in the Leicester hospitals used to exchange their minutes until, according to the market force thinking of at least one of the trusts, they became 'commercially sensitive'; but some sharing of information still happens.

Finding a bed is one example of tools for which there is a pathway and which works well, at least within the trust. Before the reforms, if one hospital in Leicester was full, the registrar on evening duty would phone the next hospital and they would take the case. Admission remained prompt. Now they do not do this. To take a case from another hospital may impair one's own ability to meet contracts or deal with one's own emergencies when 'on take'. And it is not within the contract. Why do it?

GPs told me of a letter from one hospital announcing that they were now offering coronary arteriograms in addition to their previously available services. Within two weeks, another hospital wrote a much longer letter setting out in careful detail the coronary arteriogram service which they offered, and explaining why they were better than the others.

Money well spent?

I had heard that the grant for re-engineering had been a couple of million pounds. Certainly they had used it to make changes. But why such a costly and lengthy procedure for what were after all such commonsense solutions? I was told that it had taken an initiative like this one to be able to get enough heads together to obtain consensus to do the commonsense thing. Of course everyone thought that masses of people waiting for the clinics was not very nice, but the NHS had become so used to solving everything by money, that it did take the re-engineering process to get there.

That some other hospitals have done similar things, they acknowledged and welcomed. What they think has happened at LRI is the unleashing of a process which will continue to find more commonsense solutions.

Patient choice

The above picture was a snapshot I took in the summer and autumn of 1995. I know that things have moved on. More has happened over the junior doctors' hours and training programmes, and the new cancer block is coming on. I have had messages which suggest that it is still hectic, but exciting.

Before I left LRI, I visited the restaurant for the fourth time. Was it privatised or run by in-house contracts? I had heard both. It was excellent, well signposted and open to staff and visitors. It was pleasantly appointed, had a variety of good food at several self-service counters. There were no queues. The coffee was superb. It was a good place for me to meet people. No queues?

As I was sipping my last coffee, watching the world of LRI go by and wondering where it would all end, I was thinking that it seemed to be the sort of place that many a trust management was aspiring to create. At LRI, morale appeared good. How was it being achieved so painlessly? I thought again of queues. None in the restaurant. None in the outpatient clinics. Were there no queues at LRI at all?

Then I remembered. I *had* seen a queue, and seen it several times. It was on the floor above, near one of the main entrances. It was for a drink and sandwich kiosk beside a small shop. It seemed to be run by a voluntary organisation. I walked through the corridors again. There were ten people standing in the queue. I had the urge to go up to them and tell them that there was no queue downstairs, but I stuck to my observer role. Ten people. Men and women, some in uniform, perhaps ambulance staff.

I walked around outside for a carefully timed five minutes and returned. The queue was exactly the same length, but four people had joined and four had left. I walked off again, this time travelling the corridors and checking on the restaurant, which was still buzzing, queuelessly. Five minutes later I was back again. There were now nine people standing. All the originals had gone. One more in uniform had arrived. I joined. A pleasant queue and a patient one. There was some chatting of a very general kind about the weather and journeys. I was greeted pleasantly by the lady in front of me and later responded quietly to a very civil and unobtrusive question: I was visiting someone who worked in the hospital. I was seven minutes in that queue and had good time to observe the quiet and utterly unhurried manner in which the middle aged ladies served each customer. I chose a coffee and sandwich, which were both cheap and which I took to one of the small tables. I ate the sandwich slowly and I sipped at the coffee. I marvelled at the ability of LRI to give me new experiences. I found the coffee so strange that I could not finish the cup.

The price of the undrinkable substance upstairs was 40p. My cup of coffee in the restaurant downstairs had cost me 58p, but for staff it was 37p. The walking time between the two places was one and a half minutes. What did this mean? One of my friends who attends many hospital outpatient departments tells me that there are people who get enjoyment from the queues. Such people arrive early, not to been seen earlier but to sit longer. It is part of the social structure of their week. I have not met any of them, but I wonder if what I stumbled across at the LRI coffee stall was something to do with it. Perhaps it is the only place at the LRI to have a good queue. But anyway the next time I am in Leicester, rather than worrying about purchasers, junior doctors and GPs, I will go back to LRI and go to the restaurant and the kiosk. I shall try again to understand the meaning of the two services: one efficient, good value for money, but not cheap; the other slow, with unpalatable product, cheap for visitors and worth queuing for.

Chapter 19

Occupational health, occupational hazard

I visited three occupational health departments in various stages of remaining integrated within the hospital and trust, having their services put out to tender, and wondering what was going to happen. They also represented different extents of development of the service. One department was very small and did little work beyond dealing with staff sent by management with one of two questions: 'Is this person fit to work?' or 'This person has had two weeks off sick during the past year: can you comment?' Two departments provided open access to any member of staff, except those who worked for one of the private companies which had a contract to provide services but had not 'bought into' the occupational health service.

The stories that I heard in all three places were very similar. Each department saw people undergoing difficulties when in the throes of a career change, people with chronic psychosomatic complaints and stress symptoms, and those in acute crisis.

Their stories

Workers in the ancillary services such as portering or catering experience much more isolation than before. Their offices and departments are on the service floors of the hospitals so they see less of the other staff. Domestic staff rotate more from ward to ward so get to know the staff and the patients less. Their sense of participating in patient care or the hospital team has often gone.

These departments often have new managers from outside who have not themselves worked through the discipline and are brought in for the very obvious management reason that they are uncontaminated with the past culture. They are good at initiating efficiency drives and cutting costs. The easiest way of doing both of these is often not to replace staff who leave. Those who remain all feel undervalued, but as the managers do not listen to them, it is to the occupational health departments that such people sometimes speak. Porters or domestics have described waking and feeling that they can no longer face coming to work, and their GPs sometimes wrote that they were not fit to work because of stress.

A reduced workforce leaves the managers with fewer resources to manoeuvre when staff are sick or demand is high. Many staff report managers begging or cajoling them not to go off work because they are so short staffed that day. The human and clinical consequence of such a pressure is that staff fear for their jobs and may come into work when they would be deemed medically unfit. The public health implication is that staff are in work while right on the edge of the health and safety margins. The occupational health departments are particularly concerned because of the number of people working in catering while clearly infected.

Staff say they can no longer communicate with the managers, and the departments are also becoming more reluctant to draw these concerns to the attention of management. They have been told that their job is to determine whether people are fit to work or not. If they are not, say so. All very well at one level, but the occupational health staff are well aware that the next time they see a particular person it may be for a management requested assessment because she or he has been off work ten days in the last year.

Among the administration and technical staff, the secretaries still earn far less money than they could do in the private sector (why did some people think the freedom of the trusts to decide on levels of pay would mean more money for such groups of people?). They face the ergonomic strain of word processors and computers, the increase of data collection and the production of reports, procedures and business plans. The pace of nearly every clinical department in a hospitals has increased and most of that seems to travel through the secretaries. The other change is that all secretaries have managers and some of them had, in their naïveté, expected managers to listen to their statements of despair over the work load and its nature. I was advised that the secretaries who did not seem to have experienced this were the secretaries of the junior managers. They were said to be the ones who produced glossy documents and read novels at work. (My own observations from my last years in the NHS confirm this: the secretaries that I came across with time on their hands were those in the newly created posts working with the new management departments.)

The middle managers appear to be as disturbed by their managing as their subordinates are by how they are managed. They study diagrams of new management structures and realise that their own job may go. They hear on the grapevine that it will. They hear of people going at very short notice with deals which are never disclosed. They manage operating theatres, outpatient clinics, industrial therapy units and other small departments and, if they are in their forties, may see a grim future in front of them. They are the ones whose sleep is most disturbed, who have psychosomatic disorders and are irritable or aggressive: it all gets taken out on the people they are managing.

And they have their own managers to deal with: their own performance review, the demands made upon them for change, change, change.

Who is watching whom?

Many people have reported to the occupational health department the experience of being watched. I was assured that this was not in a 'paranoid' sense. They were not putting a new interpretation on an old or repeated phenomenon. These were new signals that they were getting. Staff have been told to tell their manager when a particular person comes to work. Junior doctors, leaving an emergency in one ward and arriving late at an outpatient clinic, have noticed other staff making a note of their arrival time. Staff who have gone on management courses have visited other trusts, and some returned with a curious tale. They were encouraged to visit departments and to ask staff about their experiences working there. At the end of the day, the host manager asked them to tell him what these colleagues had said.

Pressure to work and pressure of work

From each department I heard stories of staff breaking down in the middle of work. Sometimes this is an acute psychosomatic episode such as chest pain, breathing difficulties, nausea and vomiting. Sometimes it the open expression of distress; usually crying. I heard this of very senior and of very junior people. There were, I was told, fewer of the latter: I supposed that they could less conspicuously just disappear by going home or hiding in their department protected by colleagues.

The occupational health department's role in such cases was mostly to do a patch up. Sometimes they were able to offer counselling or point to where it could be obtained. They could counsel and help devise a work programme with reduced hours and more control. Such changes were sometimes particularly difficult for senior people in clinical work, where admission and discharge decisions have become influenced less by clinical and social criteria, and increasingly by matters of management.

Conclusions

Two departments admitted the same sick 'in joke': how many people who will come to see them that day will start to cry? (Sometimes it has been three out of four.) All of them share the same wisdom: if you are over 45 and still in the National Health Service, life is tough.

Chapter 20

Bureaucracy and managing

Like the others, these stories are all true. Some I was told by other people, and some are from my own experience working in the NHS. I begin with one of the latter.

Do trusts have to make a profit?

Some friends thought they do. They quoted the National Association of Health Authorities and Trusts. Its guide for members and directors included the main financial duties of trusts as:

- to break even;
- to earn a 6% return on their capital;
- to live within the external financing limit set by the Secretary of State.

I tried reading some of the early briefings that I still had at home and I sought out a few people who had been in finance departments. None said it would be easy for me to understand, or for them to explain, but my understanding of that 6% return on capital now goes like this.

In the old days, the people running the hospitals had the buildings as an extra goody. For sure, they had to maintain them, but if they stopped being used or fell down, no one would be asking for their money back. I remember on a committee, asking who owned the hospital. Answer, 'The Secretary of State'.

The reforms changed that. And it is to do with accountability. As each trust was established, the district valuer, on behalf of the Secretary of State, went around the property (land, building, equipment, vehicles) and determined the value of these assets.

The Secretary of State then gave these assets to the trust, but on conditions.

Let's say the trust's assets were determined at £40 million. They were divided in two equal parts: government loan and public dividend capital, £20 million each. Together they represented the financial interest that the Secretary of State had invested in the trust.

On the loan, the Secretary of State could charge interest of up to 12%. On the public dividend capital the Secretary of State could charge a dividend of anything, so long as the total charge on both sums did not exceed 6%. Thus 6% on the loan would mean 6% on the dividend; and 12% on the loan would mean 0% on the dividend. Of course the figures were never as neat as that, but it was a way of taking national interest rates into account.

So the hypothetical trust with assets of £40 million could have to pay the government anything up to 6% of £40 million a year.

That is £2.4 million.

How was the trust to get that? It was to include an appropriate proportion in the charge for every service provided to a purchaser.

How was the purchaser to get that extra 6%? It was to get it from the Department of Health, which got it from the trusts.

'It keeps the thing going,' I was told. 'But don't worry, other people find it hard to understand.'

I suddenly remembered discussions regarding charges in the ward where I used to work. For weeks we had timed every telephone call, discussion, interview, car journey, report. We had calculated the hours and minutes of professional time for a consultation and for each day of a patient 'in' a bed. Whatever figure came out of the calculations was followed by 'plus 6% for capital charges'. They tried to explain often, but I always felt stupid and told them I believed them.

Making the most of the bed shortage

One of the ways of pleasing the trust and purchaser (and certainly, the government) was to reduce bed numbers. Freezing was easiest. They may be seen, but not used.

One evening a man in his fourth psychotic episode could not be admitted because the unfrozen beds were filled and the empty beds frozen.

Eight hours later, telephone calls had been made to three neighbouring trusts, four private hospitals, the social services department, the trust's consultant psychiatrist and the manager on call. Eight hours waiting for that man and his relatives. Facing the ridiculous thought that if he gave a guest a breakfast someone might demand a memo and a formal approval for it, the senior manager rang in again. It was impasse. It could be solved at a stroke, of course. Managers freeze beds. Managers could unfreeze beds. They might get into trouble but they could do it. They did it.

Up to that moment the management policy meant that it would have been preferred for this person to go to one of several psychiatric wards where he knew no staff and no staff knew him, or to one of several private hospitals, even 60 miles away.

I came across two trusts that had turned this matter to advantage.

Their mental health units were forever short of beds after closures in accordance with the optimism for care in the community. This often meant that their patients became ECRs elsewhere, with them having to pay another trust or private psychiatric hospital.

Managers, aware of the difficulties that their clinical colleagues were experiencing and of the frustrations in the social services departments, learned that the experience was widespread.

They each opened a new psychiatric ward especially for ECRs from other trusts or other parts of the country. With the extra income they would be in a much stronger position to finance the ECRs for their own patients who could not be admitted to their own wards because they had no beds free…well, except those that they were opening to admit patients from other areas in order to be able to earn more income for their trusts to be able to pay for them to go to another trust when….It seemed straightforward and simple when the manager first explained it.

Turned to advantage? Yes, I was told, but no one had said to whose advantage. The cynical response was that it was to the advantage of whichever manager had dreamed up and 'driven' the idea. Good for individual performance review.

Taking all complaints and suggestions seriously

A letter from a relative, commenting that the night staff did not seem to have much to do, suggested that needles and thread should be provided so that the nurses could do mending for the patients and their families.

In accordance with the trust's policy and Patient's Charter, the suggestion had to be considered formally and the night staff had to put in writing their objections to doing sewing for the relatives of their patients. Their case was accepted by the managers. The relative of the patient, long since gone from the ward, received a polite letter thanking her for the helpful suggestion, but saying that the trust was not wanting to implement the suggestion because it was mindful of the need to keep the night staff available at all times.

Is it a trap?

A new senior manager found people reluctant to speak their minds. They seemed bright enough but hesitant to give their point of view, even when asked. Eventually, she challenged some of them over this and responses included:

'I have had seven years of being verbally abused and beaten up.'

'I am not ready to walk out of the cage yet.'

'Please remember we are only gradually realising that when we are asked for our opinion, it means we are being asked for our opinion. It no longer means, "This is a trap".'

Quality survey

The only delays that two consultants could recall in the outpatient clinics were when every single patient was late because they had been filling in a user satisfaction questionnaire introduced as part of the contract which the trust had with the purchaser.

Spending the surplus

A small specialist department created a financial surplus through ECRs. Flushed with enthusiasm and encouraged by their manager, they decided to buy some good quality second-hand waiting room chairs. On the following day the manager rang: 'Until we know from the purchaser the preferred shape of the service, we must not spend the money.'

'But yesterday you agreed…'

'I have said that until we know from the purchaser the preferred shape of the services, we must not spend the money.'

The way in which that statement was repeated made the staff who received it conclude that their manager had become a messenger again. He had probably been told off by his own manager for encouraging something which did not fit with the master plan, and he feared for his job.

(I heard such a story in several forms. In another case the department wished to spend their savings on equipment but their immediate manager was fearful of stepping outside the trust-wide position on how long it should be before such items were replaced. Instead they spent the money on carpeting a floor which they did not want to carpet and the equipment continued to break down.)

The managers get things done

At the slightest raised tone the junior managers jumped. A young secretary was told that she had been heard laughing and the senior manager wanted her to know that she had been heard. A porter was told that it was not allowed for him to talk to other staff in the corridor. (I used to talk to everybody in the corridor.) Any good idea which the senior managers did not agree with was ridiculed, and few dared risk that experience more than once.

But the junior managers were important and were led to feel that they were 'different' from the rest of the staff. It felt quite right to be spending more money on their new offices. Ignore the fact that the other staff called it 'the palace'. Behave as if you deserve it. They noticed that the 'palace' was not big enough to accommodate all the managers and secretaries, so plans had to be changed (and more money spent), but no one mentioned it.

Moving the medical secretaries was necessary for the co-ordination of services. It cost money, time and effort. The managers were told that the real reason was to remove doctor power. It would be good for the doctors to have to walk further and to have their wings clipped.

It was an exercise in power.

Within the management suite the receptionist had no work to do most of the time.

Staff appointments

It remained exciting for the managers and they did not complain when some old colleagues of their new leader got more of the well paid jobs. Nor when some of those new manager colleagues were having twice as long for coffee and lunch breaks. And when the son of one of them was caught going off with trust equipment, well they did wonder how he knew where to get it, but then they played their part in covering the event up. After all, if that got out it would not help the main task of controlling the doctors.

Communication

Junior managers were not allowed to see reports or told when reports would come; or were not told when the senior manager was negotiating a massive change in the contracts.

Junior managers were to continue to work on some small projects, 'as a token gesture, to keep them quiet', when they knew of impending changes which would make the product of the work irrelevant.

Quality?

Within the quality department an audit assistant was appointed. One of his first jobs was to organise the procedures throughout the several hospitals brought together under the one trust. The present assortment of procedures was chaotic. In his second draft he had the total number of procedures greatly reduced and there was some co-ordination of them. However there were still spelling mistakes, contradictions and sentences which were incoherent. The job was taken off him and handed over to somebody else to finish along with several other projects. Next, his computer was taken and placed in an office which was unoccupied and was to remain so for six weeks. He was allowed to share a computer with a student, so long as 'nobody knew'. Three months later a few thousand pounds worth of laser printer and computer were provided.

Some general surgeons

This inner city teaching hospital changed from having a four-week-ahead clear booking system in which everybody knew where he or she was. I had met three of its general surgeons, who were promised annually that next year 'It will be got right.' The purchasers and trust would have agreed the volume of work to be paid for, and this would be an accurate prediction of what would happen in the following year. Each year, when the contract target had been met, they had to turn people away although they still had the capacity to do the work.

These consultants could not understand how the promise could ever be kept. The contract was a volume one which included dealing with emergencies which could not be predicted. If there were more emergencies than predicted, the contract volume would be completed before time.

They told new patients that they could not specify a date for their operations because they could not tell how the contract would be managed.

Sometimes, after the patient was in the pre-admission clinic, with the completion of 'clerking', examinations, and having seen the cardiologist and anaesthetist, the operation was cancelled.

Sometimes, patients were advised to ring and ring again. Even up to 7.00 pm the decision to admit might be made. The patient could come in for surgery the next day, not having been seen again by the consultant, but by a junior and inexperienced doctor.

Open communications?

Although not in writing, the ward staff were told clearly not to say that the cancellation, postponement, or changes in the arrangements were due to the reforms. And, when the contract had run out, they were most certainly not to say that it was because of money. Various suggestions were made of what to say.

In manager-speak it was not put down to shortage of money in itself. Managers talked of the 'total equation' of purchasers, provider, contracts, emergencies and ECRs.

Work practice and training

Consultants work faster than trainees. Senior registrars, training to be consultants, do smaller operating lists. Cases are 'managed' and operating time is used to compete in the market place where the trust must do the maximum number of operations it can. Consultants have to do more operating and less training or supervising. The next generation of surgeons, the current senior registrars who do less practising, will be less experienced.

If not money?

If, with day surgery so developed and, in theory, enough beds, why do patients get sent away for the third time? This is because the highest priority is to keep beds free for emergencies, especially ECRs or cases from GP fundholders. To that end patients are moved from bed to bed, or sent away.

In the old system the intake surgical team kept beds free. Now the 'bed problem' is left to the managers who know how much an ECR brings in and will welcome it, even if it encroaches on other wards.

Another part of the 'equation' which makes beds appear in such short supply is to do with disposal. Day surgery and modern post-operative inpatient management lead to the need for community care and this involves GPs. Over cases of the nearby patients, it had been difficult enough for surgeons and GPs to meet because both were having to put more time into administration; but in the cases of the contracts which the trust got with purchasers further afield, GPs and consultants would rarely meet.

Most internal patient moves (some within hours of the last one) were to keep 'useful' beds available. This was not money following patients but consultants following patients: they might have to visit several wards to find the patient they operated on. In a different ward patients were with different ward staff, so although seen by the consultant before discharge, they had little continuity of care. As clinicians and managers trip each other up, clinical management is lost. The people running the system, which is, after all, experimental, are learning to carry it out, and management turnover indicated the difficulty of the job.

The lack of familiarity between GPs and consultants had its counterpart in the wards, where consultant and junior doctor, junior doctor and ward staff, did not know each other as they used to. All often feel they are treading on thin ice.

Contrasting it with the drive to 'evidence-based medicine', one consultant surgeon described what was happening as a large uncontrolled experiment. Fewer nurses in the team, with a higher proportion of agency ones, means wards run by less experienced, and often less trained, staff. For many, their first training was in another country so they are working in their second language. Non-consultant doctors are increasingly supernumerary, so the consultants do more of the direct clinical work as well as administration. Frustration, restlessness among the whole team, and friction between individuals and groups, between the secretaries and clinical colleagues, between managers and others, is spilling over into home lives.

Sadly they were now accepting a three week wait for an operation on diagnosed cancer because there was so little operating time. But it met the contract. When the surgeons asked for extra operating sessions the managers said, politely, 'Use the resources you've got.' And both sides were hearing the words of the chief executive, 'Once we get it right...'

The new management and the old team: Penelope and Martin's story

The first change that Penelope noted was style. The previous hospital secretary (manager) had come up through the ranks, usually had his door open and was known to most of the staff. Penelope could walk into his office with messages or to fix meetings.

She delivered a letter, as requested, to his successor: the door was open. In silence, without a moment's eye contact and by the smallest gesture of one index finger, she was shown the way out.

Things were going to be different. In her department's own office, Penelope overheard the conversation with one of the new management team who had visited to hear of the work they did. A consultant was showing where they kept the working notes on support to patients and families. Penelope heard the manager's response.

'No. To me they are not families. They are statistics.'

But clinicians do get involved in management

A new consultant, Martin, joined the team, met the chairman of the medical advisory committee, decided to attend those meetings; and got worried.

'Big changes are happening. They are talking of contracts, costings and procedures and standards.' The hospital was split between the two trusts and everything that went on between them was being costed. Their main department was in a building belonging to the other trust, which sooner or later would charge them rent. Their own trust would have to pay (but no one mentioned out of whose budget) or move their department (but no one mentioned to where).

Clinical directorships

The chief executive needed clinicians involved in management in particular who introduced clinical directorships. Martin was asked by both sides to do it, but he did not want to be pushing himself forward (nor to become a scapegoat). No, they said they really wanted him to do it and get these things sorted out.

The first thing that the team wanted the clinical director to ensure was that the department would stay put without loss of staff. Martin seemed to think that things had already gone too far, but could not convince them.

It was too late

As clinical director, Martin soon discovered that the decisions had in fact already been made. All that could be done was what, in a curiously mixed metaphor, the operational manager described as 'fine tuning at the edges'.

The staff were informed. The local press found out.

Martin argued the case. He had been to a meeting at his specialty's Royal College and heard that other services such as theirs were being given a great deal of support by their trusts. In a meeting, the chief executive told clinical directors that they had to face the limitations of their professional peer groups, who might have academic or clinical skills, but no longer led the services. Those were now consumer- and purchaser-led, and in a different direction.

'No chain store sells exactly the same proportion of goods all over the country. There is more interest in buying thermal underwear in the north.' The clinical director had to go back to his colleagues to help them understand the reforms.

The whole department was going to move to smaller premises. Their main 'flagship' would be disbanded because that was a service no longer on the purchaser shopping list. If the families or patients asked what was going to happen to them, staff were to tell them (ridiculous though it appears here) that they were not severe enough cases.

Martin became a bearer of bad news and an impotent negotiator, and Penelope noticed among the other consultants a defiance which was sometimes triumphant. They would increase their business in ECRs to build up immunity against the managers. When a memo instructing them to take no more ECRs arrived, they decided to ignore it.

Some months later at a meeting with the manager, one of the consultants challenged him directly on the ECRs. He took it in his stride:

'No, no, that's fine. Of course you should take ECRs and of course you should build up as much business as possible. You have the full trust backing for that.'

The consultant pursued the point. 'Then why the memo?'

'Don't worry. There are all sorts of agendas being played out and some-times they cross over or intermingle. Treat that memo as a tactical move.'

The consultant was still not satisfied and asked for another memo revoking the first and giving her authority to do the ECRs.

The manager evened the score with one well delivered sentence: 'Now who is asking for more paperwork?'

What happened to the staff

Meanwhile some staff left, and there was no funding for replacements. 'Not a freezing of the posts. Mainly a pause, pending reassessment of the shape of the service required by the purchaser when you are moved into the new premises.'

The clinical staff were beginning to look tired, made cups of coffee as soon as they came to work and sometimes stopped talking when the clinical director came into the room.

There were 15 people, including Penelope, at the staff meeting. Those who worked few sessions (the occupational therapists and the two enrolled nurses) made special arrangements to attend.

They complained to Martin that it was not fair that they were not being recognised, that the work and the team they had built up was not being valued, that they were not being consulted over changes, that he did not keep them sufficiently informed and had not stopped what the management was doing. Martin, in his turn, complained that the others had let things go on too late, and were now sabotaging his efforts on their behalf by not producing figures and information he needed to argue the case.

It was one of the enrolled nurses, in the team for 20 years, who brought the meeting to its senses. She would be leaving soon, one way or another. It was obvious that her post would happen to go in whatever came out of the changes. That was difficult enough, but what she really could not bear was everybody fighting and talking of this mysterious 'them' out there.

'I don't really know if there is a *them*; but if there is, to have us all fighting among ourselves would be exactly what *they* want.'

They did start to behave better towards each other after that, but what would in-fighting be replaced by?

More changes

More staff left and were not replaced. The main team was down by one third. Rumours of the move increased. They liked the place mentioned.

Martin brought draft contracts drawn up by the purchaser and the trust's negotiators. The detail was shattering. It included the service, the types of investigations, assessments and treatments offered, the costing and the number of staff required to provide the service. Clearly it would require fewer staff.

In meetings, the management position was in a pattern:

It is too late.

These things have been decided.

These things happen.

Of course it is unfortunate that you were not more involved in discussions and decision-making earlier, but that is the reality which we must all face.

There is not time now to go over all this again.

For whatever reason, relations between management and the clinical team were such that there were not more discussions.

We can have discussions but we cannot go back over old ground.

The government is determined not to go back into history again and again.

Yes, we know things are different in other trusts and with other purchasers.

You must accept the reality of where and when we are.

That is the trust's decision.

This meant that at least one of the units was to be closed.

An entirely new unit was to be set up with staff brought from others that were being closed, or 'downsized'. It was to be in the furthest corner of the district. The social workers, employed by the social services department, would have to apply for their own posts because those job descriptions would also change. Some posts would no longer exist and staff would be given the opportunity to apply for new jobs created.

Another new service was to be developed in the heart of the urban area.

And the site for the department proper? Unfortunately the originally agreed site was going to the estates manager's directorate and would not be available. There was an old chest diseases ward on the first floor of another wing and they could go there. And the money (£14,000) they had raised? 'Oh, that is absorbed by the trust, to benefit all the patients. It's swings and roundabouts.'

To the weak outcry from the staff against the apparent purloining of the £14,000: 'Yes we can understand you feeling strongly, but please remember that other groups have also felt hard done by. We are where we are for whatever reason, but what we must do now is to work from where we are.' As usual, in the end it came down to, 'It is a trust decision'.

Their department had been privileged and then forgotten. They had thought they could go on being forgotten. They had been discovered.

A new face or a facelift?

The new services were to be marketed differently. Staff were to concentrate on assessment. A quality standard was that the average involvement was not to exceed six weeks. Locality teams and day centres were to be set up.

All the staff were to do some work at the centre. ('You see, we have taken to heart what you said of the value of team meetings and preventing people getting professionally isolated.')

They saw plans for the site in that first floor chest diseases ward and Penelope was one of the first to visit. Of the ten rooms, four were tiny and had no windows, five were small with windows, one was large with one window but not suitable for further division. Into these were to go fourteen staff who needed space to see patients and relatives, make reports and telephone calls, see colleagues from the community, hold meetings, supervision, training and staff seminars. The management would have to deal with the next accreditation visit from the royal medical college, now very strict on senior registrars having rooms of their own and certain facilities. The college could withdraw accreditation and the post.

Staff said it would not work. Martin agreed. The manager agreed but was leaving. They were getting a new business manager who would sort it out. They did not get a new business manager, but an acting business manager who said it would not work and put this to a meeting with the service manager. The service manager said: 'It may seem that it is impossible. Do what you can. We may need to wait until there is somebody in the substantive post who will have commitment and will be able to take a long term view of how those rooms are used and how the service will be developed. Meanwhile sort it out as best you can.'

Too late, the staff group was organising itself. Each discipline and the subunits or potential sub-units had monthly meetings. The total staff of the department had a meeting once a week with the clinical director, who was doing even more directing and even less clinical work.

Martin could say very little. He did not know how things would work out. Sometimes staff put proposals to him and he put them to the manager. They went to the trust and then the purchaser. Accepted by both. Sometimes the purchaser had a change of mind and it was back to the drawing board.

The managers could not take in the value of talking to patients or their relatives, or even of supervisions. Instead they needed statistics on the numbers seen, of written procedures devised and the numbers of staff who had signed that they had read them.

But the move was still in the future, four months away.

In a staff meeting the acting business manager ran through a number of arrangements and, almost in passing, mentioned a date three weeks ahead for the new teams to start and the new building to be 'operational'. Some thought the date was mentioned in passing because of fear of the response, but others thought she really did not appreciate the shock she was giving.

Because one of the small satellite units was not going to be ready for another five months, that team was going to run a day service in one of their old buildings which had recently been closed. Thus a team not trained or used to working together, but recruited in order to run one sort of service, was to run a different sort of service which another team had been running most successfully for ten years before being closed and disbanded four months earlier; but they were to do it for four months, after which they were to start for what they had been brought together for. And, the acting business manager added with obvious pleasure, there was already a waiting list.

Staff talked of restless nights, not sleeping, being irritable, getting on badly with people at home, thinking of looking for jobs, feeling disloyal and trying to be professional. One community nurse and a community occupational therapist, who worked evenings in people's homes, were to work in offices and with people from a different area. Any of their old patients who approached them were to go to other teams.

They stopped asking each other how they were lest all they got was, 'Don't ask.' Occasionally people said, 'I slept last night.'

Penelope and the other secretaries received new requests: 'Can I sit for a minute?' Or were thanked after a silence from somebody who had dropped in: 'I needed some peace.'

Martin heard that a consultant he had known for years had been reprimanded by management for not going to a meeting arranged after she had agreed to go to court to give evidence on that day. She had subsequently resigned. Martin had been shaken by that news, and said that he could not afford to resign and would not dare to quit being clinical director. Ineffective as he was, that would really be letting everyone down.

Which line to take?

In Penelope's 20-odd years in the hospital, part of it had often been a building site. It was sad to see what had become a thriving workplace revert to building site again. Other departments had been told that they were likely to be abolished next year. Penelope saw misery on their faces. In the corridors, so much sadness.

Departments had had four lots of writing paper, as the names of departments and the trust had changed.

Prettifying was occurring sporadically, especially at the times of visits by important people. Then the gardeners would produce plants in pots and boxes along the corridors and sometimes new lighting would be installed. At least part of the place would look cared for. Was the message: we are becoming more like a private hospital?

As for the changes being 'purchaser-led', Martin met one of its managers in a corridor after they had both left separate meetings. They chatted for a few moments on the stairs and Martin was asked why they had closed the day unit. When he said that he had been told it was what the purchaser wanted, his companion shook his head slowly saying, 'So they used that line, did they?'

How much paper?

From my own experience of the growth of paperwork, I felt I would be surprised by nothing I heard. Estimates were mostly that it had quadrupled. I wanted something more objective. I had been a member of a small group of consultants who had published what we thought were the first audits of doctor time (Black et al, 1974 and Black and Black, 1982). The audits were done again in the year after I retired, that is in 1995. Time spent on management or administration had gone up threefold in the 21 years.

One hundred pages of forms and reports are required to arrange community care for a mentally ill person discharged from hospital, as was described by two consultant psychiatrists, Doris Hollander and Robin Powell in a letter to the *BMJ* in April 1996.

I asked some direct questions of the chief executives I met over the past few years, or of those around them. Some spoke of it taking three quarters to one and a half hours for one person to open the post on Mondays. Others told me of it being a difficult day if the chief executive had not, the previous night, taken home a pile 'this high' with an indicated 5 to 15cm worth of papers, letters and documents.

And to estimate how much came from higher management (the regions, NHS executive, government) I asked a few people to measure post from those sources for a particular time. It was a rough investigative tool I know, but the answer worked out at a height of 5m a year.

Had they never commented on the volume, or tried to do something about it? I received several replies which boiled down to the same thing: the people who were sending it could not stop it.

The 'good news' press releases came in for special comment, in particular those not for release until one minute past midnight on a particular day. They covered notice of the distribution of new guidance; 'Rumours of the death of NHS dentistry are greatly exaggerated'; 'Groups of young people from schools across the country gather today at Planet Hollywood in London to receive prizes for their winning video entries in acting for health, drugs, smoking and alcohol misuse'; 'Primary healthcare teams' role in health promotion made clear'; and many in the vein of 'The new NHS is delivering more and better services'.

(In the week I wrote this paragraph, I received in the post a 210g package from the Department of Health on the measles, mumps and rubella vaccine. Interesting to see but I did not open it. And remember, I have never been a GP and have been pensioned for two years. It cost 55p to post second class.)

Locum doctors: William and Jessica

In some of the stories, there were references to locums or to doctors on weekend duty. I think they were all locums.

There are doctors who have 'proper jobs' which have been advertised and for which the candidates have been through a thorough ritual of selection. And there are ones who have been found to fill a gap, anticipated or unexpected. Some of these locums are selected almost as laboriously as are holders of the 'substantive' posts; some are grabbed, as at a straw when consultants panic that they might have to do the juniors' work and sleep in the hospital overnight.

In the old LCC hospital in East London, where I did my second job as house surgeon, every summer they employed a young trainee surgeon as locum for three months to help to cover for every house officer, registrar and consultant while on their summer holidays. This was the only use of a locum all year.

So what has changed?

Mostly, it is the numbers, but they are difficult to check.

Many a substantive post has become difficult to fill. The work is done, if at all, by locums. The implementation of the new deal for junior doctors, controlling hours and opportunities for sleep, has resulted in the necessity to recruit locums, without the same control of hours or opportunity for sleep, to cover the shifts. Slowness in recruitment (by the procrastination of consultants and personnel departments) has left gaps to fill as doctors leave.

Risks are taken, but locums are the easiest doctors to get rid of. Tell them to go, or put enough pressure on them so they go by themselves. The thing to look out for is preserving the relationship with the locum agency.

The locum businesses

There are now 20 or so companies that often advertise in the BMJ. A couple of them sent me their brochures direct after I retired, luring me with the possibility of an extra £50,000 a year. In 1996 their advertisements filled six or seven pages each week at the front of the classified ads supplement, which has roughly the same number of pages as the academic and news section (62). In February 1983 locum agencies had 10 column centimetres out of 36 pages of the supplement. In 1995, 584 column centimetres (5 pages plus) out of 80 pages.

And what is it like to be a locum? A radio programme in 1996 found some doctors whose negligence and fraud had gone undetected by agencies and employers alike. They found needy doctors whose hours of sleep in the days prior to starting were never questioned. I met a few locums and tell two stories.

William

William arrived at three minutes to nine for the start of his two weeks' locum as senior house officer (SHO) in geriatrics at the general hospital, as arranged through the agency he had contacted shortly after his return from a year in Canada. To his relief, the woman on the switchboard was expecting him. Two days earlier he had received a letter telling him to report to a different hospital from the one that had first been arranged. He was directed to an office on the next floor where a secretary welcomed him with a white coat and told him where to find the two wards on which he would be working.

In the wards, William could find no one who was expecting him; but no one who was surprised either. He asked to meet the patients, but the nurse manager had already done his ward round and no one had time to take him. Instead he was shown where he would find the notes of the patients and, by himself, found the computer used as part of the process of requesting tests and receiving results. The notes were scanty, but understandable. He could not work the computer and no one on the ward knew how so he phoned the secretary. He would have to speak to someone at the main hospital, but she was away until the afternoon.

William read the notes and met two of the patients. He tried the computer again and got himself a cup of coffee from a machine in the corridor.

Around lunch time, another junior doctor, not a locum, arrived. She was surprised to hear that William had been looking at the notes of all the patients on both the wards. There were three consultants and they had patients on both wards. William was to be the SHO for two of the consultants, but on the other ward alone. They had lunch together (they had both brought sandwiches) and together they tried to get William familiar with the computer. His colleague could manage it a bit, but did not use it much, because she worked mostly at the other, larger, hospital.

After lunch, when William was the lone junior doctor again, one of the consultants arrived to do a ward round. He had known that William would be there and said that he had been misinformed of his duties: he was to work for all three of the consultants, and in both the wards, but not in the other hospital. The ward round lasted ten minutes and during it they did not leave their chairs in the office. William had collected some tasks to do and was relieved when, in the middle of the afternoon, the person from the other hospital returned his call for computer help. That was very helpful and William was able to arrange for the investigations ordered by the consultant.

After a change in the nursing shift, William tried again to find someone who would introduce him to the patients. Again, the nurses were very pleasant, but did not have time. He was told not to worry; they would get in touch with him if they needed him.

Before he left, he introduced himself to those patients who were awake.

The other days were rather similar. He met all the consultants, but did not see patients with them more than three times. He was given no supervision and nor was he asked if he needed any. He was shown a folder of the trust's procedures for doctors and signed that he had read them. The feedback he received was after patients died. He was complimented by consultants on having done all the investigations, and the relatives told him that what he had said was helpful. Three patients died.

William did four nights sleeping-in (isolated accommodation) and for that he was paid his due extra. Those nights included the last but two and the last.

William went on to another locum in another trust immediately. No one asked him how many nights he had been working that week, as he started his new rota.

Jessica

Jessica needed some part time work. Through an agency, she was put in touch with a general practice which was looking for someone to do one session a week to replace time spent on fundholding by one of the partners. She met the reception staff, the practice nurses and the partners, in two informal meetings. After a formal, if agreeable, interview with three of the partners and the fundholding manager, she was appointed. She could start the following Wednesday.

Jessica did one surgery in that session. One of the other partners was always present in the building and they always met. She had spoken of her interest and experience in asthma and, as time went on, the other partners referred some cases to her. There was always someone available for Jessica to discuss cases with if she wished.

It was a comfortable relationship.

Mary, the longest serving member of staff, was retiring after 35 years in the staff canteen. The trust was to provide a leaving event on her last day and arrange a collection for the present.
Mary was told that she would be sent a bill for the postage of her invitations. So she delivered them herself.

The social workers' office or learning in a meeting

At the end of a meeting to discuss the new management structure, a psychologist said he had heard a rumour that the trust wanted to move the social workers' office to the back of the hospital. Did the chief executive realise that the people who go to the social workers often have more difficulty in getting around? They may not speak English, may not have cars and may have small children.

The chief executive's reply went something like this:

'Yes, that's quite correct. It's part of the rationalisation of resources forward plan. The social workers will have good offices and it will be more cost efficient. I understand that's how you see their clients. But you must remember that I see them as people to keep away from the main entrance, because they don't give a good impression. Try to remember that in business terms it is not good to have deprived looking people wandering around near the entrance where fundholder cases and ECRs come in. This is the world we live in.'

The non-workaholic manager: Frank's story

Managers have come from all over the place: ambulance services, builder's merchants, mail order firms, nursing, physiotherapy, pathology departments, psychology, speech therapy, admin and clerical, medicine, and elsewhere. I had heard so many bad stories about managers, that I had to find a better one.

I sought out a manager who was recommended by those managed, and yet seemed to get things done and be fairly secure in post. Frank's professional background could be any of the health service ones, and he was in his early thirties. His experience included being a union rep, so he knew something first hand of prejudices from both sides: neither gave the other any chances and he was experienced by both sides to be uncompromising.

Encouraged and supported to attend courses on time and resource manage ment, and databases, he took on more of a management role. To junior colleagues he was no longer 'one of them'. Being excluded from their talk was a learning experience not to forget.

When the first business plan was demanded, the management offered consultations with outsiders which Frank and colleagues resisted. In these discussions, he knew he appeared difficult when he spurned the teams of consultants going around the hospital. Managers challenged him directly to write the plan himself.

Realising that that he could lose his job if he failed, Frank did what he had seen others do. He negotiated the terms; two months full time, taking colleagues 'out' as required, half of secretary's time, with computer and word processor.

He did not let colleagues know of the weekend of panic, telephone calls and support from friends, before agreeing.

Frank organised the team, devised structured interviews and did it. Colleagues seemed to find the experience of one of their own group doing all this to be better than how they imagined the team of consultants would have been. Questions were answered clearly. All worked hard, Frank enjoyed it and completed on time.

His introduction to management had been exciting and, back at his old job, he was frustrated by the poor communication. No one really knew what was going on, even in his or her own work. Frank realised the lever this gave the government.

A job in management? At first he resisted, because he also wanted to continue being what he had trained for.

He was to manage excellent and dreadful (and very powerful) clinicians, often negative to each other or to change. It was not the nurturing environ ment of the old days. Status was now in making big changes and developing great ideas. Without doing that, new managers would be snuffed out. What of those who were doing a good job and letting nothing go wrong? They needed a safe environment to maintain the foundation for more exciting stuff. He wanted to support not only those rushing around and changing the world. Could he keep everyone on board?

Challenging the experience of age

With half the experience of half of those he was supposed to manage, he did not have the pessimism engendered by umpteen previous attempts at reorganising the NHS. But he had seen things he wanted not to reproduce: more paper and forms to fill in, managers so busy that they had no time to find out if staff were experiencing creative working conditions or a nightmare.

Frank remembered how people who did not get on together avoided each other. More secrecy. He decided that if there was somebody he was finding difficult or who was finding him difficult, he would seek that person out. He would even change his route in order to be more likely to have a chance encounter, or to be able to drop in to an office. He also actively telephoned, invited or requested meetings. He badgered people with attention and that became a pattern, so that sometimes, if he did not do it for a few days, he would get a message from them.

The tug of war or loss of control

Determined to avoid the consultants versus managers conflict, he appointed a clinical director. Frank made that appointment: the clinical director was not going to have an administrator as lap dog, ganged up against by an alliance of managers and clinicians. Frank, directly accountable to the chief executive, would take budget decisions.

Independent of the inter-disciplinary and inter-departmental parts of his unit of management, he could be in a position to see if any one part was dominating. He did not want to exploit instability.

Frank referred several times to instability and what he called the destabilisation introduced by the government when it had first included the strings of budgeting into the nurses' regrading pay deal. It put nurses against nurses, and heightened awareness of budget limits. Similarly with doctors: the introduction of some fundholding GPs, out of hours contracts for GPs, the time constraints of the junior doctors' new deal, individual contracts for some consultants, more openness over distinction awards and training money for consultants, have all been destabilising forces. Destabilised staff may cling to the spurious stability of any agreement, could be destabilised and stabilised again.

Frank added that some managers felt destabilised when they first realised that those who closed wards as efficiency savings still had to pay capital charges on the floor space.

Any result?

Five years ago, most staff could barely recount the number of patients seen, or their diagnoses, and certainly not their outcomes. They had little idea what helped people to suffer less. Now, not too onerously, they use a database from referral, and can account for themselves. They can give information to clinicians and managers; and to purchaser and public.

They set goals with individuals and families for discharge. They can now pick out those groups that do well with short intervention.

They use 'integrated pathways' to look at what happens between referral and discharge, and then to reduce the time between referral and response, and appointment waiting times. Clinical staff use fewer sessions and cling to patients less. Someone telephones patients to remind them of appointments and using the 'clinical pathway for average good practice' they note if things do not happen. It is not too arduous, nor too jargon-ridden.

Support groups have replaced individual follow up.

Frank does not have to face patients directly and experience the pressure to do more for them or see them more often. But to support those who do, he must be available. His secretary has a copy of his diary and he has a mobile phone, answering service and pager. It should be impossible to say, 'I couldn't get hold of you.' And that is good for keeping senior managers off his back.

Urgent message from secretary to allocation meeting: 'ECR consultation requested for this afternoon — funding agreed.'
The dilemma: The allocation meeting could postpone a patient due that afternoon from the trust's 'purchaser' authority and see him or her next week instead (after all, the money is secure); or they could turn down the ECR and risk losing the money if the patient went to another trust. *Your choice:* Which way would you vote in the meeting? And if you had been told previously that your post would not be renewed unless the department got in more cases — would that make you vote differently?

How hard does he work?

The intensity of Frank's work is intermittent for he meets people when they want it. He reads enough to be fluent in the latest buzzwords and to have the necessary information at his finger tips. He defies the workaholic appearance, refuses to be compelled to arrive before the boss or leave after him, especially on Fridays. He sometimes works from home and encourages others to do so (but checks on delivery). He delivers and is available. He may still be seen as difficult, perhaps still the buoyant challenger: 'Accept me or sack me.'

And the future? Well, he has refused the trust's offer of a higher salary without superannuation and is worried for himself and family growing old with the NHS. Meanwhile, it is exciting and enjoyable.

Chapter 21

Life with the purchasers

The purchaser/provider split is a clear boundary and clear boundaries are often useful. They allow each group to do its job. In the theory of the reforms, one group of people has the task of assessing and then 'looking after' the health needs of a community, by way of *purchasing* the best services. The other group of people *provides* the services. Several managers and clinicians had given me examples of how useful it can be.

For example, a group of people working in a department become concerned over 'unmet need' and worry that they are unable to provide everything. They are told to be specific on what they do provide, definite on what they cannot provide and accurate on what additional resources are required to do both. This can then be put to the purchaser who may challenge the figures, compare with those from elsewhere and, ultimately, make a decision.

While I was still working in the NHS I attended meetings on purchasing, read much of what the Department of Health sent out and read some of the first papers. An example of a publication which does the idea credit is John Dennis' chapter 'How does it really feel?' in Peter Spurgeon's *The New Face of the NHS*. I had heard of the old boast, attributed to somebody at Marks and Spencer, that as purchaser they had used many of the same providers for years and hoped to continue for many more.

The early meetings pushing the idea in the NHS helped me to develop a picture of a benevolent, creative and economical relationship between purchaser and provider.

In my working life I had always been a provider when I met a purchaser. It was therefore with eagerness that I met some people working in the purchasing agencies. They gave different stories, but each conveyed an identical caution to me: remember there is a difference between theory and practice. I had been expecting purchasers to be mindful of the needs of the populations they served.

In fact their minds were full of much else.

Survival: Hazel's story

Hazel's 49th birthday was in the week we met. She had seen her job disappear five times but had always applied for others, or one that was virtually the same as the one that was disappearing, and had been re-employed. This had happened three times in the last three years. She said that she had been helped when one of her friends pointed out that most top people in NHS management five years previously had not survived to retirement age. Management life was precarious. She was determined to turn it to her advantage.

Hazel had joined the NHS in what she described as the days of being looked after. The introduction of the area health authorities in 1974 was a carefully structured and regionally co-ordinated reorganisation. Redundancy was rarely heard of. There were even people taking note of those in each region who were applying for jobs and trying to co-ordinate them. While some took early retirement, the great majority ended up with something that felt like promotion. When the area health authorities were removed in 1982 and more power was pushed to the districts and the unit administrators, there was much more competition for the posts in each region. More people were displaced.

Three years later, when general management came in with higher salaries for those at the top, significant numbers of the new people were from outside the NHS. Fixed term contracts were introduced and Hazel heard the first rumours of 'Clear your desk and clear off'. Significant regional or cross-regional co-ordination of displaced people ceased. For the first time Hazel became interested in the possibilities of early retirement. A friend had noticed the circulars and had put out a tentative feeler, to discover that most of the allocation had already gone. It had been taken up by the managers who had first received the memorandum or had handled its administration. If retirement was not yet possible, for Hazel it was the start of being mindful of survival.

Two years after the reforms had started they had generated their own momentum, and in an even less co-ordinated way mergers (among both purchasing authorities and the provider trusts) were being talked of. As these mergers got under way, it was often difficult to trace their origins. A process was taking place. Those authorities outside it often seemed anxious about being excluded from the process or being engulfed by predatory take-over. Therefore there was pressure to be active to merge. The only brake was that Department of Health approval was needed.

Hazel knew that if she stayed in the service for many more months after our meeting (in the summer of 1995) she would face the government-led

merger between the district purchasers whose origins were in hospital administration and public health, and the FHSAs which managed GPs' funds. They
would become the new purchasing agencies. And she knew that these
mergers would be taking place with directives from the government that the
total number of managers must be much less.

The turmoil, tension and loss were bound to continue.

While Hazel tells herself not to get worked up by all that is happening
around her, it has an effect. She has to remind herself that she has a considerable experience of survival. Guiltily she told me how she often forgot that
the younger people whom she was managing had far less experience of
survival and were often more stressed. She has to remind herself of this, she
says, because her credibility as a manager is dependent upon the performance
of her subordinates. They have to do the work which enables her to produce
the papers and proposals and negotiate the contracts which earn her credibility in the eyes of her chief executive.

She knows that the next merger, like all the others, will be immensely time-
consuming. The organisation will still be locked into the mechanism of
application forms, interviews and appointments committees.

Hazel also realises that whoever is appointed to the new posts will be able
to feel secure only while the structure itself remains secure. Let alone what
may be dictated by government in its next breath, there are many other influences (market forces?) unleashed: the chairperson retiring and being replaced
or rumours of merger or internal reorganisation. I murmured 'short term
contracts' and Hazel said that in many places these were now a thing of the
past. But that was no reason to relax, because they had been replaced by performance reviews which gave a very sharp edge to any new contract. While the
annual objectives of the performance review may be agreed by both parties,
failing to meet them can be a disciplinary matter. She is well aware that some
people can be tempted to make sure that their subordinates create figures and
proposals which look right enough for a good final performance review.

A cultural change: a new openness

Thinking of applying for a job is usually a private matter. Often preliminary
enquiries and informal interviews are also private. Occasionally, even attendance at the final interview is not known to current colleagues. The reforms,
Hazel explained, had thrown the whole process into a very public arena.
Some people have likened it to the revolution in openness over sex. She waits
for it to be given more prominence in the Health Service TV soaps.

The disappearance of certain jobs is now publicly proclaimed, new structures are published and everyone knows what is happening. Suddenly Hazel and a group of others have become people with limits on their employment, having to apply for jobs or get out. While there was some element of mutual support, close colleagues were also competitors. When I met her, Hazel had already been through several rounds of internal interviews which had been very public.

The sorts of questions that an individual used to think through with a friend or two, went something like this:

Apply for another job, or not?

Think of 'sensible' possibilities, or very widely?

Apply for jobs that I really want but other people might want too, or for jobs that I don't want, but know that higher management is very keen to fill?

Aim high in the hope of being offered something less, or low to be more sure of getting something?

It was all very well talking through some of these when one's friends were not in the same boat. But when a department was being reorganised or, more radically, merged, everybody had the same questions. Who was there to turn to for truly independent listening or advice?

In the times this had happened to Hazel she had had a variety of experiences. Perhaps the worst had been when the senior management brought in psychometric testing to help in the decisions. This made it appear as if the senior managers had no confidence at all in themselves: had they learned nothing of the people they had been managing for many years? It had the effect of raising the already high level of fantasy and rumour: 'Decisions have already been made' or 'There is a master plan'.

Hazel hated the fine words. The chairperson and the staff bulletins spoke highly of the individual programmes created, the personal development of the dedicated members of the team, the bright futures for everybody and their wish to nurture people well. In this glowing enthusiasm for fellow human beings, and for totally unassessed and unvalidated qualities of resilience, they seemed to be missing any awareness of the hurt that was being inflicted and experienced. Word processors, which it had been hoped would make this process more humane, sometimes had the opposite effect. Every carefully composed and printed letter, giving bad news or thanks, fed the suspicion that the only personal bit was the name of the recipient. How many others were receiving an identically worded piece? At the leaving parties, the chairperson's apologies were delivered so regularly that Hazel and her colleagues wondered if he or she had even been invited.

Attempts to get the timing right

After the board had agreed one of the reorganisations, Hazel's chief executive decided that everybody should be told at the same time. Unfortunately there was so much bureaucracy installed to curtail the bureaucracy that it was very hard to control. They tried as hard as they could to get the personalised letters to everybody in the staff group simultaneously, or at least within 24 hours. When they discovered that it could not be done, some of the executive directors decided to postpone the staff meetings which they had already arranged before the chief executive had decided to co-ordinate it all. The effect was more rumours and inevitably leakage. Hazel wondered if that chief executive had ever learned how hard it was 'to delegate and control'. She smiled as she said this, telling me that the chief executive she had in mind was one who had used that phrase herself, but had used it in a criticism of the government.

Individual performance review

Hazel wanted to tell me how she had used individual performance review (IPR) to survive. Critics of the system had said that in practice it was extremely difficult to do well and that there was no validity to it. To this and any other objection the answer was always the same: if you get the objectives right, then you are well away. Of course it was nowhere near as simple as that, because so many of the very clear objectives could be picked up by the opportunistic and used to make performance look good.

It was this opportunity that Hazel claimed to have turned to her advantage. She still saw little validity in individual performance review and knew that performance related pay had little evidence to support it, at least at the levels of salary increases allowed (they are rather like the old increments that were so common). For immediate salary increases, it was barely relevant. But for survival in one job, or being ready to grab the next, IPR could be very important. In negotiating her own performance reviews with her line manager, Hazel was careful to select criteria which she knew she would be able to meet (but not all too well for she was careful to leave something for the manager to criticise).

Similarly she would be very careful in doing her subordinates' IPRs. She would support them in their work and make sure that they would be unable to let her down.

Once she had been in a performance review of a different dimension: it was for a department as a whole so everybody stood to gain, or to lose.

Staff shedding and continuing to survive

Like others, Hazel's department had to grow smaller. One of the easiest ways of managing this was to have a small reorganisation of one's own. It was always possible to justify changes for almost any number of reasons. Not only could staff numbers be reduced but it was a very good way of getting rid of people who were holding up progress. Of course the process had to be gone through very carefully and often there were formal procedures to be followed, but the path to the conclusion that somebody else's job no longer existed was now well worn. New developments with new jobs with formal interviews were very good ways of making sure that someone disappeared from view. However, the whole process of getting rid of somebody could take months, especially in the case of the more comfortably paid. Such people, being better established, may realise that it will be harder to get an equivalent salary elsewhere, so they may fight more. Every method and procedure ended with the most dreadful and difficult stage: having to tell people that they had no job and had to go. But Hazel would do it to secure her own survival.

So Hazel continues to survive. She has always had a network of colleagues and friends to talk to and, in whatever job she has been, has been able to find new ones. But she keeps on coming back to two thoughts.

When she reaches 50 she will be pensionable at a good rate. A waste of all her training and experience, but she could go. She can make the transition without disgrace, and she might even join the ranks of some of the thousands of 'consultants'.

But then she thinks, 'Do I want to go through it again?' Hazel says that there is no sign of the turmoil lessening as the government pushes on with reducing the number of managers. Fifty-year-olds are the ones most easily eased out.

Hazel's story was not very much about how to assess the health needs of a community or how to negotiate contracts, but it was, she assured me, what she was mindful of in her work.

An introduction: Keith's story

At 28, Keith was the youngest purchaser I met, but not the youngest person I interviewed for this book. He had two degrees and had been a manager in the NHS since the start of the reforms. His current job in the contracting department of a purchaser was on a one year contract. It was really a 'rolling' one, he had been informed. This meant he could go at a month's notice, at most, at any time.

'Here's one to cut your teeth on,' he was told as he was assigned the negotiations for the contract for the purchase of services for rehabilitation. It was a small budget and therefore not very significant, his manager advised him, so he tackled it confidently. He soon realised that insignificance lay in the eyes of the beholder: insignificant this contract might be for the purchaser, but not for those making bids.

With two colleagues he worked on a service specification to be presented to a meeting at the end of the month. When he suggested that they should go to meet some of the people running services, he was strongly warned off that by his colleagues who had been in the department longer. The community medicine people were the ones who did that and they might already have done so. He got that file, studied it and, by the end of the first week, his first draft was on the manager's desk.

It was nearly all wrong. 'No, that's not how we do things here.' He was given a couple of old contracts for other services that had been agreed in the first round last year and advised to produce something that looked more like them.

His rewritten draft was, in content, almost identical to the first. Its shape was different. A number of key phrases had been added. It was much longer. His manager thought it was much better. When Keith wondered how appropriate the quality criteria (which he had lifted from the contract for an acute service of the previous year) would be for rehabilitation, he was told not to worry. What they were doing was negotiating. They were saying what service, with what sort of quality controls, they were interested in purchasing. If a provider came up with a refinement or an improvement so much the better. That seemed a good argument, but when he was out of his boss's room Keith did wonder what would happen if the providers came up with no improvements and the contract was agreed, together with meaningless quality clauses. He had learned to wait and see.

The meeting approved the proposed service specification, the chief executive said to go ahead, and Keith had landed the job of publishing the document, managing the consultation process, and organising a panel for the purchaser to make the decision.

The pace quickens

Within two days of the service specification going out, the first telephone calls came. They did not come to Keith, but straight to his manager or to the chief executive. Keith realised that some of the key players knew both of them well when he received a note from one and a summons to go as soon as possible to the office of the other. What had he sent out? No, he had not been expected to send out the document exactly as it had appeared at that meeting, Of course, some tidying was expected. No great matter, for it was not a very significant contract.

Keith drafted brief explanatory letters for the manager to send out to the telephone callers.

Keith's department was the 'lead purchaser' of a group of purchasers who were jointly negotiating the contract. So far so good, but now he had to have some representation from the other purchasers at the evaluation meeting (called a 'shoot-out'). The people 'heading up' the corresponding sections in the other authorities were easy enough, but when it came to proposing more specialist members of the panel, he discovered that some of the callers had already been assured that one particular person would be there. And the date? Some people in the department told him to fix one of the dates which the purchaser's team could manage, regardless of requests from two of the bidders for certain dates to be avoided; some said to accommodate them

He began to wonder if his job was to get to best service in rehabilitation, or to win a battle.

Before the meeting

The date and the panel were fixed. The ex-adviser on the specialty to the old regional health authority, a doctor from the public health directorate, Keith's manager, Keith's opposite numbers from the other two purchasing authorities, one of his immediate colleagues and himself.

Five bids were received from five different trusts in the near neighbourhood, the one nearest making a feature of proximity and the others making features of separateness. A manager from one of the bidders complained to Keith that the ex-adviser to the old regional health authority had worked with some of the bidders on similar proposals a year ago: his impartiality was in question. Keith's manager said he would make the change and have the chairperson of a more impartial medical sub-committee instead. 'Leave it to me.'

Keith realised that most of the people who were making these protesting calls, or at least the consultants, were old enough to be his parents and that did not help him to feel confident handling the rest of the contracting. There were many more telephone calls on the composition of the panel. Some claimed to have been told 'by the purchaser' that neither the ex-advisor to the region nor the chairperson of the sub-committee would be available. Keith, who was now getting most of the calls, tried to be reassuring and to sound confident.

The shoot-out

9.30 am was the time to start. At 9.25, the chairperson of the medical sub-committee had not turned up, and Keith's mobile phone rang. It was Dr Brown, the ex-advisor to the old regional health authority, to say that he had arrived at a different building. He would be a few minutes getting across. 'Start without me,' he added. On impulse Keith handed the phone over to his manager. When his manager put down the phone, she told Keith that he had better tell the first provider team, already waiting outside, that there would be a few minutes' delay before they could start their presentation. Keith had the presence of mind to ask what to say about the 'other' doctor coming. 'Manage it,' he was told.

Keith tried to do his best. He told the waiting team that he was sorry to say there was going to be a delay, because Dr Brown was held up. They would start in a few minutes. He thought that he had got away with it as he turned round, but the manager from the visiting provider team said, 'Hey, wait a minute!' and said that they had been told several times that specialist medical contribution would be from the chairperson of the specialists' sub-committee. In his desperation, Keith employed a tactic he had seen managers use time and again. He lied and denied that they had ever said that.

Ten minutes later and the missing doctor had still not turned up. Keith's manager suggested that Keith or his colleague go out again and say to the waiting team that they were considering starting anyway. 'And see how they react.' In despair, Keith looked at his colleague and she offered to go. She reported back that the provider team was worried they might be interrupted by a latecomer and wondered if it would be within the spirit of equal opportunities. (She later told Keith that she had a very rough time.) Keith's manager said to explain that it was not a formal tendering process in itself. She told them to negotiate with the visitors and, 'Let's get started.' It fell to Keith to do that and somehow he managed it. At the start of the formal meeting his manager reassured the presenters that their concerns had been noted.

Ten minutes into the first presentation, the door opened and the ex-medical adviser to the old regional health authority walked in. He looked flustered and sat alongside the purchaser team.

The presentation continued and after another ten minutes the door opened again. This time it was the chairperson of the medical sub-committee. They all seemed to have forgotten him. He sat on the other side of the table alongside the presenters. He moved over when asked by the manager.

That presentation went long over time, with the panel being accommodating in the extreme and the manager asking if the presenters needed more time. Every one of the subsequent presentations passed and finished late Keith had the opportunity many times to practise giving explanations in a reassuring and increasingly confident manner about something that he never did understand.

The decision making

Keith did not know how the purchaser panel made the decision. Certainly it was nothing like what he had experienced at, say, appointment committees at which all members of the panel had a say and a table of rankings for each candidate was constructed. Plainly it was nothing like the 'SWOT' analysis (strengths, weaknesses, opportunities, threats) he had learned in training for business planning. He suspected that the final decision made by his seniors had much to do with behind the scenes negotiations, with what other contracts the purchaser was wanting to finalise with which trust, and with a history of relationships between managers far too senior for him ever to have much to do with. He was told it was 'managing'.

Keith had sharpened his teeth.

How the community physician made it work: Lydia's story

Lydia had been a community physician for many years and, with the reforms, was appointed to a post of director of public health in a purchasing authority. She was on the whole an enthusiast for the reforms but contented herself with telling me one example of how the power of the purchaser/ provider split could be used constructively.

She was not a community physician who isolated herself from other doctors: she continued to meet medical colleagues in the trust which was their main provider.

One of the doctors, who was clinical director of a substantial group of services, mentioned a problem. Most of the units were developing well, had improved their efficiency and made changes in line with common 'good practice'. One had not. This one was still led by a senior consultant who was very resistant to change. She had run her department as she had for many years and seemed set on continuing that way until she retired. The minimum of reform had been done, so that at least GPs were receiving summaries in better time. All suggestions made by the clinical director were thwarted. The consultant attended no medical staff meetings and replied very late to any memo from the clinical director. She went on in her own way, writing articles in the tabloid professional journals, but in her treatment methods and way of relating to hospital colleagues and GPs she had become an anachronism.

When the clinical director had raised the matter with the chief executive, he was told, 'Well; these are not capital offences.' The clinical director knew that. It was not blood or a life that he was after. He was wanting a considerable sum within the directorate's budget to be used more effectively, to bring all parts of the services in line with each other and, through more sharing of resources, really to be more cost effective. Other managerial colleagues obviously considered that particular consultant to be untouchable because for a long time she had had the ear of the chief executive. None dare challenge that.

The worst happened when the directorate put on an open meeting. It had been agreed that each team or department would present in a way which demonstrably utilised grassroots contributions: junior nurses, physiotherapists, occupational therapists and technicians were to share in the presentation of the work. All went well for each presentation. The team that the clinical director was worrying over was last. It was known that some of the ancillary workers had been practising what they were to say. When their time came — to the surprise even, it seemed, of the team — the consultant did it all. And no one challenged her. The clinical director sensed that in the eyes of many of the professional visitors the credibility of the directorate was severely damaged.

Audit, grievance procedure, appeal to the trust's chief executive, public confrontation — all were considered carefully. None would be effective. Lydia tried always to think of the partnership of three: purchaser, provider/managers and provider/clinicians. But a threesome is easily rocked. When children's services are being discussed in one particular area a trust chief executive plays on vicars, school staff, parents and the education department so that they are mobilised as an awkward pressure group. Here she thought she could be more helpful.

As director of public health for the purchaser, Lydia wrote directly to the consultant expressing concerns over how slow her department had been in implementing some of the changes that had been discussed two years ago in one of the big 'pre-reform' meetings. She sent a copy of her letter to the chief executive of the trust and to the manager of the clinical directorate, as well as to the clinical director himself.

The consultant met the manager, so there was some change at least. But then there was no more. In her next letter, Lydia specified certain changes that were required by the purchaser. If they were not in place within two months, there would be a reduction of nearly £100,000 in the sum allocated to the trust for those services.

The consultant did not make the required changes so the purchaser insisted that the money was redirected. It went into the general budget of the clinical directorate, so colleagues were able to take over some of the services to make the developments which were in line with modern practice.

Perhaps, Lydia concluded, an example of power being used without too much bloodshed.

GP power, or how to get money to follow patients

In one part of the country, before the reforms came in there had been a small specialist unit which took cases from a wide area. Visiting government repre sentatives and senior civil servants assured the local community health council and general practitioners representatives that there was no reason in the reforms why this should not continue, because 'money would follow patients'. They quoted letters saying that valued existing clinical services would not be damaged.

So the unit started by getting more referrals.

The GPs, who were the main referrers, suggested to the purchaser that there should be a block contract with the specialist unit. The purchaser refused, saying that they had another, much larger, provider unit with which there was a contract. The GPs, not pleased with this because they did not find the service from the larger unit satisfactory, challenged the purchaser but without success.

The referrals continued by the manoeuvre of ECRs, and the ECRs continued to be paid. The GPs, in keeping with the drive for community devolvement, had arranged for a consultant in the specialty to do a clinic session at one of their practices. All cases that any of the GPs wished to refer to the small specialist unit were then referred to that consultant who put her pen to the ECR consultant-to-consultant form.

The GP who told me this story was somewhat shy about it and wondered if it was almost the 'black market' of the NHS reforms. But the consultant got no money for herself. As the discussion went on, my informant concluded that this was a way of making the system work.

Chapter 22

Regional authorities and the NHS Executive

I knew that, unless someone at the top decided to write his memoirs, there would be no 'personal' story on this subject. That is no sexist misprint: there are very few women at the top of the NHS. No, the most I would be able to do would be to visit a few places and get some people to talk to me in general terms and then, taking what was in the public domain anyway, create a story of the ideas, the organisations and what it felt like to have been there.

It is the best I could do. Here it is.

Walk out of the Town Hall or City Art Gallery in Leeds, turn left up Headrow, over the top and then down Eastgate. The horizon is dominated by Quarry House, headquarters of the NHS Executive (NHSE, called NHS Management Executive until April 1993), a massive building on a traffic island (Quarry Hill) at the end of the road. It is made of three different shades of brick, there is a ramp going up to the grand glass entrance and a number of closed-circuit television cameras recording the outside.

My quest for this chapter was to find out what it was like to work in that building and what life had been like at the tops of the regional organisations. There had been 14 regional health authorities in England and they were reduced to eight in 1994. Their role in Scotland, Wales and Northern Ireland was performed by the relevant Department of State.

With so much turmoil and so many people leaving jobs, it was not difficult to find some who would talk.

I met some civil servants and heard of the long civil service tradition of independence, neutrality and integrity. This has changed with the reforms. Briefings for ministers could no longer be objective and they coined the new expression, 'defensive briefing'.

As the reforms gathered pace, the level of excitement in the government department and the NHSE rose. An evangelical fervour took its grip, with some officers publicly expressing enthusiasm for the reforms. The change of prime minister in 1991 and talk of an early election led to an urge to get the reforms through as quickly as possible. An election lost, the good work of the department might go by the wayside.

The tradition of pre-general election neutral briefings was firmly dropped in 1992. Briefings were even supplied before party meetings; a big shift. I was reminded that civil servants are supposed to work for government, not for political parties.

The government had taken on various groups with vested interests. Now it was the turn of those in the health service, especially the doctors. It was a campaign to be fought with passion: some senior politicians believed the original siting of St. Mary's, The Middlesex, and University College hospitals in London was linked to the ambitions of consultants to work near Harley Street.

Professional representation in the higher NHS management was reduced. Career civil servants and managers were given more power. This new administrative class of executive director was to put doctors in their new place. Opposition to the reforms was routinely interpreted as self interest.

Dealing with the clamour for more resources

In the quest to get the NHS off the political agenda, levels of provision had to be tackled. Other ways had to be found of dealing with waiting lists. Already some of the more assertive regional health authority leaders had been challenging the idea of a right to everything. They were not afraid to make statements which could be interpreted as favouring rationing. Nobody had argued that varicose veins had the same priority as cancer, so it was not too difficult to question whether everything should be on the NHS and not difficult at all to find sceptical clinicians to cast doubt on some procedures.

The first discussions with clinicians and managers were easy. Money was taken. It was called the Waiting List Initiative. Some waiting lists were reduced and the ideas of purchasing and priority had become acceptable. Decisions were no longer made only on a clinical basis.

One more step and uniformity could go. Purchasers' priorities could differ. Local managers could decide. They could hear how MPs' constituents also differ in their priorities.

Life at the Department of Health and the NHSE

The higher echelons of the Department of Health and the NHSE were exciting places to be. Up to half a dozen times a week, briefs to ministers, some at less than 48 hours' notice.

What proportion of hospital staff are directly involved in patient care and what was the figure for 1990? A definition of that question. Can we call medical directors (doctors who used to be full time clinicians, now doing only one or two weekly outpatient clinics) 'hospital staff directly involved in patient care'?

Think of the hidden agenda of the questioner, or of other people who may put a supplementary.

Think of efficiency questions that may be included in a supplementary, or efficiency answers that could be useful in parrying.

Look up the last tally of number of patients treated. It may be too soon to announce it again.

Ministers and sometimes the Secretary of State were met and debates in the House of Commons were attended (a special seat). Ministers might be pleased (yes, Kenneth Clarke did take people out to the pub); or not, and demand a meeting, or give a dressing down.

The excitement of being near the government. The 6.00 am call for the personal briefings, the last-minute ride in the taxi to go over the briefing with the minister before the radio or press interview. Knowing that the briefings and reports are deposited in the House of Commons Hansard library. They may be dug up years later by researchers.

All this excitement plus, for some, the use of an office in the Department of Health's Richmond House which is the William Whitfield designed light coloured, modern, gothic looking building opposite the entrance to Downing Street. (Kenneth Clarke and I shook hands there at the start of one of the early meetings.) Life could be high.

The government was telling the Department, which was telling the NHSE, which was telling the regions, which were telling everybody else, to *get on with it.*

The executive moved to Leeds

Cost effective government departments review their accommodation needs. A very good deal could be got in Leeds for the NHSE to be. Once this idea caught on, nobody noticed London rentals dropping fast in the recession. The 'mobile' grades, middle and senior civil servants, were encouraged to agree to the move.

It was going to be the building for the centre of thinking. The powerhouse, leading the way for other departments to shake off dependence on London.

The move was heralded with slogan talk:

Get out of London.

Get rid of fragmentation and all be in the same building.

Drive to work.

Be able to open the window in your office.
Find cheaper housing.
Live in the countryside.
The city of Leeds will welcome you.

Miscellaneous relocation expenses were generous. In addition to removal allowances of the usual sort, there was the possibility of five years' London weighting as a (taxed) lump sum.

Many staff at the lower end of the hierarchy were to be recruited locally

The building was designed, accepted, planned, started. It was to be shared between the NHSE and some sections of the Department of Social Security: the Benefits Agency (BA) and the Central Adjudication Service (CAS) which considers legal and medical criteria for social security payments.

Teams were set up and the move started in 1992. Floor by floor. Staff had to go through 'hard hat' areas to get to work

Housing was attractive, with many buying in the Yorkshire Dales. The countryside was marvellous. Journeys to and from work were easy. Welcome parties and celebrations, as new teams arrived. Breakfast welcomes for those making their first trip on the early morning train from London. A camaraderie unknown in the London offices. Staff had a buzz.

A team of 1,000 was built up. The vanguard of the NHS reforms, the National Health Service Management Executive. They were the younger end of the age profile of the London set, plus younger people brought in from Leeds. Even when all the floors were ready, the outside of the building was still 'hard hat' and the landscape gardens were still unfinished at the beginning of 1995.

This was not all of the NHSE. At least the London Implementation Group (LIG) and some parts of personnel or human resources remained in London in Hannibal House, Euston Tower and elsewhere.

Rumours of manpower reviews started almost as soon as the first floor was occupied.

Tackling the management of management difficulties

Those who still had responsibilities in the south of England had to travel there fairly often. Some kept offices in both London and Leeds. Occasionally a start in Leeds, to London for a meeting and return to Leeds to continue that evening.

Committees which used to meet in London, attracting people from along the spokes of the rail network, became more difficult to service in Leeds. Bills rose for travel and subsistence.

Travelling long distances several times a week, part of the early excitement, became arduous. Families and relationships changed: 'How many nights are you going to stay at home this week, Daddy (or Mummy)?'

One of their main tasks was dealing with public consultations on every proposed hospital closure. Every one of these was processed by the NHSE. I was told that in every case the objections submitted in the consultations were disregarded, after lengthy and detailed consideration. They had to be seen to have been taken into account. One of the people who talked to me about this spoke ironically of how suited they were to the task of tactfully disregarding the feelings of objectors after their experience of 'consultation' over the move to Leeds.

But the excitement continued. Faxes, internet and video links ensured that. (Video links were popular with those politicians who liked sitting still.)

Medical director: 'Transferring patients to shorter waiting lists as formally encouraged by the NHS Executive helps many people. The trust with the longer waiting list can claim to be reducing it. The trust with the shorter waiting list can claim to be increasing business. Whether the patient is in fact dealt with any sooner (we do not know what else might have been done to that waiting list by the trust) remains an open question. Perhaps an opportunity for evidence-based management?'

The cut and the new strain

The move was in 1992. In April 1993 the government decided on a manpower review of the civil service. There was to be 24% cut over two years.

People had moved house, the property market was askew, and they contemplated losing massive sums of money. There were rumours of the NHSE becoming an 'agency'. Like separation and divorce, with which the experience was compared, people do not realise all the financial implications until they are upon them. The five years' London weighting lump sum, and the generous miscellaneous relocation expenses, had to be paid back pro rata if staff retired within five years of the move. Some would have to pay back £5,000 if they opted for early retirement.

The uptake was greatest from the lower ranks who saw fewer promotion prospects in the slimmed service with its individual contracts. In fact far more applied for early retirement than anticipated and no criteria had been set to deal with this. They had to be invented.

Information on the 24% cut was obtained in the usual way: rumour, press leak, memoranda and meetings. To their credit it seems that those who ran the meetings to confirm the decisions, and to take some of the flak, did their job well. Nonetheless, staff own the imminent splitting of their departments and cutting of their links. Inevitably they were more vulnerable,

Being at the centre of one of the government's prime strategies — driving unwilling departments into action and dealing with problems and complaints — was so exciting that anxiety, tension and depression were often pushed aside. Tell people, with little warning, that having been at the centre, they are now to be on the scrap heap, and those protective forces no longer apply. Feelings of panic, fury, tension; psychosomatic complaints, heart trouble and depression gave the staff support systems of Quarry House a lot to do.

A summary of optimism, cynicism or ineptitude

The strains on marriages and relationships grew: I met people who told me of serious mental health breakdown and physical illness in themselves and their families.

In the early stages, when it was all very exciting, most people managed to continue to work well by working harder and longer. They did not notice the ones who were cracking up. Spouses and close friends noticed first when they stopped talking or, worse, would talk of nothing else.

Some people said to me that they could not decide whether it was optimism, cynicism or ineptitude that summarised how a government department had moved 1,000 people 200 miles to a new building in one year, announced redundancies for a quarter of them the next, and a year later, made a bid for the Investors in People Charter Mark.

The regions

The top of the English RHAs

Many of the highly qualified and experienced people at the top of the regional health authorities (RHAs) had been head-hunted: by leaders at the RHAs, by members of the boards, by people at the NHSE, by politicians. They were the cream and they had a job to do in leading the reforms and trimming staff numbers.

They were uncomfortably near the political centre, increasingly working for government and politicians rather than as public servants, no longer expected to do what they thought was the best, but to do what those at the very top wanted. They led the reforms in the regions and they reduced staff, some dramatically by nearly half.

They managed much of the transition to community care, they audited audit, they trouble-shot, they supported many people struggling with the

Duke of York marching his troops up to the top of the hill, and marching them down again.

Then the rumours started. The RHAs were to have the axe wielded over them. In October 1993 the announcement was made: the fourteen English RHAs were to be replaced by eight NHS executive areas. The job of the regional general manager or chief executive of those sentenced RHAs took on some aspects of running a hospice. How long will people stay? How long was there to go? Will there be a life hereafter?

From October 1993 to March 1994 was the time of intense jostling for position. Surveying the field was done from all sides. Those in the really senior jobs in the NHS were considering flight, retirement or open competition for what jobs were left. Who was competitor and who was friend? As they were jostling, so the rules were being straightened out, refined, redefined; anticipations and expectations postponed. Some pacts were made between colleagues not to 'cross-apply'.

At the end of 1993 Duncan Nichol, the NHS chief executive, was coasting out as his successor Alan Langlands was appointed. Alan Langlands had a busy quarter-year inauguration, carrying most of the NHSE load as well as arranging individual meetings with the fourteen heads of the RHAs. Who was looking after him in this difficult time?

In those individual interviews with the regional general managers (a few already being called chief executives) their potentials were explored. Some expressed an interest in one particular job; some in several. Some considered moving to the purchasing side.

Formal applications. Psychological tests at the NHSE.

Spread over ten days near the end of the financial year, the interviews were conducted by a senior civil servant of permanent secretary grade (Graham Hart), Alan Langlands, the chairperson of the regional authority concerned and Duncan Nichol. Each candidate had tests with a psychologist and an hour-long interview; and a formal two-hour interview with the panel.

The number of people interviewed for each of the eight posts varied. For some it was up to four. Over that time the three full time managers (the permanent secretary, the chief executive and the retiring chief executive), together with the eight part time, but remunerated, chairpersons from the regional authorities, met twenty candidates for intensive interview. Thirty people were involved in this process altogether.

The candidates were told that they would be informed within two weeks. They were reminded that for some posts such as those at the NHSE headquarters itself, Cabinet approval was required.

By the Wednesday of the second week they were told that they would be informed during the coming week-end. In fact the first phone calls went out in the afternoon of the Friday. Some were told that they had been appointed to the job which was their first choice, or to another one. Some were told that they had not been appointed but somebody else had. Some were told that they had not been appointed for the job they had applied for, and that no one else had either.

I am sure that Alan Langlands made all the phone calls well, and especially the ones that gave the news to these senior, primed, groomed, highly trained, highly paid leaders of the NHS reforms that they were not wanted: not that they were not wanted because somebody else was better or fitted the bill more precisely, but that no appointment had been made. They were not wanted. I am sure that he used all the correct formulae: 'This is a phone call I dread to make… this is the most difficult one… weighing up all considerations… we did not think it was the right job for you… we need more complementarity between chairperson and chief executive… there are differences between different regions… we need a heavyweight player… we need a lightweight player… what you have done so far in the groundwork for the next stage of the reforms is excellent and we have no fault to find in that… it needs a different person now'.

Some, during that phone call, were given advice on other possible jobs. I am sure that he made the reality point that the future jobs were different from the old, that the new regional offices were in a civil service context.

Whose decision had it been? How much say did the outgoing chief executive of the NHSE have? He was the man who may have known the candidates for longest and have heard and seen them perform in front of government ministers. Had they said too much or had they said too little? He was also the man who was leaving the Department of Health within days, had recently been knighted and was shortly to take a post in the private health sector. Who had the veto? I expect that the local chairperson of the health authority could veto the appointment of anybody if in no other way than by resigning him or herself. But I expect that one or other of the chief executives, the retiring or the new, could veto the other way round. And because one of the spoken but unwritten changes which was taking place was from public servant to civil servant, I expect that Graham Hart as the senior career civil servant present also had, at least in effect, a veto.

In the end this process failed to identify, out of the cream of the NHS management, anyone to do one of the jobs. Seven were filled. It ended with eleven of the most senior NHS management people, who had been driving the reforms, being discarded. Sure, they were discarded with financial settlements more generous than those received by domestics or care assistants, but nonetheless they had recently been chosen carefully and now saw the jobs for which they had been chosen disappear.

Of the seven appointed, over the next two years one left publicly discredited, one retired and one moved to Glasgow. Or, put another way, of the eight posts to be filled in the spring of 1994, only half were still held by the committee's choice two years later. Not necessarily an indictment of the decision making (I was reminded of all those 'When we get it right' statements), but a sign of uncertainty and change continuing in 1996.

And then?

So how did they cope? Many of their close colleagues were enraged and in tears. There was much telephoning, meeting, seeing. The people on the appointments committees had a tough time too. There was an active bereavement process going on. They saw friends, they saw family. They used faith or they used agnosticism. Weekend meetings took place. Ports in a storm were offered to some: something quickly to go and do while they quit the post that was to be taken from them and whose even temporary tenure was untenable. Rumours abounded: the telephone calls would have been put off further if various people had not put pressure on the executive to get on with it; who would be brought in as acting chief executives while the newly appointed could not yet join and the organisations had not yet been fully brought together?

Some had a busy next week with many formal management engagements fixed a long time ago. There were chocolates, flowers, letters, cards.

Much personal support was forthcoming from the chairpersons of their regional health authorities and their many colleagues there. Redundancy settlements, when arranged with the NHSE, took six months. Six months of uncertainty. Meanwhile some could try a turn on the consultancy circuit. In the relative isolation of independent work they had little reflective time with colleagues, rarely saw things through and they missed implementation. They did not use their skills in leading, developing and managing change.

I wondered who wrote the letter to the whole of the region, telling them what had happened? The departing chief executive, the incoming chief executive, somebody from the NHSE or the chairperson of the board? How could it be couched in positive terms? Could it be sent out by a region on its own, or had it to be agreed, supported or sanctioned by the NHSE? There did not seem to be a procedure for this: practice varied.

Tears and bad nights and preoccupation continued. They rang each other. Answerphones were great sources of support. I heard twice of more than a dozen messages on a machine in a day.

How were the 'ports in a storm' organised? It was ad hoc. Some senior people knew of jobs that had to be done that could absorb a person for a few months. I had come across this when working with trusts: a senior person who had lost a job was taken on as a short term manager of a project. I was told that it was to the benefit of both sides: the casualty is supported and the trust (which pays) gets a piece of work done. (It was sometimes difficult to convince other people in the trust, especially those whose departments had been denied money for development or who had seen jobs go; and all in the interests of efficiency.)

For some, it meant temporary (or perhaps permanent) retirement; becoming a visible parent, or going to classes at the local institute. For most the realisation that they could never again have the same loyalty to any organisation.

Friends were angry and assumed that the decisions had been political, but I found no evidence of this.

Had they said too much?

What was the difference between the candidates who were given those new regional jobs and the ones who were not? Nobody I spoke to seemed to be clear on this but several people voiced the same uncomfortable question: had some said too much? I heard vague stories of government ministers asking what it was really like working at that stage of the reforms. After giving the standard answer ('exciting, challenging') managers had sometimes been pressed again: 'No, I really mean it. Tell me what it's like.' Occasionally the question had been answered and a number of the difficulties which I have recorded were relayed to the government minister who heard them with no outward sign of disapproval. However, somebody else in the room later expressed concern, worry or disapproval, in gesture or in words; or, at least, the story got passed on and eventually came down to me. I think that amounts to the same.

Alan Langlands offered each unsuccessful candidate a meeting. A humane, sensible, caring act but inevitably, in a climate of suspicion and despair, an opportunity to compare what was said in the initial telephone call with what was said in a cooler mood, weeks later. Some felt they were given two different opinions, 'before' and 'after'. Had new information really come to light on these, the highest profile, best known people in the NHS? Had they really changed that much? Or had the NHS?

It may have been more difficult for the men because the traditional masculine role of not crying and keeping a tough exterior was so much part of the new macho image. It may not have been so easy for them to have been given or to have received flowers.

How have they coped? There is always unfinished business in being rejected and there was always unfinished business from previous jobs. After several months of shock or hibernation, they are starting new jobs, or not. Some said they should be in a good position to counsel people who were distressed by work in the NHS, and might even notice the plight of the cleaners who lost their jobs or got re-employed at £2.40 an hour. Others thought that they might not notice.

Back to Quarry House: a splintering

All sorts of parts of the original NHSE have been or are being market tested and set up with sub-agencies. The restaurant is now privately run and said to be cheaper and mushier. To begin with it was not mushier but there has been a gradual, steady deterioration. This may have been due to changes in the staffing necessary to cut down their costs in line with the contract negotiated.

After testing and granting a contract for a sub-group or outside agency to run a service, there has to be a monitoring team to check that it is being done right. In some cases the people who used to do the job become the monitors checking other people doing it. In some cases the total number of people involved in the service has not gone down.

The monitoring team is not responsible for what happens. Responsibility lies with the holders of the contract. Crown immunity is a thing of the past so there is potential for lawsuits against the new, smaller organisations.

What 'cost effectiveness' often means in the new contract is that there is built into its life (usually three years) such a reduction of total cost that 25% of the staff must be shed, or have pay reduced. Who should be thrown off the life raft first?

Those with their heads in the lion's mouth seem to last the longest. They dare not give up. They have to stay on, they must cope. They drag everybody along with them right down to the bottom of their own pyramid. The people who are so bullied by managers that they cannot say no. They also have to work longer hours for no more money.

What's it like to work there?

I had first heard of Quarry House when photographs of this gigantic building appeared in the newspapers. There were predictable outcries over money being spent on management when there were so many crumbling hospitals. Much was made of its palatial swimming pool and I had seen photographs of that too.

I went in the building three times. I walked around, looked at the notice-boards, went up and down in the lifts, got undressed, swam in the pool, got dressed, observed and listened. (I often worried what to wear when visiting an informant for my researches. One of my old consultant suits or not? The nakedness of the swimming pool changing room took all that anxiety away I could be bolder in my questions and no one seemed to mind me.) Anyway, the army of leavers or those who had already left provided me with many willing informants.

Quarry House is an oval building. The point facing the centre of the city has the entrance I described earlier and on the slope down to the traffic at the roundabout I passed the famous West Yorkshire Playhouse. The other point faces east out of the city and has St. James's Hospital three-quarters of a mile to the north. That is the entrance for the swimming pool and fitness centre.

Many offices are open-plan, so people make corridors of them. They cannot open the windows (so much for that promise when they were all in London). They can use the car park on a one in three rota. They often cannot book rooms for meetings because there is no free accommodation, and they then have to go to one of the satellite places in Leeds, or out of the city altogether.

They complain of pressures from deadlines and projects, and the 'promotion board' to which civil servants are subject.

I heard a story of one person's job disappearing during her maternity leave.

Any new legislation increases the work, because it is the task of some staff to produce research to back the legislation and to prepare ministers for questions. At these times they are all the more aware how many fewer of them there are.

I heard that staff can be observed muttering to themselves in lifts, breathing heavily, fidgeting, walking up and down and even, in some places, chain smoking; and I saw most of those behaviours for myself.

Those that talk often say that others are in a worse state.

People often talk of having given up. Given up walking, given up their families. They talk of the strain on relationships and family life. No one tells them not to work like this for the exaggerated work ethic is the new norm. Some have had breakdowns or been very ill.

The pulse of the building

Everybody in this building is suffering from the double major organisational change: relocation, followed by cuts. What is it like?

Stress seminars (avoiding and managing it) have been well received. Staff were invited to have checks on their blood pressure and other signs of stress related strain. The results did not look healthy for the building, so the management told the occupational health department to provide something.

This seemed like so many organisations. When stress starts to show they organise help (did they think of another contract?) rather than look at how it was caused.

It is as though the people with the power to change the way things are, think of sub-contracts to prevent them from having to do anything. And no one dares challenge them.

Throughout the building there is a tension and a sense of life being short. For example there were three different occupational health nurses in each of its first three years.

The paradoxical joke I was told twice was to try to think it's all rational and then you'll really go crazy.

Twenty-four hour changes in contract? If an outside organisation wins a contract, existing staff are usually kept on, but contracts can be changed within 24 hours. In fact, this very rarely happens but more subtle changes can come later. No one I spoke to liked the story of cleaners being paid £2.40 an hour by the contractors, but there it is.

There are several first aid rooms. It is part of managing stress.

Stressed people with headaches, tearful, feel their panics coming on and say they are struggling with changes in their role, or their room, or the telephone number of their project.

Health promotion includes leafleting and notices on the boards which are on every floor. There is a reflexologist and aromatherapist, for which people have to pay although the use of the room is free.

HASSRA (Health and Social Services Recreational Association) in Leeds is an active staff association. It provides trips at reduced rates to the theatre and other places and organises a lottery, fitness centre activities etc. Was there some suspicion that people working in the contracted organisations are happier than the civil servants? In a strange way they may feel that they know more of what is happening than their colleagues still directly employed by the state, who are fearful of what may happen to them next in the privatisation process.

I did not contact HASSRA, in accordance with my own 'policy and guidelines' which kept me away from professional or staff organisations for the purposes of this book.

The Intelligence Unit of the NHSE is there to collaborate with the regions, purchasers and trusts in presenting effectively to the public a positive account of the health care services… and the code of practice on openness in the NHS. I was curious but did not try to call in.

A further walk around the building, inside more than out

Outside, for every flight of steps, there is a ramp for wheelchairs. The gardens, which I had noted on my first visit as being imaginatively landscaped and promising looking, appeared much the same. Still promising.

The restaurant had closed at 3.30, but in the shop by the pool I bought a packet of biscuits and a bottle of water.

The building is oval on the inside too, with a hollowed out centre with a thick bar of corridors across the middle. Trapped in the middle are the two internal gardens separated by the central corridors which go transversely, on several floors, between the sides. The gardens are Japanese style and look little attended or used: even before 4.30 in the afternoon the doors were locked. The central area on the ground floor of the transverse bar is around the lifts. It is vivid and can be viewed from many of the high vantage points on the inside of the oval. It is covered with a brightly coloured carpet in a design representing the rivers and hills of Yorkshire. It has wide bands and shapes in blues, yellows, greens and reds.

It has a thick pile which paralyses wheelchairs.

Chapter 23

Sexism in NHS management

I was not looking for this chapter. The subject appeared before me so often that a chapter grew.

It reminded me of the last thing I published in the *BMJ* with my colleague Sandy Bourne (1982) from the Tavistock Clinic. We had written over half a dozen papers on distinction awards for consultants, criticising the allocation by committees in secret of up to the equivalent of an extra whole salary in addition to the basic one every year until retirement. We had examined all sorts of factors: age and specialty of recipients, specialty of members of committees, collection of data. Suddenly, as we were working on what was to be our last paper together, we realised that most of our very bright female fellow medical students had vanished. Women were grossly under-represented both on the committees and as recipients of awards.

I knew that of the 30 or so people interviewing and being interviewed for the jobs of leading the eight English NHS Executive areas, there were four women. But I start with a story of my own.

The BMA meeting

A couple of years before I retired, I was at the first meeting of medical directors of trusts to be held at the BMA. For political correctness, the literature, the notices, the acceptance letter and the handouts were impeccable.

To open, the chief medical officer of the Department of Health addressed all 100 of us with a message from the Secretary of State, Virginia Bottomley, whom he had met at 8.30 that morning. I recall the opening three words of the message: 'Tell the chaps...'

As the day wore on I heard that word 'chaps' again and again from speakers, most of whom, like the majority of those present, were male. I know dictionaries give different meanings, but the Shorter Oxford clearly has 'chiefly of young men', and 'men' does seem to the common understanding.

When I mentioned it, I was applauded and the chairman, acknowledging the point, said the literature was so good because it was edited by a woman.

Sporting and military metaphors

The policies have to be kicked in.

The referee's decision.

Get it done by close of play.

Loose cannon.

Keep your powder dry.

Rules of engagement.

Scatter gun approach.

Getting your ducks lined up (for shooting at).

Rapier, not blunderbuss

Women and how they are referred to

Identifying women in terms of the men with whom they had sexual rela-tionships. (The senior manager, who sleeps with X.)

'Ladies' as mode of address, if the group is women.

Women's hair and clothing referred to more than that of men.

If women do as men do

The women's group, stimulated by the women's unit of NHSE, met in the evenings and then decided to meet in the daytime. The chief executive asked why there was such a meeting. They organised a meeting with an open invi-tation to women in the trust. Forty to fifty attended. They agreed to have two events per year.

An executive director asked publicly who had been the leader in setting up those meetings and why so many managers were unavailable for that time without him being told. (When other groups of managers were not available, the chief executive and other executive directors were often not told.) An observer noticed the telling-off manner in which this was said and, when his gaze was returned, 'Don't eyeball me, lady.'

Negotiating in the style modelled by the male leaders was, when tried by a woman, called 'going for the jugular', or 'hitting hard'.

If the numbers of women increase

When the number of women in a regional group of 15 representatives got up to three, it was described as a 'take-over by the ladies'.

Body language and groups

On Friday evening the men went to the pub where many decisions were made.

Men, before meetings started, leaning back in their chairs with their feet on the table. Or tipping right back on their chairs, with their legs stretched out, groin up.

At the top table

Regular dinners for the general managers or chief executives of the regional health authorities were held in London, attended by the previous chief executive of the NHSE. A feature was sexist jokes. Then one month, the joker alluded to a need to protect the ladies and changed the emphasis to smut.

How to get a job

One middle manager boasted that she had been told that she was appointed because she was the one who opened her legs. And she said it got her more than the job.

It is typical for many of the mixed sex management groups, all at the same level, to be one older woman in her mid forties amidst men 10 to 15 years younger.

I was told that mostly it was certain types of women who succeed. The 'feminine', younger women who do not challenge the men and who clear up and pour the coffee, and the older ones who have given up dressing for a fashion parade.

It is not all in men's favour

At the appointments committee, the young woman is appointed over the older man with the comment, 'What's taken him so long to get there?'

The ability to show, share and accept emotion is to do with many things, but often women tend to embrace emotion more readily. Where a man and a woman have both not got jobs, it has been suggested to me that the woman is more likely to have felt surrounded and supported by a great many people, whereas the man will have felt isolated and deserted. I heard the usual difficulties were encountered by any who challenged these practices.

Challenge is going on, within the BMA and the Department of Health. There is an educational programme for the BMA's own committees. Its Career Progress of Doctors Committee has produced interesting guidelines, especially on patronage (1993), in which it identifies informal references as a major tool of patronage and sexism, and recommends forbidding them.

Chapter 24

How many patients?
'I'd rather die at home'

Philip and David had been friends at school but had barely met again until they were thrown together in a coronary rehabilitation unit five years ago. They had both had coronary bypass surgery. They both did fairly well but they both had some complications. When worried they were able to telephone the cardiac surgery unit and any crises were discussed with them directly. Their GP could refer them there and they would be seen.

When Philip moved to live with his daughter Alison in another part of the country, his specialist in the cardiac hospital sent his notes to the 'sister' establishment serving the area in which Philip was going to be. Even the check up date was transferred and Philip and his daughter were both reassured when a reminder of the appointment came from their 'new' hospital.

The check up confirmed their worst fears. All was not well and one of the bypasses was choking. This was the cause of the distressing sensations which Philip had had in his chest since the move. He might need another bypass. They would watch him closely, do further investigations, but if there was any trouble meanwhile, they said:

'You must get yourself admitted here immediately.'

The real test came six weeks later.

Day 1

Friday evening Philip collapsed with severe chest pain and sweating. He and his granddaughter, who was with him at the time, both recognised the signs. She telephoned for an ambulance. The ambulance and Alison arrived at the same time.

'You know to take him straight to 'X' hospital for the cardiac unit, don't you?' said his daughter, as Philip was taken on the stretcher into the vehicle.

'On no, we can't do that. We have to go to the trust hospital first.'

'No it's been arranged. We saw the specialist six weeks ago and he said admit immediately to their unit.'

'I'm sorry, we have our orders. We have to take everybody to the trust hospital. Then they can be transferred to the cardiac unit. That's the order.'

Philip was in no position to argue and Alison gave in, but accompanied him in the ambulance to the trust hospital's accident and emergency department.

Six hours later Philip was transferred to the cardiac ward of the trust hospital. It was not six hours' idle wait but six hours' activity of investigation, drips and medication. It took them over into:

Day 2

In the cardiac ward Alison thought the staff worked hard and were dedicated. But she had not seen her father in so much pain before and the staff seemed to have difficulty in alleviating it. She began to wonder what difference it would have made if he was back in the unit with which he was familiar in his own part of the country. Or if she had managed to persuade the ambulance driver to go straight to the cardiac hospital, as they had been led to expect.

This was a six bedded ward. People seemed to be admitted and discharged every day but neither Philip nor Alison could work out where they went.

Day 3

Still in pain.

Day 4

Still in pain, but less so. The consultant visited Philip, looked at all the test results, agreed that he should be transferred to the specialist hospital and said that he would speak to the consultant whom Philip had already seen there.

Day 5

Philip was told by one of the nursing staff that the consultant at the specialist hospital was away and nobody else could change the priority waiting list. Therefore they would discharge him and transfer him to the medical ward. Why talk of discharge and transfer in the same sentence? Philip and Alison both wondered this when all that was happening was a move down a corridor. They came to understand more later.

Day 6

'We are going to do some tests on behalf of the specialist hospital, so we can speed things up later on.'

Day 7

'The tests confirm the need for the bypass so things should be quite smooth now.'

Day 8

Telephone call to Alison.

'Please would you come to collect your father and take him home? Well, we need the bed. He is off his drips and therefore he could as well be at home while he is waiting to go into the specialist hospital. But do remember, because he is on the priority waiting list for the specialist hospital, he could be called within the next 48 hours.'

Days 8 to 13

Philip at home. Alison off work to be with him. A few telephone calls with the specialist hospital.

'Don't worry. You will be called any time.'

Day 14

11.45 pm. Sudden attack of chest pain. Ambulance to trust hospital accident and emergency department.

Day 15

First five hours in the accident and emergency department. Admission and investigation procedures.

'But he has just been discharged from your medical ward. Why not get his notes from the ward?'

'We must treat him as a new patient and go through all the investigations.'

'But could I go and get the notes?'

'The notes won't be in the ward now.'

'Well they might be in the medical records department. Why don't you get his old notes? They have done all these tests.'

'We must treat him as a new patient and go through all the investigations.'

Admitted to the trust's own six bedded cardiac ward again.

Day 16

Pain being controlled more effectively this time. Philip more comfortable.

Day 17

Alison goes back to work. Visits in the evening. Four beds full. Two empty. No father. He has been discharged.

'Discharged? But I am his daughter. Where is he? Nobody has told me.'

'Did the ward have your phone number?'

Alison resisted the impulse to count the number of times she had given her telephone number to various clerking staff and limited herself to saying 'Yes'.

Another nurse walking by heard some of this and interrupted to say:

'No. He has not been discharged. He has moved to...' and she named another ward.

Alison went, but he was not there. Back to the cardiac ward.

'Sorry. No, he is not in that ward. He has gone to a different bay. Come, I'll take you.'

Down the corridor, round a corner, through swing doors, past more beds, into the side bay. Empty.

'Sorry, he's not there.'

Alison had noticed.

'We'll do a search.'

Together they walked down a wing of the hospital; by piles of stores, trolleys and furniture; through two wards with space for three six bedded bays in each, but containing packing cases and cleaning equipment; down a corridor with many closed doors and a bathroom, with door open, stacked almost to overflowing with babies' nappies, into a two bedded room where Philip and a fellow patient were lying in beds.

Philip was subdued but clear in his mind. He had been told that he and his companion had used up 'their' five days in the cardiac ward and had therefore been transferred to two separate six bedded medical bays. Among the other occupants of Philip's bay, there was one woman who looked as his own mother did shortly before she died, and opposite her was another one who reminded him so much of his wife before she had died. He said very quietly that it was the first time he had done it, but he had made a terrible fuss. So had his companion. The other medical bays were full, so they had been discharged. That's why they were now geriatrics.

Philip was 73.

Day 18

The geriatric consultant saw Philip and telephoned the specialist cardiac hospital. 'Yes, the consultant has agreed to take you in.'

Day 19

Further tests show that this attack was 'angina only'. 'Yes, you still need to go to the specialist cardiac hospital.'

Day 20

The consultant discussed transfer with Philip.

Day 21

Comfortable.

Day 22

Philip was introduced to the nurse who would accompany him in the ambulance on the following day. He was told that because the tests had already been done in the trust's hospital, he could expect to be operated on during the day he arrived. He was very positive and asked Alison to bring in some special clothes. Optimistically anticipating the next day.

Alison had noticed on the nurses' noticeboard her father's transfer and the name of the accompanying nurse, both in red, against the next day.

Day 23

Alison telephoned the specialist hospital from work, but whoever she managed to speak to knew nothing of her father. She telephoned the trust's hospital and was told yes, he was still going.

'Don't worry. We are waiting for the transport to arrive. They are sometimes delayed because they have to deal with emergencies.'

At 7.00 pm someone from the hospital telephoned Alison at home:

'Sorry, but please would you take your father home. We are discharging him to your care. This is all unofficial and it won't affect the transfer to the specialist hospital. We are keeping it all unofficial, well, in case what happened last time happens again. That is in case the specialist hospital sees him as no longer a priority. He is still a priority. This is a paper exercise and it really doesn't affect that. Please would you take him home now.'

A very deflated Philip went home. At least he would get regular meals. On at least three days they had not given him his lunch.

Day 24

Alison stayed at home and received a phone call from the trust's hospital in the early morning:

'Please would you tell us where your father is? We had a phone call for him and couldn't find him here. Do you know where he is?'

She answered the question but for once did not tell her father what the call had been about.

Instead at 9.30 am she telephoned the specialist hospital and learnt that they had been told that her father had been discharged and he was therefore again off their priority list. She telephoned the local hospital.

Day 26

In despair, Alison telephoned the doctor who had done one of the more complicated tests (the angiogram) at the specialist hospital. He had listened before and might do so again.

He did listen, and then said very clearly that what had happened was exactly what they had been told would not happen: they had lost the bed there for her father, because of the discharge home.

'The system is one in which we take patients in a very critical condition and somebody who has gone home is deemed to be no longer in a very critical condition.'

When she persisted and pointed out that her father had not seen a heart specialist after this last episode, he suggested that she could:

- complain to the local trust;
- get hold of the secretary of the surgeon at the specialist hospital and try to fix an appointment;
- try to understand (he did say 'please') that so many consultants are having to see him because that is now part of the system.

She did telephone the local trust to complain and was asked, 'Is it an outpatient or an inpatient and if it's an inpatient, is it medical, surgical, or what?' She told the story and said that she was not wanting to complain about any particular person, but about the system. 'OK, I will speak to Dr X and he will give you a ring.' The manager added some words which implied that an apology would be made. Again, Alison said, 'I am not complaining about a person. I am complaining of the system.' Then she was told: 'Well, it really can take five hours to find a bed in hospital because you have to arrange to discharge others, move people from one place to another. All that waiting in the accident and emergency department is not staff idly sitting around. They are waiting for something to happen. If your father did have an emergency they would act very quickly.'

She telephoned the specialist hospital again, spoke to the surgeon's secretary and got an offer of an outpatient appointment in a week's time.

Alison tried to understand that seeing so many consultants and being in so many wards was part of the system. She started by counting the number of consultants that her father had seen, at least while at the local trust hospital. They seemed to come from:

(i)   the emergency team;
(ii) the cardiac ward;
(iii) the medical team (down the corridor);
(iv) the geriatric ward;
(v)   the cardiac surgery unit in the other hospital (two).

Day 30

Outpatient appointment. 'Well, things have changed. We don't now recommend a second bypass operation for somebody of your age. We will see you again in a month. We might do a simple procedure to help remove the clot that has re-formed.'

Day 31

The GP called and she, Philip and Alison reviewed what had happened and what they could do next.

The GP knew that the six bedded acute cardiac ward in the trust hospital worked on a five day 'turnaround'. Following the recent merger of the trust with its neighbour, the ward was serving a population double that for which it was set up a few years ago.

They discussed their rights for a second opinion under the Patient's Charter, but the GP was pessimistic. 'They would say that you have had a second opinion already, even a third, fourth and fifth opinion. You see, I am really not confident that we can get out of this system unless you move back to your old home town. I know that's not what you want.'

It was clear to them that their GP was in as much despair of the service as they were. And as tired out too.

Alison told the GP how a week into the second admission to the trust hospital when the staff wanted to transfer Philip to the geriatric ward, she had noticed that the written details were as if he had been admitted only the night before. She had wondered if this was a slip, or if it was to give it the appearance of discharge and readmission?

The GP explained to them that the most important statistic was the 'number of patients treated'. This applied to hospitals, to units or departments, and especially, she added, it mattered to politicians.

They showed the GP the drug box supplied by the hospital. They had been alarmed to see that a change had been made to a complicated prescription given by the people at the specialist hospital, but the nurse had said the change was perfectly satisfactory and they should not worry. The GP inspected the drug box and concluded that they were the same medicines, but in a different preparation. She did not know why the nurse had not told them that there was no change at all.

If it happened again, the first thing that Alison said they would do differently would be on no account to leave communication between the professionals, to the professionals. They would do it themselves every time they could. An example of this was the very first appointment at the specialist hospital. Alison arranged this while the staff at the hospital said, 'We think we can do it. We'll get on to it right away.'

The next thing they would do would be to take food with them every time they visited in case Philip had been moved to another ward and his food had been forgotten.

Philip closed the discussion by saying that he would never go back to the local trust hospital again. He would rather die at home. At least he was not going to be 'another patient treated' again.

The friend's phone call

David telephoned. He had had a few troubles of his own, but was still very pleased with the staff at the specialist hospital in the other part of the country. And there were not even rumours of trust mergers where he lived. Responding to Philip's story, David said his son had told him of 'finished consultant episodes' and 'numbers of patients treated'. He was sure that Philip's experiences of transfer and new case notes must have had a pay-off somewhere. As for himself, he said that he was not ambitious. He was quite prepared to stay at being one person, or rather one patient.

Chapter 25

Conclusion

This is the end of the book, but not of the story. That seems to be continuing as fast as ever. I still see it in the papers: 'Go-ahead for trusts to sell private health plans', 'Trusts banned from selling private health plans'. 'Thirty casualty units should be closed'. 'Casualty closure unlawful'. '£500,000 perks scandal'. 'Second rate only for NHS cancer cases'.

In July 1996 the Association of First Division Civil Servants issued a press release on the increasing pressure from government departments to compromise their political impartiality. In August 1996 a trust in Swansea made its clinical director and a dozen others redundant when they lost the elderly care contract, and within a week withdrew the notices for four months.

I still receive messages from people. (Have I interviewed an occupational therapist or a catering manager?) I still hear from people who say they have stories. I have had to refuse. Market forces in the world of producing, selling and buying books (how big a book would you buy?) persuaded me to cut much from my manuscript.

And I had to stop.

Stress at work and its effects

You will have heard of 'cohort studies' when for example a group of children all born on the same day are followed up for years. Some effects of young children going into hospital, or of people smoking (causes of deaths among doctors were being examined) came to light in this way.

The Whitehall 11 study is following up 10,000 civil servants and it so happened that over 600 members of one department were up for special change: privatisation. The study took into account 'health related behaviours' (smoking, drinking and exercise patterns), baseline screening and follow up over four years. A sound scientific study. The conclusion, published in the *BMJ* in November 1995 by Jane Ferrie et al., was that being privatised was not good for you. It was not the sort of work that has often been done, but it did confirm the findings of a prospective study on the effects on the health of the workforce of a factory closure in Michigan, published in 1977.

The latest publication from the Whitehall 11 study prior to this book going to press was in February 1997 (Bosma et al). It concluded that low control at work carries an increased risk of future heart troubles.

In April 1996 the *BMJ* carried an editorial, 'Overwork can kill' (Michie and Cockcroft), and the BMA launched its stress counselling service with a 24 hour helpline for doctors. (I have tested the helpline and it is still working.)

What is happening at the NHS Executive at Quarry House in Leeds, let alone what is going on in most of the NHS, would make excellent subject matter for further research.

The 'league tables'

In the month when the 1995/6 hospital figures were published, all 262 pages of which I got, Edward Pilkington, a *Guardian* journalist, described (3 July 1996) his visit to a five star casualty department where 99% of patients were assessed within five minutes of arrival. The five stars had an upward pointing arrow indicating improvement on last year's figures. A bandage was put on his bleeding face wound and he was lifted on to a trolley within the first five minutes, and it was done impeccably. Ten hours later, he was X-rayed by a radiologist who said she or he could have seen him hours earlier if asked. In the next hour he was stitched up; as were the figures, because he had been 'seen' within the first five minutes.

Secrecy

The Nolan Report (*Standards in Public Life*), published in May 1995, got much attention at the time, but mostly for what it said about quangos and secrecy. People did not seem to notice that much of it was on the NHS: even the BMA library had no copy until I requested it. On 'whistleblowing', its recommendation (no. 116) was that each NHS body 'should nominate an official or board member entrusted with the duty of investigating staff concerns about propriety raised confidentially. Staff should be able to make complaints without going through the normal management structure, and should be guaranteed anonymity.'

In the same year *Whistleblowing in the Health Service*, edited by Geoffrey Hunt, was published by Edward Arnold, and in 1996 the *BMA News Review* reported in August that 83 of 120 doctors who had been suspended over the past ten years had been reinstated. Harry Jacobs (1989) and the Society of Clinical Psychiatrists had already published a supplement (*Suspensions: A Blot on the NHS*), and a paper by Peter Tomlin and Harry Jacobs, bringing the concerns up to date, will be published in 1997.

I have often wondered what difference the Nolan proposal would have made to many of the stories I heard, and how many NHS bodies have implemented it.

I know it had not been implemented in the trust where, soon after that date, a consultant did write to the chairperson on how a particular investigation had been handled (hostility to nurses, no offer of support to staff, no acknowledgement of distress and subsequent staff illness). The consultant received a quick response by telephone: 'We had better meet.' They met and the chairperson addressed him with raised finger, saying that a letter like that was not wanted again. The consultant was told that he was considered like a shop assistant at the high street chemists, his job was to give out the medicines as he was told by the pharmacist and the branch manager (the medical director and the chief executive of the trust respectively). The consultant was to do what he was told. (The consultant resigned and another left soon after.)

Sometimes discussion on openness has become polarised and adversarial. Under the title *The Rise of Stalinism in the NHS*, the BMJ published three papers in December 1994. The first of these was Naomi Craft's *Secrecy in the NHS*, which listed 30 examples. One was that of Dr John Spencer (see Chapter 17) who signed an agreement not to speak publicly on what had happened. A few weeks later Alan Langlands, the chief executive of the NHS executive, responded. He suggested that the anecdotes did not bear objective scrutiny. He deplored the bugging of the telephone, but complained that the 'prompt' departure of the chief executive was omitted from the account. Well, in fact, the consultant was suspended at two minutes to midnight and the chief executive did not go until a couple of weeks later. On the point that Naomi Craft was making, namely that a doctor signed an agreement to talk no more in public, he said nothing.

Sometimes discussions on openness fizzle out. No letter was published pointing out the omission.

May there be peace at last?

I dwelled on the management of change at the NHS Executive in Leeds, realising that something similar has been happening in many places. One example that has received considerable press cover, including in the management press itself, has been Cardiff. The usual thing of bringing together hospitals and groups, having to reduce costs, finding which things could be cut, amalgamated and so on. Done in much the usual way as I have described already. I wondered if the bad vibes I had picked up were deserved, until I heard a new acronym in common use there. It was FIFO, which stands for Fit in or...

The frequency of new publications seems to be increasing. In 1996 Hadley and Clough produced *Care and Chaos: Frustration and Challenge in Community Care*. A dismal picture. On a more constructive note came a suggestion from Stephen Harrison and Peter Lachmann, *Towards a High-Trust NHS: Proposals for a Minimally Invasive Reform*. In ending this commendably brief, 25-page work, they consider possible resistance from what they call 'hard line' managerealists, noting that such a style 'thrives on low-trust relationships'.

The new Health Secretary, Stephen Dorrell, saw the beginning of April 1996, the date of the amalgamation of the GP and health authority sides of the purchasers, as a point of consolidation. The reforms are here to stay. David Brindle, writing up an interview with Mr Dorrell in *The Guardian*, headed his article, 'After the revolution, a time for peace'. I hope there will be; but peace, too, may be costed.

Another bid for peace came three months later from Karen Caines, Director of the Institute of Health Services, in an open letter in *The Guardian* to Jane Richards, chairperson of the BMA's representative body. In acknowledging the frankly political pressures on the NHS, she muses how much more effective doctors and managers could be if they stood 'shoulder to shoulder'.

Back to Leeds and Quarry House

It was raining heavily on the day I returned to Leeds for my last visit. For the first time I got a taxi to Quarry House. It took nearly ten minutes, which is not much less than the best time I had managed the distance on foot. The driver talked.

He told me that for a year or more after the new building opened, the first train from London would disgorge 20 people who took 20 different cabs through 30 minutes of rush hour traffic to Quarry House. On the ramp they had to queue to get through the machine for the security passes. One passenger forgetting a pass could jam the whole line, because the queue of taxis behind prevented any single one from reversing. My driver did not know if there were fewer people making the morning journey from London nowadays, or if they were taking more exercise, but there were not the lines of cabs going to Quarry House. He hoped it was because they were getting on better and could share cabs.

I thought of the good things that had come out of Quarry House and out of management. Alan Langlands has denied that there is a 'conspiracy' in the executive to destroy the NHS and I believe him. I agree with him that he and his colleagues aim to work for the best interests of patients.

I thought of endings. I have seen several resignation letters, and the replies received from senior management. Some of the leavers wrote eloquently of their frustration with the pace of changes, of demands for more efficiency with fewer resources; and they felt the managers, or others driving the reforms, had little idea of what it was like to do clinical work, facing sick or dying people. Some of the managers wrote back acknowledging that they had too little experience of the work. Some wrote regretting the pressure which the need to balance books forced them to place on staff.

NAHAT (National Association of Health Authorities and Trusts, my last acronym) publishes a series called *Speaking Up: Policy and Change in the NHS*. They are occasional 'think pieces' by senior people. In *Minding Our Own Business* (1995), Ken Jarrold, who is the director of human and corporate resources at the Executive, writes of more skilled and experienced managers being more likely to deal with change sensitively and less likely to behave in a macho style. By using the phrase 'indulge in' for the latter, he seems to acknowledge at least an undesirability in it. His main appeal is for those in the NHS to 'mind' each other. Bottom lines have to be bottom lines, but Ken Jarrold still wants managers to care for the NHS and to be demonstrably doing so.

I hope he is heard.

Leaving and beating

I am a passionate swimmer and never travel without the necessary trunks, goggles and the smallest useful towel. Collecting stories for this book I have swum in ... well, all sorts of places. My last swim was in Quarry House. As usual, I was told that I may use the swimming pool as a visitor. I paid my £2.40 and swam. A long pool, with a small paddling pool. It is the sort whose water comes right to the top of the sides and is drained away through grills in the tiles immediately round the edge. (The modern style, it looks smart and a swimmer's bow wave goes right over the top rather than bouncing back: timed lengths may be faster.) In this particular pool the edge tiles themselves are the same colour as those under the water, but some 20 or 30cm further out is a line of dark ones. From my position as a swimmer, that line looked like the edge. I was not wearing my spectacles, but ordinary swimming goggles. Head banging is a risk which I discovered to my cost.

For my last length I often do back stroke. As I neared the end of the pool,

I glanced over my shoulder, saw the black line of tiles, and treated that as the edge. I am a strong swimmer and have little hair.

As I was recovering in the changing room I thought that how my visit had ended might be the nearest I shall ever get to banging my head on a brick wall. It is a modern pool, efficient and fast track, high-quality; and I got hurt. Perhaps a metaphor for all sides in the NHS.

And two subjects, mentioned by more than one person, kept on coming back to me.

One was of business people who became non-executive directors of trusts: this led some to comment on how many presentations to the board opened with an emphasis on money, and others to remark that no large company would embark on so great a reform of itself without doing a 'pilot' first.

The other concerned origins. I am not keen on 'linear' ideas which often attribute blame to one person. I think we are too complicated for that. But I was directed to a story that appeared in the *London Review of Books* (20 October 1994). I call it the story of Mrs. Thatcher's beating.

> Christopher Hitchens, journalist and writer, described meeting Mrs. Thatcher at a book launch in the House of Lords. It was in 1977, so she was leader of the Conservative Party, but not yet Prime Minister. He wrote that he was 'bewitched' by her presence and got himself introduced. After seconds, they got into an argument, and on one point (he was right and because I now know more of the story, I know he was right) they faced an impasse. After a turn or two, he used the social device of making a slight bow. When he resumed eye contact, she held it and delivered what, in the context of this book, I call a managerial directive: 'Bow lower.' He did, a bit, but was further directed, with stronger emphasis on the first word, '*Much* lower.' He described his following mental state in terms which reminded me of a hypnotic trance: he lost his sense of independent volition. He did go lower and then, after a few moments, was hit hard on the behind with a rolled up paper which she had produced from behind her back. He struggled upright and saw her making for the door as he was addressed over her shoulder, 'Naughty boy.'

I was so curious after reading this story, which two of my informants had mentioned, that I rang Christopher Hitchens himself. Yes, it was as he had written (and as I describe).

I asked what the other people did. It seemed that there was a strange silence with rather embarrassed looks, but no one mentioned it. And no one wrote about it after he had made it public in 1974. He had of course taken the matter no further. He had co-operated in the experience, although he had not known what was going to happen next. Not what you could call 'informed consent' He agreed that the episode could be seen as a metaphor for much of what happened to the country under her rule, and under the changes in the NHS.

The last thing to look at in Leeds

The sun had come out when I left the NHSE by the city side and walked through the gardens down Quarry Hill.

I went past the West Yorkshire Playhouse, across the one way system of the roundabout, up Eastgate, over the top and down Headrow to the City Art Gallery on the right. Upstairs was a massive work composed entirely of memorial plaques. It is pale bluish-green, rectangular in shape, with writing in blue.

Mary Rogers, stewardess of the Stella, Mar 30th 1889 self-sacrificed by giving up her lifebelt and voluntarily going down in the sinking ship.

Harry Sisley of Kilburn aged 10 drowned in attempting to save his brother after he himself had just been rescued. May 24 1878.

Alice Ayres, daughter of a bricklayer's labourer who by intrepid conduct saved three children from a burning house in Union Street, Borough, at the cost of her own young life. April 24, 1885.

It is entitled 'Monument'. It is not always there. The artist is Susan Hiller, who based it on Geoffrey Watts' memorial plaques in Postman's Park, Little Britain, near St. Paul's Cathedral.

I thought of those who had been made redundant, been suspended, seen their jobs disappear; who had been ill, taken drugs, antidepressants and tranquillisers; seen their GPs and specialists, had breakdowns or major physical illness. I thought of those who had felt bewildered, worried or had lost their reasoning; who had not kept up with the paperwork, had not slept, who cried and trembled, woke in the night, lost friendships, relationships, or their souls; who said that telling their stories was like a therapeutic session.

I wondered if there would be a monument for those caught up in the NHS reforms.

Probably not, but I hope the NHS survives and that you continue to work in it or to use it. Whatever the encounters, I hope you will wonder what story lies behind them.

APPENDIX I

Just a bit more paperwork

Here are a few examples from all the memoranda, letters, notices and leaflets I have seen. As usual, I have made changes to safeguard sources.

INFORMATION FOR PROFESSIONALS

My attention was often drawn to the *Patient's Charter*, particularly (under Rights and Standards Throughout the NHS) over access to services:

*You have the **right** to:*
* *be referred to a consultant acceptable to you.*
* *receive detailed information on local health services*
*You can **expect** the NHS to make it easy for everyone to use its services.*

In her foreword to the last edition I was sent (in February 1997), Virginia Bottomley wrote, *'More and more information is available to the public about their local health service.'*

I thought about this as I travelled to one specialist department which was having a drive to streamline its procedures and inform patients and referrers about financing. By the time I visited, they were working things out less clumsily in a brochure to stimulate business from professional referrers.

We have now streamlined our referral procedure for your convenience.
Non-urgent cases
Referral letters must include the patient's postcode. The postcode enables the business manager's department to identify the potential funding health authority as soon as possible.

In those cases where the health authority has an existing and active contract with our department, an appointment will be sent, by return, to the patient and a letter will be sent to the referrer.

If the contract is no longer active, usually because it has been 'completed', then a request will be processed by our business department to the health authority for approval (i.e. funding) for us to see the patient as an extra-contractual referral (ECR).

If the health authority has no contract for our department's service, the same process is initiated, so as to have the necessary funding arranged as soon as possible.

As soon as approval for an ECR payment is confirmed (usually by fax), the patient is sent an appointment and the referrer is advised accordingly.

However, if no approval is forthcoming, no appointment is sent, but the referrer is informed immediately. The referrer may then arrange for a re-referral to a provider for which the appropriate health authority does have an active contract, or appeal to the original health authority for a reconsideration of the case on the grounds, usually, of lack of alternative specialist facilities provided by any provider with whom the authority does have a contract. A final appeal may be on the grounds of need for the special excellence of this department.

We, ourselves, would not normally be involved in any such appeal or negotiation. And, of course, in accordance with the guidelines of the Department of Health, the patient should not be involved in any way, or even be aware that the process is under way.

If you have a patient whom you are wanting to refer to us and are having any difficulty with the process, please do not hesitate to contact our business manager's department on...

HELP FOR CHARITIES AND THE VOLUNTARY SECTOR

For years many voluntary organisations have done some work within the NHS. They have included counsellors, befrienders, visitors. It was inevitable that the NHS would want a more formal arrangement with a service specification drawn up. Among the things which the managers in the voluntary sector were having to make sense of, I found the following excerpts:

1. The word 'support' to be justified.

2. The provider shall be liable for and indemnified for the commissioner (sic) against any liability or loss from any action, suit or claim arising out of or in connection with any work carried out by or on behalf of the provider or those authorised to act on its behalf in the relation to the provision of services covered by this contract. Equally the provider will be responsible for any loss occasioned by action arising out of or in connection with the construction, maintenance or use by the provider or those authorised to act on its behalf of the works or services constructed, operating or used by it or the plant, apparatus or equipment installed in that connection.

3. The organisation will ensure all clients are

(a) seen in a clean and safe environment, appropriately furnished and that any food and beverage received therein will be of an acceptable standard

(b) ensure that all counselling takes place in a private environment and is carried out in a responsible, dignified and reasonable manner.

WHO SHOULD GO TO HOSPITAL?

One trust and purchaser had a discussion on quality standards for the following year's contracts. The proposals circulated included that no patient should be admitted with asthma, ischaemic heart disease or strokes.

INDIVIDUAL PERFORMANCE REVIEW (IPR)

Staff appraisal has been mentioned several times and I obtained the written guidance from a couple of trusts. Reading each document gave me the feeling that my eyes were glazing over. Several sentences I simply could not understand and yet they were from documents that people were really using. For anonymity, I have made changes, but preserved the style of both in creating the following hybrid.

XYZ Trust Individual Performance Review

1 IPR — What It Is

IPR or individual performance review is a new system for the performance appraisal cascading throughout the NHS. It is intended to be 'user friendly' to those people using it. That is the individual whose performance is being reviewed and the manager who helps him or her in that review.

It is an annual process for both individuals and teams. Its intention is to reinforce the sense that an individual has of his or her contract for the team's success and towards the common aims of the team and the trust. It supports both the individual in his or her individual development and it supports the team.

It is a continual process with annual cycles. Each cycle of a year involves each individual in:

- *Work objectives setting at the beginning of the year;*

- *Drawing up a personal development plan;*

- *Having regular one-to-one meetings with your manager, throughout the year. These meetings are to pick up and to smooth out any difficulties as they arise and to monitor and review objectives;*

- *A special performance appraisal meeting at the end of the year. In this meeting all achievements over the year may be recognised, both performance ones and performance development ones.*

Our trust has an agreed policy for all staff to share in performance appraisal. Obviously, however, it will take some time for IPR to be available for everyone. In this, the first year, the trust has decided to use IPR in, among others, the XYZ service.

2 Setting the Objectives

At the start of each year in the HR cycle all individuals will set out their work objectives for the coming year. This will involve a careful review of the job description and their team's service priorities, aims and objectives and service standards. It will also need to be looked at alongside a list of clients' needs so that individuals can identify exactly what it is they are aiming for as an achievement for work.

Individuals are advised, when writing their individual objectives, to look also at those of close colleagues and of the managers so that clear, compatible goals are established, with co-ordination of roles and responsibilities.

The objectives should of course cover all areas of work (see job description) so that anything done at work during the year can logistically be integrated into the review. It is accepted that some objectives may focus more on maintaining the ongoing services and others more on management or development.

Whatever objectives are chosen they should be qualitatively or quantitatively measurable.

In the first instance, we are concerned that people try to take on too much and do advise that the total number of objectives should be in single figures.

Each objective has its own list of key targets and action points. These also should be clear so that it is clear what has to be achieved in order for the objective to be attained.

Timescales are important, but don't put too many of them too late!

When the objectives and action points are agreed between individuals and their manager, which may take two or three meetings, they can produce a final individual action plan showing a shared commitment to the achievement of the individual work goals and the way to get there.

3 Documentation

The objective setting documentation is called the Performance Plan for the objectives for the team. Normally individual objectives are written uniquely and specifically for that individual and their situation, although they also focus on the service objectives of others in the team. In particularly intense team work responsibilities may be shared and it may not be possible to identify all the individual contributions of one individual from other members of the team. Some individual objectives may be team objectives. This means that team members must join in the work together to have systematised programming of what each individual, as a member of the team, is aiming to achieve.

4 Personal Development Plan

Development is different from performance. For some of the performance objectives *new knowledge of skills, or a development of present knowledge or skills, may be required in order to achieve them. In such cases the* personal development need box on the performance plan should be ticked.

A Professional Competencies List, *as required for specific tasks, is often a very useful addendum to producing a comprehensive personal development need. The plan which shows how these development needs are to be met will be included in the personal development plan. This involves writing down clearly each learning objective which is connected to each performance objective with a* brief statement of how they will be met *(observing, reading, training etc.).*

Individuals may include other learning objectives for the wider or longer-term personal and career development, as agreed with their personal manager and set out in their personal development plan (PDP).

At all times individuals should maintain a clear distinction between performance objectives *and* learning objectives. *The first are in the performance plan and the second are in the personal development plan. However they may be functionally inter-dependent, they should, for monitoring purposes, be separated in the* objectives.

5 Individual Meetings (one-to-one)

Each job holder will have three different sorts of IPR meeting with their manager:
i) Job Clarification

These meetings are at the start of the annual cycle. Two or three may be required. At the end of this process not more than ten individual performance objectives and learning objectives will have been clarified and agreed for the coming year.

ii) Monitoring and Reviewing

Probably four monitoring and reviewing meetings between job holder and manager will be used throughout each year. These meetings help the job holder by reviewing performance and reviewing the priorities which may then be changed. Any difficulties or other snags which may be preventing objectives and targets from being actioned, may then be looked at and resolved.

Changes may or may not be necessary in the objectives and, as appropriate, new options for targets for action can be considered and chosen.

iii) Personal Development Plans

These may also be modified as work holder and manager get more experience in the IPR process.

iv) Major Performance Review

This meeting is at the end of the annual cycle. It is the opportunity for the job holder to share his or her overview of the year with the manager. The job holder is expected to say what he or she feels pleased about in both performance and personal development. Disappointments are also noted. The manager also gives his or her view.

This is a meeting which should not have surprises in it and should enable the year to draw to a close with a sense of satisfaction on both sides

6 Training

Effective IPR requires not only the commitment of all involved but also the skills. Training, as appropriate, will be available for everyone so that a comprehensive shared understanding can be developed, for everyone *to maximise this opportunity.*

COMMUNICATION: THE LAST WORD

Memo from senior manager to the sector multidisciplinary management team.

'Please put 'communication' on the agenda of the next meeting.'

The senior manager did not arrive for the start of the next management team meeting, so after 15 minutes one of them telephoned him. The receptionist at the managers' offices (the third new suite in two years) said that all managers were on a training day at a hotel.

APPENDIX II

Bibliography

Black, Dora; Black, Michael and Martin, Freda (1974). 'A pilot study on the use of consultant time in Child Psychiatry'. *British Journal of Psychiatry Supplement, News & Notes,* 3-5, September.

Black, Dora and Black, Michael (1982). 'The use of consultant time in Child Psychiatry - 7 years on'. *The Bulletin of the Royal College of Psychiatrists,* 116-117, July.

Bloomfield, Kenneth (1992). *Fundamental Review of Dental Remuneration.* Department of Health.

Bosma, Hans; Marmot, Michael G.; Hemingway, Harry; Nicholson, Amanda C.; Brunner, Eric and Stansfeld, Stephen A. (1997). 'Low job control and risk of coronary heart disease in Whitehall II (prospective cohort) study'. *British Medical Journal,* **314,** 558-565, 22 February.

Bruggen, Peter and Bourne, Stanford (1982). 'The distinction awards system in England and Wales 1980'. *British Medical Journal,* **284,** 1577-1580, 22 May.

Bunbury, Tony and McGregor, Angus (1988). *Disciplining and Dismissing Doctors in the National Health Service.* Mercia Publications.

Caines, Karen (1996). 'Time to raise the Titanic'. *The Guardian,* 3 July.

Career Progress of Doctors Committee (1993*). Patronage in the Medical Profession.* British Medical Association.

Craft, Naomi (1994). 'Secrecy in the NHS'. *British Medical Journal,* **309,** 1640-1643, 17 December.

Dean, Malcolm (1995). 'A second opinion'. *The Guardian,* 3 November.

Dennis, John (1993). 'How does it really feel?' In *The New Face of the NHS,* edited by Peter Spurgeon. Longman.

Dorrell, Stephen (1996). 'After the revolution, a time for peace'. (Interview with David Brindle.) *The Guardian,* 3 April.

Enthoven, Alain C. (1985). *Reflections on the management of the National Health Service.* Nuffield Trust.

Ferrie, Jane E.; Shipley, Martin J.; Marmot, M. G.; Stansfeld, Stephen and Smith, George Davey (1995). 'Health effects of anticipation of job change and non-employment: longitudinal data from the Whitehall II study'. *British Medical Journal,* **311,** 1264-1269, 11 November.

Glennerster, Howard; Matsaganis, Manos and Owens, Pat (1992). 'The origins of the idea'. In *A Foothold for Fundholding.* Research Report No.12. The King's Fund Institute.

Improving NHS Dentistry (1994). Green Paper. HMSO.

Griffiths, Roy (1983). *NHS Management Inquiry: The Griffiths Report.* DHSS.

Hadley, Roger and Clough, Roger (1996). *Care in Chaos: Frustration and Challenge in Community Care.* Cassell.

Hansard (1994), **250,** 1051 -1058. 28th November. The Stationery Office.

Harrison, Stephen (1991). 'Working the Markets: Purchaser/Provider Separation in English Health Care'. *International Journal of Health Services,* **21,** No: 4, 625-635.

Harrison, Stephen; Small, Neil and Baker, Mark (1994). 'The Wrong Kind of Chaos? The early days of an NHS Trust'. *Public Money and Management,* **14,** No 1, 39-46. (January-March).

Harrison, Stephen and Lachmann, Peter (1996). *Towards a High Trust NHS: Proposals for Minimally Invasive Reforms.* Institute for Public Policy Research.

Hitchens, Christopher (1994). 'On Spanking'. *London Review of Books,* 20 October.

Hollander, Doris and Powell, Robin (1990). 'The 13 steps to community care'. *British Medical Journal,* 312, 913, 6th April.

Hunt, Geoffrey (1995). *Whistleblowing in the Health Service: Accountability, Law and Professional Practice.* Edward Arnold.

Jacobs, Harry (1989). 'Suspension: a Blot on the NHS'. *Supplement to British Journal of Clinical and Social Psychiatry,* 6, number 4.

Jarrold, Ken (1995). *Minding Our Own Business: Healing Division in the Health Service.* National Association of Health Authorities and Trusts.

Klein, Rudolf (1995). *The New Politics of the NHS.* Longman.

Langlands, Alan (1995). 'NHS Chief Executive wants a culutre of openness'. *British Medical Journal,* 310, 189, 21 January.

Malleson, Andrew (1973). *Need Your Doctor Be So Useless?* Allen and Unwin.

Malone, Gerald (1995). 'The NHS — a secret service!' *The Guardian,* 17 February.

Maynard, Alan (1980). 'Performance incentives in general practice'. In *Health Education and General Practice* (edited by Teeling Smith, George). Office of Health Economics.

Michie, Susan and Cockcroft, Anne (1996). 'Overwork can kill'. *British Medical Journal,* 312, 921-922, 13 April.

Nolan, Lord (1995). *Standards in Public Life.* HMSO.

Pillkington, Edward (1996). 'Ten-hour treatment wait added insult to injury at top-rated casualty centre'. *The Guardian,* 3 July.

Robinson, Ray and Le Grand, Julian (1994). *Evaluating the NHS Reforms.* The King's Fund Institute.

Swift, Lew and Scotland, Alastair (1995). *Disciplining and Dismissing Doctors in the National Health Service.* Mercia Publications.

Teeling Smith, George (1985). 'Should GPs hold the purse strings?' *Health and Social Service Journal,* 1338, 24 October.

The Patient's Charter and You (1995). Department of Health.

Tomlin, Peter and Jacobs, Harry (1997). 'Disciplining Senior Hospital Doctors as Practised in the National Health Service'. *British Journal of Clinical Psychiatry,* awaiting publication.

Working for Patients (1989). White Paper. Department of Health and Social Security.

Index

'Accept me or sack me' 255
Access to Information Act 13
Accreditation visit 96
Administration and technical staff 233
Administrative error 126
Advice, no 20
Agency staff 199
Alan 182, 184, 193
Alcohol 186
Alison 203-209, 285-292
Allitt, Beverley 206
Amanda 148-151
Andrew 102-109
Angela 38, 42-49
Angina 5
Anne 152-162
Annual report 13
Anonymity 17
Anti-depressants 14, 215
Anxiety 145, 273
Apathy 96
Application 34; for jobs 173; for own post 245
Appointment cancelled 107
Appraisal 21
Area Health Authority 3
Art therapists 178
Association of First Division Social Servants 293
Audit 103, 11, 12, 53, 167; assistant, 239
Authority 15
Auxiliary nurses 225

Babies, seriously ill 201
Back, covering own 132
Bank loan 152
Beds 33; blocking, 134; closed, 200; finding, 32; as management task, 228; for ECRs and GP fundholders, 241; management, 49; shortage, 236-237; none, 167; useful 241; vacancies juggling, 166
Befrienders 302
Benefits Agency 271
Bevan, Aneurin 2
Beverley Report 217

Bills, for travel and subsistence 271
Black, Dora 248
Black, Michael 248
Bloomfield Report 155, 159, 160
BMA 1, 61, 63, 65, 74, 97, 98, 210, 211, 282
BMA News Review 294
BMJ 1, 2, 17 194, 294, 295
Bottomley, Virginia 17, 282
Boundary, work and recreation 59
Bourne, Sandy 282
Brain tumour 5
Breakdown 14, 95-96, 234, 280
Bridget 171-175
Briefing before party meetings 269
Brindell, David 296
British Dental Association 153, 159, 161, 162
Budget 4, 9, 20, 45, 131; control, 6, 29, 51; cut, 112; devolved, 222; separate, 109
Bunbury, Tony 15
Bureaucracy 6, 42, 67, 235-255
Burnley Citizen 66
Burnley Express 66, 72
Business plan 2, 111; jargon ridden 196
Business, build up difficult 73, 74
Buzz words 255

Cabinet approval 274
Calman, Kenneth 98
Capital charges 236
Capitation fee 153
Cardiac hospital 285; resuscitation, 5
Cardiff 295
Care and Chaos: Frustration and challenge in community care 296
Care assistant, unqualified 129
Care for the NHS 297; deficit

of, 170; plans, 163; shared, 142; to and fro, 143
Career change 232
Carer 172; power 208-209
Casualty department, 24 hours 107
Catering 232
Central adjudication service 271
Chairman 28, 29, 41, 211-212
Chaps 282
Charities 302
Charity collect 174-175
Check ups 9
Chief executive 14, 28, 32, 39, 41, 77, 181; appointment, 223
Chief medical officer 13, 282
Children's nurse 203-209; ward 194-209
Clarke, Kenneth 9, 162, 270
Cleaners, £2.40 an hour 280
'Clear your desk' 5, 36, 53, 64, 61-76, 257
Clients, some don't give good impression 252
Clinical, contact 166; director 4, 50, 69, 219, 243;
Clinicians, controlling 36; split 36
Clough, Roger 296
Co-operation, immediate 190; none, 195, 197
Cockcroft, Anne 294
Colleagues also competitors 259
Comments, negative 19
Communicate, encourage not to 84
Communication 306; improve, 217; we must improve our, 100, 195, 196; worse 131
Community care 108, 136-143, 194; GPs pick up pieces, 119; team, 171-175
Community Health Council 3, 4, 71, 84

Community Psychiatric nurse
164

Complaint 21, 54, 132, 142,
182, 205, 207-208; about
the system 290; verbal,
176

Compliment 128, 142; and
support, 149

Computer system 147

Conduct, personal and
professional 62

Confidentiality 17; clauses,
216

Conflict being both manager
and clinician 98

Conflict, stirred up 55

Confrontations 91

Constraints 29

Consultancy circuit 270

Consultant posts, readvertise-
ments 104

Consultant psychiatrist 13

Consultants, resistant to
change 265, ability to
manage eroded 94;
passive, 178; protected
right, 10; work load 228

Consultation 272; no time,
204

Consumer 13

Continuing care responsibility
154

Contract 78; lost 80; out for
tender 79

Contract, consultants, 10;
fixed term 4, 11; individual,
10; six month, 21, 35; time
limited 17; unique 68

Control, trying to take 24

Coronary bypass surgery
285

Cost effectiveness 278

Counselling 21, 35, 189, 234

Counsellor 19, 24, 302

County boundaries 123

Craft, Naomi 295

Crown immunity, past 278

Cry 1, 93, 185; crying 234

Cut of 24% over two years
272

Cuts 43

Cystic fibrosis 197

Danckwerts 2

Data collection, spurious 196

David 285, 292

Dawn 55-58

Dead wood? 15

Dean, Malcolm 73

Debriefing 174

Decision-making 89, 265;
informed 90, delayed 11

Deficit 219

Deidre 121-127

Delegate and control 260

Dennis 38-42

Dennis, John 256

Dental charges, 25 major
changes 152; time restriction, 153; clinic 102; fees
cut, 154; income, average,
152; list, 153; Practice
Board 159;

Dental Practice 160

Dental services, cost limit
155; fee narrative, 156;
market force pressure,
156; number of patients
seen, 156; purchaser
provider? 155; quid treatment 157 158

Dentists 152-162; over paid,
154; waiver, 162

Department of Health 83,
103, 159

Department of Health &
Social Security 3, 4

Department of State 269

Depressed 19, 164, 273

Destabilisation introduced
254

Devalued 143

Diary sheets 147

'Did I tell you that?' 175

Difficult decisions 29

Directives 165; the lion's den,
165

Director of corporate affairs
30; finance, 28; human
resources, 30; Public
Health, 126, 265; execu-
tive, 14; non-executive, 14

Directorate 8; credibility
damaged, 266

Discharge 8; unofficial 289

Discipline 96, 177, 179, 209;
boundaries crossed 222

Discrimination, race 37; sex
37

Disillusionment 91

Distinction awards 17, 68,
282

District General Hospital 7

District Health Authority 4, 11

District nurse 102; bought in,

138; ownership of cases,
141; work lunchtimes, 142

Division is power 269

'Do not disturb' 211

Doctor power 62, 181;
removed 239

Doctors' health 86; quarters,
6

Doctors 7, 14, 178; division
among, 6; discipline, 15;
getting to go, 15; put in
their place, 269; split, 62;
suspended, 15; trouble
caused by, 181

Domiciliary visits 11, 167

'Don' (eyeball me) lady' 282

Donald 58-60

Doris 49-54

Dorrell, Stephen 296

Douglas 152-162

Downgraded 90, 171, 174

Dreams 35, 90, 50, 100, 201

Drugs, illegal possession 14

Early retirement 41, 171, 257

ECRs 82, 108-109, 125,
135, 180, 209, 221, 243-
244, 267; ward 237

ECT 167

Efficiency savings 43

Efficiency 277

Eileen 128-135

Emergency bed service 106

Emergency referral 145-146

Enthoven 6

Equal Opportunities policy 32

Ergonomic strain 233

Euston Tower 271

Evidence-based medicine
241

Executive directors 28, 29

Families, influence 9; friction
88; as statistics 242

Family Health Services
Authority 7, 8, 9, 111, 117,
122,

Family Practitioner Committee
3, 4

Family problems 14

Family therapist 12

Fantasies 19; revengeful 175

Fantasy 93

Fay 28-35

Fear 16, 17, 143, 183, 190,
212; for jobs 199

Ferrie, Jane 293

FIFO, Fit in or ... 11, 296

Finished consultant episodes
200, 292
First names, confusion
caused by 150
Fit to work 232
Frances 18-27
Frank 252-255
Friends 172; lost 38
Fundholding pressure 123;
invisible, 116; first thought
of? 9
Funds 13

Gagged 1, 216
Gate keepers 8
General management 4
General management initiative
36
General practice 3
General practitioners, GPs 9,
65; angry, 81; commission,
8; find their voice, 177;
fundholders, 8, 12, 56, 82;
fundholders, influence,
112; muscle, 57; fund-
holding 7, 110-120, 224;
leadership, 10; not fund-
holders, 102-109; power,
6, 267; status, 6; country
doctors 121-127
General surgeons 240-242
'Get out ' 19, 24
'Get things done' 33
Glennerster 9
Goals, lower 24
Golden hello 68
Goldfish bowl 20
Good for business 9
Good news press releases
248
Goodbye, no 18
Goodwill, lost 46
Gossip 191
Graham 199-202
Grapevine 70
Grievance 24, 25, 174
Griffiths Report 218
Griffiths, Roy 4, 11
Guardian 17, 73, 294, 296
Gulf War 50, 212
Guy's Hospital 218

Hadley, Roger 296
Hammer, Michael 219
Hannibal House 271
Hansard 75; Library, 270
Harriett 181, 183, 184, 186
Harrison, Stephen 15, 296

Hart, Graham 274, 275
Hazel 257-261
'He is not there' 288
Head banging 297
Head hunted 42, 55, 273
Headaches 24, 280
Heads of department 18
Health Advisory Service 172
Health and Safety margins,
on the edge, 233
Health and Social Services
Recreational Association
280
Health Authority 7
Health visitors 102, 144-51
Hidden agenda 184
Hierarchical relationship 8
High-tech 5
Hiller, Susan 299
Hip replacement 114
Hitchens, Christopher 298
Hollander, Doris 248
House of Commons 270
Human resources department
22
Humiliation 185
Hunt, Geoffrey 294
Hypnotics 187

Immigrant children, immu-
nising 111
Improving NHS Dentistry
155, 160
'In case you are guilty' 184
In vitro fertilisation 106-108
In-fighting 42
Incident 193
Independent review 215
Indicators for good practice
11, 2
Individual Performance
Review 134, 260, 303-306
Infections mean more busi-
ness 213
Infectious diseases 130
Informants 15-16
Information technology 60
Information, income depen-
dent on 103; more
available 301
Inquiry 170
Instant dismissal 212
Intelligence Unit 281
Interest rates 152
Internal inquiry 187-188, 190
Internal market 115
Interpreters 151
Investigation 179, 192

Investors in People
Chartermark 273
'Is it a trap?' 237
Items of service 153

Jacobs, Harry 294, 295
James 163-169
Jane 136-143
Jarrold, Ken 297
Jean 102-109
Jessica 251-252
Job, application very public,
258; apply for own, 31;
assured, 58; description,
18, 22, 149; disappear five
times, 257; ending next
day, 144; exchange, 58;
first, 18; lost, 35 none for
them, 57; what job will
there be? 41
Judgement, ability eroded
192
Junior doctors 202; hours
69, 194, 226

Keith 261-265
'Kick her into shape' 20
King's Fund Institute 9
Klein, Rudolf 2

Lachmann, Peter 296
Langlands, Alan 17, 72, 274,
275, 277, 295
Law suits 132
Leeds City Art Gallery, 268,
299
Le Grand, Julian 15
League Tables 294
Leaks 70
Learning difficulties 42
Lecture theatre 28, 33
Leicester 73, 218-231; Royal
Infirmary 213, 218-231
Lewis, Kevin 160
Lies 35, 85, 90
Life and death 202
Life being short, a sense of
280
Limitation of professional peer
groups 243
Line manager 19
Locum advertisements 250;
locum doctors 86, 249-
252; easiest to get rid of
249
Logo 44, 110
London Implementation
Group 271

London Review of Books
188
London Weighting, five year's
271
Loyalty 277; gone 107
Luton and Dunstable Hospital
212-217
Lydia 265-267

Macho management 21;
undesirable, 297
Mahady, Ian 61-76
Malleson, Andrew 10
Malone, Gerald 17, 61, 161,
162
Management; block., where is
it? 46; crisis, 51;
expanded, 56; initiative, 11,
55; learning 224; paper,
13, precipitated into, 10;
restructuring, 136; strong,
10, structure, 10, 20; tasks
proliferate, 45; support
you, 128; three different,
144
Managers, 4; confused, 168;
frightened, 145, 168; get
things done 238-240; good
experience, 168; managing
235-255; messengers,168,
178; non-workaholic 252-
255; passive, 178; total
number must be less, 258,
261; turnover, 169
Margaret 144-148
Market 11, 127; forces, 8,
12, 36, 43, 84, 258, 293;
power, 208-209; pretend,
46
Marks & Spencer 256
Martin 242-248
Martin, Freda 248
Mary 77-84
Matsoganis, Manos 9
Mawhinney, Brian 160
Maynard, Alan 9
MBA 38
McGregor, Angus 15
Medical cover 177
Medical director 85-101, 13,
15, 63, 196, 218,
Medical profession, inward
looking 13
Medical records 18
Medical staff committee 71,
196
Mental health 163, 178, 273
Merge 49; pressure to 114

Merged 7, 32, 36, 37, 38,
47 53, 141, 180, 181, 257-
258
Metaphors, military and
sporting 283
Migraine 21
Minding Our Own Business
297
Ministry of Health 3
Mistake; in paperwork, 130;
no-one allowed to make
201
Mitchie, Susan 294
Money 8, 95,135; follows
patients, 81, 198, 200,
267; ran out, 124,
emphasis on, 298; extra
12; in the first sentence,
164; leakage to private
sector, 116, 117; leakage
to private sector 117;
warning list 12
Money's worth 70
'Monument' 299
Morale 52, 53, 93,128, 145;
meeting for, 205
MPs 43
Muddles 149
Multi-skilled people 220

Naftalin, Nick 218-222
Named nurse 129; responsi-
bility with 133
National Association of Health
Authorities and Trusts 235,
297
National Union of Public
Employees 183
Near patient testing 220
Needs assessment 119
Negative feelings 201
Negotiated terms 253
Neo natal ward 199-202
Network, now competitors
201
New management structure
22
New patient 147
NHS Executive 17, 268-273,
278-281, 294; eight areas,
274; move to Leeds 270
Nichol, Duncan 216, 274
Nightingale, Florence 4
Nightmares 201
Nights, how many at home
this week? 272
No case to answer 171, 190
No confidence 215

Nolan Report 294
Non-confrontational 223
Non-executive directors 298
'Nothing to worry about' 172
Nuffield Institute for Health,
Leeds 15
Nurse 19, 21; at board level,
33, 217; general, 128-135;
manager, 31; role
expanded, 26; nurses, 7,
70, 170
Nursing assistant 19
Nursing care, interpreted 137

Obstetrics 62
Occupational health 233, 234;
department, 19, 280
Occupational therapist 164
On call 02, 52, 67
'Once we get it right' 242
Open door 72
Openness 17, 37, 61, 87
Operating time, run out 104
Operation cancelled 240
Out patient department 18
Over-perform 124
Overwork can kill 294
Owens, Pat 9

Package of care, wrong
department 139
Paediatrics 7, 194-209
Panics 21, 53, 280
Panorama 5, 6
Paperwork 244, 248-249
Paranoid? 87, 118, 185, 234
Patients 35, 66; choice 230-
231; distressed, 20; new,
287; should not be aware,
302; time, down, 199;
threatening, 20; number
treated, 105, 200, 285-292
Patient's Charter 13, 54, 65,
81, 104, 123, 132, 208,
237, 291, 301
Patricia 191-193
Payment, extra 11
Penelope 242-248
Pension 37, 261; deals, 35
Performance related pay 17,
221; 37, 258; targets, 21,
61
Permission 15
Persona non grata 60
Personal attacks 21; capital,
117; file, 88, 146, 148;
support, 276
Personnel officer 30, 183

Philip 110-120, 285-292
Phone tap 210 - 217
Photograph for name badge 129, 193; use of, 135
Physical illness 14, 273
Pike, Peter 75
Pilkington, Edward 294
Pilot study 162, 298
Planned discharge 139
Planning blight 42
Plans, revise 44
'Please take your father home' 289
Police 186-187
Policy, already made 89; that is our 113
Political correctness 282; interference 43; sensitivity 60
Politics 52
Porters 232
Postman's Park 299
Posts down-graded 201
Powell, Robin 248
Power balance 11; liked, 196; without accountability 89; without too much bloodshed 267
Practice Charter 123
Prescribing activity 122
Press release 215
Preventive 5
Prices up 112
Primary care 5
Private treatment: dentistry 154-159; Health Insurance 114; hospitals 12, 46, 106, 237; secretary 21; sector, 113; services 216
Productivity increase 125; up 10% 121
Profit 235-236
Promotion 27, 136
Protests disregarded 89
'Prove it ' 83
Provider 6, 7
Psychiatry 163-178
Psychological tests 259, 274
Psychologists 178
Psychosomatic complaints 1, 232, 234, 273
Public ritual 131; reprimand 191
Publishing 13
Purchaser(s) 8, 11, 41, 42, 176 256-267; allowed to purchase, 43; as referrer, 198; money, 176; not

speaking to trust, 78,79; not to be dictated to, 195; priorities could differ, 269; required changes, 266; singular or plural, 7; wants it, 147
Purchaser/provider split 256
Purchasing 6; authorities, 14

Quality control 13; of care, 86; standards, 13; survey 238
Quarrry House 268, 294, 296-299
Queues 230-231

Racially abusive 170
Radiologist 210
Re-draft 79
Re-engineering 213, 219-222, 229
Re-instated 215
Receptionists 7
Redundancy 134, 173, 31, 32, 36, 61, 74; compulsory, 64; photocopies, 58; settlement, 276; voluntary, 63, 64;
Redundant 39, 42, 52, 73, 213
References, good 40
Reforms 2, 6, 15; excited by, 129; urge as quickly as possible 269
Regional Authorities 273-278
Regional Health Authority 3, 4, 10, 14
Regional Hospital Board 3,10
Registered sick children's nurse 209
Reinstated 171, 189
Relationships 36; with neighbouring colleagues, 80
Relatives 172
Relocation expenses 271; to be paid back 272
Removal expenses 11
Reprimanded by management 247
Requirement, new bureaucratic 125
Research 13
Residents, temporary 111
Resign 15, 26, 101; resigned, 80, 97, 131, 168, 215; could not afford, 247
Resignation 68

Resource management 11; initiative, 4
Resources 4,39; clamour for more 269
Respect 178
Restless nights 247
Retirement 214; dates, 127; early, 134, 272
Rheumatologist 77-84
Richards, Jane 296
Richmond House 270
Rita 176-178
Robert 121-127
Robinson, Ray 15
Royal College of General Practitioners 6
Royal College of Nursing 183
Royal College of Obstetricians and Gynaecologists 69
Rule, thirty year 217
Rules, changed 86, 214; new 51
Rumours 34, 37, 182, 244, 271, 274, 276

Sacked 18, 55, 215
Said too much or too little? 275
Salaries 4; and wages, 10; increment 11; negotiated 68
Savings without knowing costs 132
Savings, allowable 116
Scapegoat 19, 20, 42, 165, 174
Scotland, Alastair 15
Scotland 268
Screening advice 103
Seamless service 142
Seconded 42, 48
Secrecy 37, 254, 295
Secretaries 18, 87, 174, 181, 233
Secretary 7, 21
Secretary of State for Health 6, 10, 13, 17, 43
Security 17
Seen within first five minutes 294
Self esteem, lost 83
Self-fund 107
Senior house officer 164
Service specification 302
Services, itemisable 138
Sexism 282-284
Shadow trust 59
Shared care 197

Short term contracts 258
Signed responsibility 130
Silent industrial trouble... 77
Single visit clinics 220
Skill mix 134, 137, 145, 166,
207; positive, 226
Skilled clinical nursing tasks
138
Sleep 37; badly, 53, 88, 199;
disturbed, 234; through the
night, 101; together 59
Small budget, not significant
262
Sobbing 1, 166
Social services 134
Social work aides 140
Social worker 12, 164, 182;
office, 252
Society of Clinical
Psychiatrists 294
Soul 54, 161
Spencer, John 211, 217, 296
Spending the surplus 200
Splitting staff 214
Sponsorship 216
Spurgeon, Peter 256
St. James's Hospital 279
Staff, turnover 44
Stakeholders day 168, 171-
172
Standards in Public Life 294
*Statement of Dental
Remuneration* 161
Stephen 197-199
Stories, how I got 13-17
Strategic 31, 34; direction
219
Strategy 26; express enthu-
siasm 175; is wonderful,
94; saying fine 146;
survival, 92
Stress 21, 109, seminars,
280; symptoms, 232
Student nurses 130
Summaries 13
Supervising, stopped 86
Supervision 19, 20, 194
Support, preventive 133
Surgeon 9
Surgeons, next generation
less experienced 241
Surplus 112
Survival 24, 257; principles,
37
Suspend 183; suspended 1,
2, 128, 131, 170, 176,
211, 215

Suspension 171, 179-193,
184, almost as reflex 192
Suspension out of view
NHS 294
Sweats 53
Swift, Lew 15
Swimming pool 279, 297

Talking to patients, any good?
109; value of? 246
Tantrum 13
Tape recorder 211
Tattersall Report 160
Tears 14, 19, 26, 35, 83,
185, 277, 280
Teeling Smith, George 9
'Tell us where your father is'
289
Tension 140, 270, 280,
headaches, 101
Tertiary centres 197
Thatcher, Margaret 5, 6, 11,
298
The New Face of the NHS
256
*The Rise of Stalinism in the
NHS* 295
Therapeutic experience 14
Threat 8; theatened, 190, 20
Tom 85-101
Tomlin, Peter 295
Top leaders 36
Total fundholding 119
Totalitarian state, like living in
212
Tough 189
*Towards a High-Trust NHS:
Proposals for a Minimum
Invasive Reform* 296
Training 125
Tranquillisers 14, 65, 187,
215
Treatment delayed 126
Trouble maker 41, 189, 203
Trust, confidence 32; deci-
sion, 169; not speaking to
purchaser, 78, 79; power
to appoint, 10
Trust, improve 217
Trusts 14
Truth, distortion 99

Uncontrolled experiment 241
Union 35, 172, 183; repre-
sentative, 188-189, 252
Upgraded 27
Useless? 10
User friendly 72

Users 9, 170, 171

Valium... 10
Vested interests 269
Video links 272; recordings,
12; tape 58
Violence, alleged 182; history
of 20
Visitors 302
Voluntary: organizations 54;
redundancy, 136, 169;
sector 302
Vulnerability 97; vulnerable
101

Waiting list 10, 82, 115; initia-
tive, 12, 269; advised, 13
Waiting rooms nearly empty
220
Waking 53; in the night 88,
101
Waldegrave, William 9
Wales 268
Ward consultant 191-193,
manager 224-226
Watts, Geoffrey 299
'We have our orders' 286
'We need the bed' 287
Weighed unnecessarily 103
Weight lost 189
Welcomes 271
'Well done' 28
West Yorkshire Playhouse
279, 299
Whistleblowing 294
*Whistleblowing in the Health
Service* 294
Whitehall 11 Study 293
Whitfield, William 270
Whitley Council 175
William 250-251
Women, few at top 268
Work, taken home 59, 88,
214, 221, 228
Working for Patients 5,6
World at One 17
Worried, talking to me 214
Written policies 176; proce-
dures, 246

X-ray film envelopes 219

'You'll have to manage' 203
'You misheard me' 169

Abbreviations

'Before we start, let's have an agreement on whether we use FWAs or TWAs during the course of this one day seminar.'

Joke or serious, these are the words with which one chairman started the day: FWA stands for Four Word Abbreviation, TWA for Three Word Abbreviation.

BDA	British Dental Association
BMA	British Medical Association
BMJ	*British Medical Journal*
CHC	Community Health Council
CT Scan	Computer Aided Tomography
DGH	District General Hospital
DHA	District Health Authority
EBS	Emergency Bed Service
ECR	Extra Contractual Referral
ECG	Electro-cardiogram
ECT	Electro-convulsive Therapy
FCE	Finished Consultant Episode
FHSA	Family Health Services Authority
FIFO	Fit in or...
IPR	Individual Performance Review
LIG	London Implementation Group
LRI	Leicester Royal Infirmary
MRI	Magnetic Resonance Imaging
NAHAT	National Association of Health Authorities and Trusts
NHSE	National Health Service Executive
NHSME	National Health Service Management Executive
PDP	Personal Development Plan
PRP	Performance Related Pay
RMN	Registered Mental Nurse
RSCN	Registered Sick Children's Nurse
SHO	Senior House Officer
TLC	Tender Loving Care
TOP	Termination of Pregnancy
UGM	Unit General Manager